Herbert A. Otto, Ph.D.,
and
James W. Knight, M.D.,
Editors

Dimensions in Wholistic Healing:

New Frontiers
in the Treatment of
the Whole Person

Herbert A. Otto, Ph.D.,
and
James W. Knight, M.D.,
Editors

Dimensions in Wholistic Healing:

New Frontiers in the Treatment of the Whole Person

Nelson-Hall *nh* Chicago

Library of Congress Cataloging in Publication Data
Main entry under title:

Dimensions in wholistic healing.

Biography: p.
Includes index.
1. Therapeutic systems. 2. Mental healing. I. Otto, Herbert Arthur. II.
Knight, James William, 1927-   [DNLM: 1. Parapsychology—Essays. 2.
Therapeutic cults—Essays. WB890 D582]
R733.D53   615'.5   78-27071
ISBN 0-88229-513-6 (Cloth)
ISBN 0-88229-697-3 (Paper)

Manufactured in the United States of America

10   9   8   7   6   5   4   3   2   1

Contents

Part I
The Basis of Wholistic Healing

Part II
Evolving the Framework of Wholistic Healing

Part III
Western Approaches to Wholistic Healing

Contributing Authors

ALFRED A. BARRIOS, PH.D., is currently director of the Self-Programmed Control Center in Los Angeles (P.O. Box 49939). He was formerly visiting professor at the University of California, Los Angeles and consultant for the City of Hope. He is the author of a number of articles on hypnosis and self-actualization. His theory of hypnosis is considered by many to be the most advanced and comprehensive of the current theories. He has been involved in the psychological approach to cancers since 1961 and is currently involved (at UCLA) in one of the first controlled studies testing this approach.

DAVID E. BRESLER, PH.D., is currently director of the UCLA Pain Control Unit, the UCLA Acupuncture Project, and Adjunct Assistant Professor of Anesthesiology, Gnathology and Occlusion, and Psychology in the UCLA Schools of Medicine, Dentistry, and the College of Letters and Sciences. Dr. Bresler has lectured and published extensively on the subjects of Oriental medicine, pain control, and integral medicine. His newest book, *Hurting*, will be published by Simon & Schuster in 1978.

EFFIE POY YEW CHOW, R.N., PH.D., is president of the East-West Academy of Healing Arts. She is the conceptor of center project on Holistic Health/Cultural Practices; Project Director of San Francisco Health Services/Educational Activities (HS/EA); Consultant to Western Interstate Commission on Higher Education, Boone, Young and Associates on National Family Planning (HEW); Advisor to American Nurses' Association Minority Doctoral Fellowship program; Vice Chairman of the Steering Committee (National Heart & Lung Institute of the National Institutes of Health) for Hypertension in Minorities.

NORMAN S. DON, PH.D., is director of the Laboratory for Psychophysiology, in Chicago. He was formerly on the research staff of the Department of Psychiatry, the University of Chicago. He currently does research in the psychophysiology of altered states of consciousness, and is a consultant and lecturer. Results of his research have been published in a number of scientific and scholarly journals.

NORMA ESTRADA, has been involved in psychiatry and hospital administration since 1956. She has collaborated with Dr. Arthur Gladman in organizing symposia, writing papers, and developing a rationale and philosophy for the clinical application of biofeedback. Mrs. Estrada is working with the treatment of psychosomatic problems using biofeedback and psychotherapy and is currently a Doctoral Candidate in clinical psychology.

PATRICIA GARFIELD, PH.D., is a lecturer in psychology for the University of California Extension system. She travels widely, presenting special dream seminars, is actively researching dream consciousness and control, and publishes in professional journals, including *Psychotherapy: Theory, Research and Practice* and *Sleep Research*. Her personal dream record, in its twenty-eighth year, totals more than ten thousand separate entries. Her books include *Creative Dreaming* (Simon & Schuster, 1974, Ballantine, 1976) and *Patty and The Dream Tiger* (Delacorte Press, in press).

ARTHUR E. GLADMAN, M.D., is the co-founder and medical director of the Everett A. Gladman Memorial Hospital, an open psychiatric hospital in Oakland, California. In 1972, with his cotherapist Norma Estrada, he studied biofeedback with Elmer and Alyce Green at the Menninger Foundation and began treating chronic psychosomatic illness with biofeedback and team therapy. Currently, he is the President of the Gladman Psychosomatic Medicine Center and is involved in the development of a Cancer Counselling program.

DAVID A. GOODMAN, PH.D., is a psychobiologist with fifteen years' experience in experimental and futurist brain science. Since 1971, he has been affiliated with the Newport Neuroscience Center as researcher and forecaster. Author of more than a dozen experimental and futurist papers and reports that appeared in such journals as *Nature, Behavioral Biology,* and *Human Behavior,* he is currently at work on *The Future and the Human Brain* for Bantam Books.

BERNARD RAYMOND GRAD, PH.D., is currently an associate professor at McGill University. A researcher, lecturer, consultant, and administrator, he has published about ninety papers, most of them in such professional journals as *Journal of Gerontology, Cancer Research, American Journal of Physiology,* and *International Journal of Parapsychology.* He is a member of the American Association of Cancer Research, Sigma Xi, the Canadian Physiological Society and the Canadian Association of Gerontology.

R. D. GRISELL, PH.D., is currently doing research in the fields of biophysics of excitable membranes, biological phototransducers, and the baroreceptor component of human blood pressure control at the School of Medicine, the University of Texas. He is coordinating editor of *Multidisciplinary Research* and founding member of the International Multidisciplinary Research Association. He has taught mathematics and physics in Iran, Lebanon and other countries. His books include *Hierarchical Field Theory: A Theoretical Framework for Extrasensory Phenomena* (Khalsa Publications, 1976) and *Ultrasonic and Optical Data Processing* (Multidisciplinary Publications, 1974).

H. LEONARD JONES, JR., M.D., is former Executive Vice-president of the Association for Holistic Health in San Diego, California. He has traveled extensively, studied, taught, and done research in internal medicine and related subjects. He has lived in China, Egypt, Nepal, and Afghanistan and has held professorships at Jefferson Medical College in Philadelphia and at Kabul University. Jones is the author of over thirty scientific papers in leading American medical journals and in the foreign literature.

MORTON KELSEY, B.D., is Associate Professor in the Department of Graduate Studies in Education, University of Notre Dame. He is Rector Emeritus of St. Luke's Church, Monrovia, California, where he established a psychological clinic. He is a lecturer, writer, and consultant and has contributed to many professional journals. His books include *God, Dreams and Revelation* (Augsburg, 1974); *Healing and Christianity* (Harper and Row, 1974); *Myth, History and Faith* (Paulist, 1975); *The Christian and the Supernatural* (Augsburg, 1976); and *The Other Side of Silence* (Paulist, 1976).

JAMES W. KNIGHT, M.D., is director of the Center for Wholistic Healing, Salinas, California. For fifteen years he has integrated in his practice various healing modalities, including mediation, creative imagery, autogenics, and more recently biofeedback concurrent with traditional medicine. An intensive study of Eastern philosophies prompted recent travels around the world to explore in depth cultural health practices and integrative belief systems. Dr. Knight is president and founder of Systems for Medicine.

DOLORES KRIEGER, PH.D., R.N., is currently Professor of Nurse Education at New York University. As a teacher and researcher she has been cited in *Who's Who of American Women* and *Leaders in Education*. Since 1970, her research has centered about the healing process. Dr. Krieger has written widely on her findings and has lectured and held workshops at universities and for professional organizations throughout the country. She has been on several national television programs for NBC, CBS, and ABC.

RICHARD J. KROENING, M.D., is Medical Director of the UCLA Pain Control Unit and Assistant Adjunct Professor of Anesthesiology, and Medical Director of the Temporomandibular Joint and Facial Pain Clinic of the UCLA School of Dentistry. Dr. Kroening is a writer and lecturer of acupuncture and other less conventional forms of medicine currently being investigated in this country. His articles have appeared in numerous magazines and professional journals. He is the Director of Professional Training, Center for Integral Medicine, as well as a member of the State of California Board of Medical Quality Assurance and the Advisory Committee to that board.

WILLIAM S. KROGER, M.D., is currently director of the Institute for Comprehensive Medicine in Beverly Hills, California. He is Clinical Professor of Anesthesiology, UCLA School of

Medicine. He is a pioneer in psychosomatic medicine, hypnotherapy, and sexual dysfunction. He is a writer, lecturer and clinician. His contributions have appeared in numerous professional journals. His books include *Psychosomatic Gynecology, Obstetrics and Endocrinology* (C. C. Thomas, 1962), *Clinical and Experimental Hypnosis* (Lippincott, 1963, revised edition 1977), *Hypnosis and Behavior Modification: Sensory Imagery Conditioning* (with W. Fezler) (Lippincott, 1976).

LAWRENCE LESHAN, PH.D., is currently engaged in a research project in parapsychology. He is an experimental psychologist who has taught at Roosevelt University, The New School for Social Research, and elsewhere and was, for fifteen years, chief of the Department of Psychology at Trafalgar Hospital and The Institute of Applied Biology. He has published over sixty professional papers and is the author of *The Medium, The Mystic and the Physicist* (Viking, 1974), *Alternate Realities* (Evans, 1976) and *You Can Fight for Your Life: Emotional Factors in the Causation of Cancer* (Evans, 1977).

CARL LEVETT, PH.D., is a writer, group leader, and practicing transpersonal consultant. As a pioneer in the human potential movement he conducted various workshops on "Freeing Creativity." In recent years Levett has specialized in exploring dimensions of consciousness relative to the scientific and the mystical, the logical and the intuitive. His efforts have led to an interest in the "Essence Connection" as a grounding source for expanding consciousness realizations. His books include *Crossing: A Transpersonal Approach* (Quiet Song, 1974) and *ZOT* (Quiet Song, 1975).

EVARTS G. LOOMIS, M.D., F.A.C.S., received his M.D. at Cornell University and interned at Newark City Hospital. He spent five years on the Hospital Staff at the Grenfell Mission in Northern Newfoundland. He worked with a Friends ambulance unit in China during World War II and later joined an UNRRA team as a surgeon in Algeria. He is now in private practice, serving as director of Meadowlark (a Wholistic Health Center), lecturer, and writer. His latest book, *Healing for Everyone* was written with J. Sig Paulson (Hawthorn Books, 1975).

VICTOR M. MARGUTTI, D.O., M.D., is a practicing physician,

specializing in homoeotherapeutics and psychosomatic medicine, a part of internal medicine. He is a member of the American Institute of Homoeopathy, a past president, and a member of its council on drugs. He is a diplomate in homoeotherapeutics and a fellow of the Royal Society of Health, London. Margutti has contributed numerous professional papers to the *Journal* of the AIH and is listed in *Notable Americans of the Bicentennial Era*, and *Who's Who in America*.

E. STANTON MAXEY, M.D., F.A.C.S., has practiced general surgery for twenty years and acupuncture for five. His articles in the fields of biophysics and biometeorology have appeared in many languages. His medical inventions include an automatic tissue processor and an electric/hydraulic operating table. He is a certified flight instructor and has developed a blind landing system and an electronic moving map/collision avoidance system for aircraft. His biophysical research confirmed a terrestrial magnetic wave versus brain rhythm correlation which explains the transient incapacitation observed in many "pilot error" air crashes.

JOHN COSTON MCCAMY, M.D., specializes in the field of preventive medicine in St. Petersburg, Florida. He is a member of the American Medical Association, works actively with the American Academy of Metabology, the International Academy of Preventive Medicine, the Southern Academy of Clinical Nutrition, the Association of Humanistic Psychology, and the International Society of Biological Medicine. He is the author with James Presley of *Human Life Styling* (Harper and Row, 1976).

WILLIAM A. MCGAREY, M.D., is director of the A.R.E. Clinic in Phoenix, Arizona. He has been director of the Medical Research Division of the Edgar Cayce Foundation since 1965. A writer, lecturer, and consultant, he has published articles in a variety of magazines and professional journals. His books include *Edgar Cayce and the Palma Christi* (Edgar Cayce Foundation, 1970), *Edgar Cayce on Healing* (Paperback Library, 1972), *Acupuncture and Body Energies* (Gabriel Press: Phoenix, 1973), *There Will Your Heart Be Also* (Prentice-Hall, 1975).

CLAUDIO NARANJO, M.D., once a practicing psychiatrist, research psychologist, professor of psychology of art, and Guggenheim

Fellow for studies in values at the Institute of Personality Assessment and Research, University of California at Berkeley, was a trainee of Fritz Perls and Associate-in-Residence at Esalen Institute. At present, he is Visiting Professor of Psychology at the University of California, Santa Cruz, meditation instructor at Nyingma Institute in Berkeley, member of the planning council of the Roman Catholic Diocese of California, and member of the editorial board of the *Journal of Humanistic Psychology*.

HERBERT A. OTTO, PH.D., is a psychologist, therapist, and marriage and family counselor. An early pioneer in the wholistic healing and human potential movement, he published a chapter entitled "Toward a Holistic Treatment Program" in 1967 in *The Active Psychotherapies*, Harold Greenwald (Atherton Press, 1967). He is an internationally known author, lecturer, and trainer, has published over sixty articles in scientific journals, and sixteen books, among which are *Guide to Developing Your Potential* (Scribner, 1967), *Group Methods to Actualize Human Potential* (Holistic Press, 1970), and *Marriage and Family Enrichment* (Abingdon, 1976).

JAMES PRESLEY, of Texarkana, Texas, a professional writer specializing in medicine/health, is author of eight books and more than 100 articles. He received the Anson Jones Award (Texas Medical Association) in 1971 and was formerly a consultant, Red River Regional Council on Alcoholism (Texas). His books include, as co-author, *Please, Doctor, Do Something!* (Natural Food Associates/Devin-Adair, 1972); *Vitamin B₆ The Doctor's Report* (Harper & Row, 1973); *Human Life Styling* (Harper & Row, 1975), and *Food Power: Nutrition and Your Child's Behavior* (St. Martin's Press, 1978).

ELIZABETH PHILIPOV, PH.D., currently visiting professor at the University of Tübingen, Germany, is teaching and researching at the University's Center for New Learning Methods. International lecturer and consultant, field faculty at Humanistic Psychology Institute, San Francisco, and formerly professor of psychology at Pepperdine University, L.A., she organized and chaired the I. International Congress of Psychology of Consciousness and Suggestology, Los Angeles, 1975. She researches into areas of

Wholistic Education and Health, developing new learning and therapeutic methods and pioneered suggestopedic research in the U.S. and Germany.

C. NORMAN SHEALY, M.D., is currently director of the Pain and Health Rehabilitation Center, La Crosse, Wisconsin. Formerly a neurosurgeon and professor of Neurosurgery at several universities, Shealy for the past five years has restricted his practice to management of patients with chronic disease—primarily those in chronic pain. He has published 100 professional articles and a number of books; his primary interests are in voluntary self-regulation and health maintenance. The books include *Occult Medicine Can Save Your Life* (Dial, 1975); *The Pain Game* (Celestial Arts, 1976), and *90 Days To Self-Health* (Dial, 1977).

HAROLD STONE, PH.D., is currently a psychotherapist in private practice in Brentwood, California. He was originally trained as a Jungian analyst, but his journey led him into explorations of many healing modalities. The outcome was the founding of the Center for the Healing Arts, for which he currently serves as executive director. He is the author of a number of articles, has taught widely in university extension programs, and in recent years has been teaching consultant to the Department of Psychiatry at Mount Sinai Hospital, Los Angeles.

WALTER S. STRODE, M.D., is currently co-coordinator (with wife, Nancy) of the Hawaii Health Net, a communications network exploring health as human wholeness, and finding ways to encourage personal responsibility in health. He is also a urologist at Straub Clinic and Hospital, and assistant clinical professor (surgery) at the John Burns School of Medicine, Honolulu. He is author of over fifty articles in the medical and wholistic health fields.

DR. CHANDRASEKHAR G. THAKKUR (of Sind Ayurvedic Pharmacy, 375, Kalbadevi, Bombay) is a doctor of science in Ayurveda. He is an honorary fellow of the Royal Asiatic Society, London, and the East-West Foundation, Boston, and president, the Indo-American Astrological Association. He holds the highest medical qualification, Ayurvedacharya, and is graduate of ancient and modern medicine. Author of numerous works on

Ayurveda, he combines medicine with astrology. An internationally famous herbalist, Ayurvedia acupressurist, and Indian physician, he has toured abroad extensively, and has given lectures and appeared on TV programs.

WILLIAM A. TILLER, PH.D., is a professor in the Department of Materials Science and Engineering at Stanford University, was chairman from 1966 to 1971, is a consultant to government and industry, and serves as associate editor of two scientific journals. He has published over 130 scientific papers and was awarded a Guggenheim Fellowship in 1970–71.

MICHAEL P. VOLEN, M.D., is currently in private practice of medicine in northern California. He was until recently clinic medical director of the Pain Control Unit and Acupuncture Project at U.C.L.A. School of Medicine. He has lectured and written in the areas of acupuncture, pain management, nutrition, and preventive medicine.

Preface

The unusual way this book came together gave us the impression that the time for its advent had arrived. We would like to share these circumstances with the reader. One day in November 1975, on the basis of a spur-of-the-moment decision, the senior editor of this volume (Herbert Otto) decided to stop work on another project and begin work on this book. As is his practice, he had set up a file folder for this book about eight months before November, 1975, when he first thought about editing a volume on wholistic healing. He decided at the outset to seek as coeditor a physician who had been active or involved in the wholistic healing movement. However, due to time pressures, he chose not to seek a coeditor until after a rough draft of the outline of the book had been prepared.

On the day work was spontaneously started on the book outline and chapter headings, the senior editor received a phone call. It was from a person (Kenée Knight) who said she had read one of his books and that she and her husband, a physician, were in San Diego and would like to meet and talk with him. Although he usually has no time for visitors when working on a book project, for some reason he made an exception and set an appointment for Dr. and Mrs. Knight for early in the afternoon. Subsequently the Knights phoned and said they would be delayed for a couple of hours. This news was most happily received, for it provided the time to finish the first rough draft outline of the book.

Shortly after Dr. and Mrs. Knight arrived, we established that Dr. Knight had been fully involved in the wholistic healing movement for quite some time, used psychic healing in his own practice (and was in fact a gifted healer) and *had been thinking of doing a book on wholistic healing*. We found that our files, as well as knowledge and acquaintance with people in the field, largely complemented each other. Both of us had the very strong impression that elements other than chance were at work in this fortuitous meeting.

Thanks to Ms. Kenée Knight for her help, also to Ms. Mary Hoffman of Mill Valley for her very thoughtful suggestions and to Ms. Linda Littler for her dedication in the preparation of the final manuscript.

Part I

The Basis
of
Wholistic Healing

1

Herbert A. Otto and James W. Knight

Wholistic Healing:
Basic Principles and Concepts

THE CONCEPTS and principles that underlie wholistic healing are by no means new and are traceable in the writings of various healers and physicians dating well into antiquity. Wholistic healing deals with the totality of a person's being: the mental/emotional, physical, social, and spiritual dimensions. It is this totality as an integrative and synthesizing force, so perceived and utilized by the healing person or team, that constitutes wholistic healing.

Wholistic healing then, means treating the whole person, helping the person to bring the mental/emotional, physical, social, and spiritual dimensions of his or her being into greater harmony, *using the basic principles and elements of wholistic healing* and, as much as possible, placing reliance on treatment modalities that foster the self-regenerative and self-reparatory processes of natural healing.

When a person is ill and is seeking health, the entire person needs to be treated—the psyche, mind, and body. In this sense, *wholistic* denotes an attitude traceable to the early Greek physician Hippocrates, who believed that every person must be understood as a whole. Today, we would add that each individual needs to be understood as a whole person within the context of the total environment in which he or she functions. From the wholistic perspective, health is viewed as the quality of life instead of the absence of disease. Wholistic healing is a global concept, which includes the disciplines of orthodox medicine as a component. Wholistic healing means utilization of both the orthodox and unorthodox disciplines in the healing process and involves the emergence of a NEW medicine.

Wholistic healing may be briefly defined as follows: *Wholistic healing is the treatment of the whole person. It helps to bring the mental/emotional, physical, social, and spiritual dimensions of the person's being into greater harmony and employs wholistic principles and the elements of a total, integrated treatment program, with emphasis on any therapy or treatment that stimulates a person's own healing processes.*

The term *holistic* is originally derived from an early twentieth-century philosophy called *holism*, which states that the determining factors in nature, and particularly in evolution, are wholes such as organisms and not their constituent parts. The originator of this philosophy, Jan Smuts, observes that

> the creation of *wholes*, and ever more highly organized *wholes*, and of *wholeness* generally as characteristic of existence, is an inherent character of the universe. There is not a mere vague indefinite creative energy or tendency at work in the world. This energy or tendency has specific characters, the most fundamental of which is *whole-making*. And the progressive development of the resulting *wholes* at all stages—from the most inchoate, imperfect, inorganic *wholes* to the most highly developed and organised—is what we call Evolution. The *whole*-making, holistic tendency, or Holism, operating in and through particular *wholes*, is seen at all stages of existence, and is by no means confined to the biological domain to which science has hitherto restricted it.[1] [Emphasis added.]

The editors have chosen to use a variant spelling of holistic, adding a *w*. This was done to emphasize the subtitle of the volume, ". . .treatment of the *whole* person." It is of interest in this connection that the word *health* has an etymological relationship to the word *wholeness*. It implies that all aspects of the total system are in balance with each other.

Many persons today realize that they are not functioning optimally, and although they do not seem to be suffering from any specific illness, their health status could be improved. Such a person may also, for example, eat a sweet, starchy diet, smoke heavily, take no exercise, have few interests, and appear to be glum and emotionally repressed. To biologist René Dubos, this person is a carrier of what he calls "submerged potential illness." Such persons are increasingly seeking out physicians and other healers, but to assign the label of "patient" to those who simply seek optimal health would be confusing. Since wholistic healing is as concerned with this segment of the population as with the clinically ill, use of the term patient has been avoided in this chapter.

Isolated principles dealing with wholistic healing can be found scattered in many published works, and various individuals have tried to formulate wholistic programs based largely on their own experience with specific healing practices and methods. However, there is no history of a major effort to bring together and synthesize such principles and practices or to formulate a comprehensive set of concepts that, in their totality, constitute a wholistic treatment program useful to the practitioner regardless of his or her speciality or particular predilection for certain healing disciplines. *It is the purpose of this volume to furnish a basic conceptual framework of wholistic healing applicable to a wide range of treatment programs, and to provide an introduction to some of the promising new or neglected modalities that can make an important contribution to wholistic healing.* All but four of the contributions were originally written for this volume.

Emerging today is a refreshing openness, an eagerness and willingness by practitioners to learn from the experience of others in the health sciences and the broad field of healing. This openness to new ideas and approaches distinguishes an increasing number of contemporary professionals and practitioners in the field of healing. Significantly, it is marked by a notable reduction in the internecine warfare, the insistence on orthodoxies, doctrines, and absolutes, that has been one of the dominant characteristics of the field of healing for the past one hundred and fifty years. This new and growing spirit of openness, tolerance, and search appears to be a hallmark of those involved in the wholistic healing movement.

Although the wholistic healing movement has entered an accelerated phase of growth and expansion, what psychiatrist Roy W. Menninger calls the resistance of physicians "to practice a genuinely holistic medicine that integrates knowledge of the body, the mind and the environment," is nevertheless a reality.

Why do these resistances persist? At least one possibility is the fact that there are several fundamental conceptual polarities in medicine, established in the physician's perspective by his training and reinforced by the hyper-specialization of current practice. They are the mind-body dualism, and the separation of health from illness. Both dualisms are characterized by a tendency to separate the extremes, segregate the opposing elements, and assign them to separate disciplines. Both seem to work at preconscious levels, affecting the behavior of practicing physicians in subtle ways that may be obvious to an observer, but pass beneath notice of the practitioner. So established are they that, in a real sense, they have become part of the background of our medical system. . . .

Breaking the grip of these dualities will permit medicine to recapture the whole person as the focus of attention and reduce those dehumanizing preoccupations with the disease alone, the psyche alone, the liver or the pancreas alone, the psychosis alone. This is holistic medicine for a society that needs to learn from the medical profession how to be an effectively caring society.[2] [Emphasis added.]

Psychosomatic Medicine and the Wholistic Healing Movement

Findings and concepts from the field of psychosomatic medicine make an important contribution to the understanding of wholistic healing. Psychosomatic research clearly pinpoints the dynamic role played by emotions in the onset of illness and pathogenic processes.

Such research spans more than four decades. In 1932 the psychiatrist Franz Alexander and his associates at the Chicago Institute for Psychoanalysis found that patients suffering from certain organic ailments had similar patterns of emotional conflicts. The doctors felt that such conflicts offered clues to what would subsequently be called *psychosomatic disease.* Alexander (often called the "father" of psychosomatic medicine) and his associates soon confirmed that specific configurations of emotional factors accompanied particular disorders. For example, individuals suffering from hypertension had difficulty handling hostile impulses; those with duodenal ulcers had conflicts involving their dependency needs; and asthma sufferers appeared to fear loss of their mothers.[3] The work of Alexander was subsequently enriched by the pioneering studies of Flanders Dunbar, M.D., who contributed one of the early basic texts in the field.[4]

Many physicians now recognize that emotional factors play an important role in a large number of disorders or illnesses, if not most of them. There is an increasing awareness of the highly complex interplay of emotions and organic disorders.

> . . .the factors that are significant forerunners of psychiatric and psychosomatic disorders—namely repressed hostility, dependency, anxiety, guilt, feelings of inadequacy, and isolation, to mention only a few—are common to *all* emotional disturbances, though they may differ in degree and duration. Moreover, multiple disease states may coexist. A person may suffer from two or more psychosomatic diseases, or a psychiatric and a psychosomatic disease, or an organic and a psychosomatic disease. *Psychological factors in illness are therefore more complex and subtle than the general medical model of disease.*[5] [Emphasis added.]

It is significant that one of the pioneers of psychosomatic medicine, Flanders Dunbar, M.D., by the quality of her contribution, still remains in the forefront of contemporary thought on healing.

> On the whole, the physician can judge the results of his treatment in this way: If the bodily symptoms are cured, the job has been fair. If the patient's susceptibility to disease has been decreased also, the job has been good. If the patient furthermore has reached the point of understanding himself, the job has been excellent. . . .
> Psychosomatic treatment usually qualifies the patient to help himself afterwards. . . . The patient who has reached the point of applying a psychosomatic treatment to himself has had more than relief from the bodily symptoms. *He has achieved a cure of the whole man;* he has become sound both in mind and body.[6]

Psychosomatic concepts and findings are of particular significance to wholistic health because they clearly point up the unity or wholeness of the person by clarifying that emotional and physical factors, in their interaction, and with the help of microbes, viruses, or other disease agents, result in a certain set of symptoms which are then defined as dis-ease, or illness.

The Academy of Psychosomatic Medicine, established in 1954, joined together professionals with various experiences in the disciplines dedicated to give special attention to the management of patients from a generally wholistic point of view. In an era of partial or incomplete medical care brought about by the rapid increase in specialization, the concept of *total medical care* of the physical and emotional needs of the patient became the philosophy of the academy.

Although definitions of psychosomatic medicine differ with the expert, the model developed by the physician C. Alberto Seguin is among the most comprehensive. "We speak, not of a psychosomatic medicine but of a *psychosomatic tendency in medicine, which has as its aim the study of man as a whole, a totality, considered as such in health and in disease* and the application of the conclusions of such study to diagnosis, prognosis and treatment."[7] [Emphasis added.]

Many of the more sophisticated physicians today are aware that seventy to eighty percent of patients seen by the general practitioner have presented problems that are functional in nature or of psychosomatic origin. These figures by themselves are the clearest indication of the paramount need for a wholistic approach as the preferred framework for prevention and treatment of illness as well as the maintenance of wellness for the whole person.

Basic Principles and Concepts of Wholistic Healing

A number of principles and concepts form the basic framework for the practice of wholistic healing. They are applicable regardless of the particular treatment modality of preference, or the type of therapeutic program used. Each of the principles will be discussed briefly and significant underlying elements described.

1. Recognition that every human being has vast untapped potentials, resources, and powers is inherent in wholistic healing.

From the human potentialities hypothesis that we are using less than ten percent of our capacities,[8] it follows that up to now we have not learned how to help a person use more than a fraction of his or her potential (the human potentialities hypothesis is widely accepted by behavioral and other scientists of many nations). Despite our accumulation of knowledge, then, *every human being remains essentially a mystery* with much as yet to be actualized and to be discovered. It is important to be aware of this because, regardless of the condition of the human organism at any moment in time, this recognition introduces the element of hope.

Since every person has vast unused resources and capacities, *the paradigm of the human being as an energy system* with tremendous latent powers is especially appropriate. From this perspective, the human being emerges as a very complex configuration of interlocking and interacting electrochemical subsystems. An imbalance in these subsystems can then be seen as a cause of disease. Each individual human energy system in some manner interacts with other human energy systems and the total energy systems referred to as the universe. From this point of view, individual human energy systems can also become conduits of therapeutic power and healing.

2. The fostering of self-awareness and self-understanding can play a vital role in the healing process.

The human being is best understood as basically striving toward health and vitality. The presenting symptom or disease is a part of this basic thrust toward health and often has strong symbolic overtones. The disease fundamentally functions as a sign language or communication that may point to an imbalance in life. The essense of this communication is "I cannot cope (with my life situation), and I am in need of help/love/caring at this moment in my existence." The person has reached a point of crisis. At the deepest level, the symptom or disease represents a way of reaching for health. In the crisis of disease, there is also the greatest potential for the resolution of the life crisis facing the person. *Gains in self-understanding and self-awareness at such times can have a profound and positive effect on the healing process.* Therefore, it is important for the person who facilitates healing to help the person with the disease to acquire increased self-understanding and awareness of his or her functioning. Disease presents a singular opportunity for synthesis and personal growth. In this sense, it can result in more adequate and creative functioning of the personality.

3. Placing reliance on the capacities and resources of the person seeking health is a key factor in mobilizing the healing processes.

There needs to be a clear awareness at all times by everyone concerned *that the healer is merely a facilitator of the healing processes*, that despite the skill of the healing team, attaining health and wellness is in the hands of the person who is seeking healing. It is important to point out that *the healing team does not make the person well, but helps the person to make himself or herself well.* The responsibility for attaining health is thereby placed where it belongs: it is *primarily* the responsibility of the person seeking wellness. In this connection, *as much as possible the person striving for health needs to be actively involved in the processes designed to foster healing.* (The person who is encouraged to walk shortly after an operation, and who thereby recovers faster, is in fact an active participant in a process which fosters healing.)

The healing team, then, needs to know the person sufficiently well to help tap those motivational wellsprings or aspects of his or her being that will reinforce the thrust toward health. Finally, wholistic healing places major emphasis on the utilization of psychological factors in the healing process and in the maintenance of health (see also principle 8).

4. The interpersonal relationship environment is an integral part of the treatment program and is of outstanding importance throughout the period of healing.

Since the need for caring and love is particularly pressing at a time when a person is disabled by disease, and since love and caring can hasten the process of healing, the person seeking healing needs to be consistently aware that *all healing personnel are giving abundantly of their warmth, empathy and understanding and are furnishing the type of emotional nurturance particularly needed at a time of illness.* The relationship environment provided by the healing team is of fundamental importance in this connection. It creates a climate of healing that fosters an optimum recovery process.

At times of illness, most persons have a tendency to become increasingly dependent and to some extent regress to earlier modes of relationships. During this process, members of the healing team tend to be perceived and related to as compassionate, authoritative parent figures or "significant others." This in part is due to a recognition by the person suffering from a disease that love and caring given to him or her by others is a dynamic force that fosters healing. It is also important for the healing team to use this "regression dynamic" to challenge the person *to assume the power of his or her own healing potential and not to remain excessively dependent upon others to facilitate the healing process.*

Wholistic healing recognizes and values the unique individuality of each person and is opposed to the dehumanization inherent in a perspective where the focus is on the treatment of an organ (a "kidney case" or a "heart case") rather than treating the whole person. Included as a part of wholistic healing is also an awareness of the importance of the physical environment in which the healing takes place. A person's room and other surroundings can affect his or her attitude and can play a supportive role in the healing process.

5. Maximal use needs to be made of self-regulating processes and therapies within the dynamics of a disease process before that process reaches the point where major chemotherapy or surgical treatment is required.

The use of self-regulatory processes (such as meditation, relaxation, and Autogenic Training) builds on and utilizes the potential for self-healing and the thrust for health that are present. It is well known that with some basic therapeutic support by the healing team, many conditions "yield to the passage of time." In effect, with adequate support and encouragement, the person often heals himself. *The emphasis in wholistic healing, then, is on nurturing the natural healing processes of the body.* Often the healing process can be accelerated by helping the person activate his own healing resources and by helping him or her take a greater responsibility for activity to promote healing. *The self-regulatory therapies tend to restore health in the sense of bringing harmony to the organism and reestablishing a more fully conscious equilibrium within the whole.*

6. Wholistic healing makes optimum use of the dynamic and therapeutic forces inherent in group interaction and group work.

Properly conducted, group sessions can make an important contribution to the healing process by furnishing a support network, enhancing motivation, and providing positive reinforcement in relation to the optimal utilization of healing programs and regimes.

As the author and former *Look* editor George Leonard points out, wholistic medicine is also concerned ". . .with all the tragic and ingenious ways we have learned to abuse the gift of life."[9] The group provides the best possible environment for unlearning habits and attitudes that abuse health. Under the guidance of trained facilitators, the group can become a potent medium for helping participants explore underlying emotional forces or elements that play a role in illness or dysfunction, *or that block or impede healing*. Wholistic healing recognizes that anomie—people's estrangement from themselves and each other—is pervasive in contemporary society and that groups can be so conducted as to diminish anomie. In such groups the nature of the relationship structures favors the formation of friendships, and is characterized by deep caring and the creation of a group climate that enhances the process of healing.

7. Recognizing the integrative aspect of life, wholistic healing also addresses itself to the quality of a person's life by fostering exploration of the personal lifestyle, to bring values, goals, aspirations, and personal functioning into increased harmony.

The lack of consonance among beliefs, values, and a person's behavior and functioning often creates inner conflicts, devisiveness, and tension. There may also be interpersonal conflicts within the family or in relation to the vocation, which can cause or contribute to dysfunction and disease. Added to this are often other social and interpersonal forces and pressures which, in a similar manner, can cause or contribute to pathology. Improper nutrition, lack of exercise, or other habits inimical to health (for example, excessive smoking or drinking) may also play a role in the disease process. Therefore, and as an integral part of the treatment program, *wholistic healing is also concerned with the treatment of the underlying causes or cause of a disease, i.e., the primal cause*. All of the preceding factors need to be recognized and dealt with to foster optimum healing. In this connection, it is important to be aware that social forces and the very structure and function of society can and do affect the health status of the individual member. In recent years, the environmental origin of many diseases has been increasingly recognized. For example, according to one recent estimate, up to eighty percent of all cancer results from exposure to carcinogenic agents in the environment.[10] *Regeneration of society in such a way as to foster the optimum health of its members is thus acknowledged to be an aim of the wholistic healing movement.*

8. Utilization of a person's spiritual resources or belief structure is an important aspect of the wholistic healing process.

The spiritual or religious resources, the element of faith, including the nature of the individual's relationship with his or her God, the Ground of Being, or the Universe, can play an important role in fostering healing. Thus the quality of faith can be of utmost value through the establishment of greater harmony between the person, the self within, and God or the Universe without. The quality of faith can enable the person seeking health to discover the nature of those spiritual forces that open the pathways or flows and harmonics necessary to unfold the channels of the self within the body and the self within the world, the Universe, and God. From this perspective, then, the minister, priest, shaman, or spiritual guide is considered to be a vital contributing member of the healing team.

It also needs to be understood that, regardless of the religious faith of the person seeking health, through *adequate exploration of the belief system* this faith can make an important contribution to healing. (For example, a person suffering from a disease may have no religious faith in the generally understood sense of the term but may believe that everyone is part of a larger system and that through such means as the laying on of hands a particular individual can channel energies that foster healing.) Research psychologist Dr. Kenneth R. Pelletier further clarifies the function of a person's belief system.

> In the modern sciences ranging from the neurophysiology of consciousness to a quantum physics, it is evident *that the structure of an individual's personal belief system concerning the nature of himself and his universe governs that person's experience.* Inherent in any system of belief is the self-fulfilling prophecy that what is expected is observed and what is observed confirms the expectations. . . . An immediate implication of this principle is that it is possible for an individual to completely reformulate his belief system and become aware of a vast realm of new possibilities.[11] [Emphasis added.]

The belief system of a person who is striving for health represents a valuable resource that can effectively be utilized in healing. Finally, it must be emphasized that *suggestion* (sometimes called the placebo effect) plays a very powerful role in human affairs. With a good understanding and utilization of a person's belief system as a base, positive suggestion can become a dynamic force that fosters the healing process.

Some Notes on the Implementation of Wholistic Healing

Innovation and advancement in any field of human endeavor inevitably are confronted by the roadblocks of (institutional) tradition and human resistance to change. Wholistic healing programs are no exception. One effective way to minimize the resistance to change is to organize a wholistic healing center—a path chosen by a number of pioneers in the movement. Others work effectively within the framework of institutions and are bringing change and growth to these institutions. The following notes on the implementation of wholistic healing programs are offered as an initial contribution toward the building of a foundation for program development.

First and foremost, training opportunities need to be created to help practitioners explore the theoretical base and acquire a more thorough understanding of the principles and elements of wholistic healing. Closely allied are the practical (as well as theoretical) aspects of the four key components of wholistic healing: (1) the wholistic functioning of the healing team (2) wholistic diagnosis and the selection of appropriate healing modalities (3) the optimum active involvement in the healing process of the person seeking health and (4) creating the healing environment. Each of these key components will be briefly discussed and major factors in each component summarized.

1. Wholistic Functioning of the Healing Team

To function wholistically, a healing team must have certain characteristics. Of primary importance is a *consensus or general agreement about the basic principles and elements of wholistic healing.* Since different people define or understand terms differently and semantic difficulties are frequently encountered, members of the healing team need to develop their own framework of principles and elements that underlie wholistic healing.

The composition of the healing team may vary, but generally an effort is made to have an equitable ratio of men and women on the team. Besides the physician, the nurse, the psychologist, the social worker or paramedical person (whose special task is to mobilize emotional support and nourishment—see also section 4 below), and the minister, there are the other practitioners of the healing arts, including natural healers and psychic healers. The composition of the healing team is based on both the needs of the person seeking health and the general philosophy, orientation, or specific commitment to healing of the team and its members.

Of basic importance is the selection and *clarification of function of the team members.* A healing team functions best when the unique individual quality of each person on the team, as well as the contribution each can make, is understood and deeply respected and valued by all the team members, who consider each other as coequals in the common task of wholistic healing. In order to ensure optimum functioning of team members, it is desirable that the team use democratic leadership principles (shared and rotated leadership responsibilities) and avoid hierarchic, authority-centered functioning.

In view of the significance of the emotional climate during the healing process, as well as to obtain a better understanding of and develop a comprehensive treatment program dealing with the root causes of an illness, the presence of a psychologist, social worker or paraprofessional with special skills for helping people help themselves as members of the healing team is of particular importance. Another function of these members is to explore how family and friendship relations can contribute to the wholistic healing program. Two additional functions of such team members are (1) to furnish training in relaxation techniques prior to elective surgery and to help the patient develop a psychological attitude most conducive to the regaining of health and (2) to furnish follow-up services. These latter are especially important after major surgery and/or dismissal from the hospital and in instances of stress-induced illness where a change of lifestyle or alleviation of primal causes is indicated.

Although the addition of such team members may result in some increase in cost, this is outweighed by savings in treatment and recovery time. It can also be expected that some physicians will object to the emphasis on building a supportive relationship with the person seeking health, on the basis that this takes too much time. It should be made clear that training courses are available that can equip the physician with relationship-building skills that will actually save time.

To ensure the wholistic functioning of the healing team, frequent meetings are scheduled to establish and maintain open communication about both the healing program and team member relationships, as well as to foster personal and professional growth. In this connection, sophisticated healing teams are aware that the use of skilled outside consultants represents one of the best ways to help a team function more effectively. This is also the most economical and effective way to deal with significant problems and difficulties that may arise within a team. (It must also be recognized that a group of people who have already been working together for some time, and who wish to form a wholistic healing team, can profit greatly from the assistance of a skilled outside consultant.) Finally, it needs to be emphasized that an effective wholistic healing team not only functions to facilitate healing in others, but also gives emotional nourishment and support to its own members.

2. Wholistic Diagnosis and the Selection of the Appropriate Healing Modalities

Wholistic diagnosis involves a readiness or openness on the part of the healer or healing team to use the total range of diagnostic means or techniques available including those not commonly accepted. (For example, various forms of paranormal diagnosis by "psychic diagnosticians" have been increasingly utilized over the years by physicians both in this country and abroad. Unconventional diagnostic systems such as the acupuncture system are increasingly used as well.) As an integral part of wholistic diagnosis, the person seeking health is also encouraged to contribute as much as possible of his or her own impressions and knowledge about both the causes and the nature of the dysfunction or pathology. Recognizing the value of personal intuition (sometimes also referred to as clinical judgement), members of the healing team both foster and utilize it in the diagnostic process.

As previously mentioned, the wholistic healing team is concerned with primal-cause therapy, i.e. the diagnosis or determination, and correction, of the underlying or root causes that are ultimately responsible for the illness, dysfunction, or lack of optimal functioning of the human organism. In this connection, an understanding of underlying emotional factors *and* the lifestyle (including the familial, vocational, and social environment) of the person seeking health is indispensable.

From the perspective of wholistic healing, the selection of the appropriate healing modalities, or means utilized to bring about healing, *is based on the guiding principle of treating the whole person, including the physical, mental/emotional, social, and spiritual dimensions.* In the selection of healing modalities, emphasis is on the fostering of the natural healing processes, on self-regeneration and the self-regulatory therapies; the use of major chemotherapeutic and surgical intervention is avoided whenever possible. It is recognized, however, that if traumatic or disease processes have passed a certain point, chemotherapeutic or surgical intervention may be the only alternative.

Many physicians today are utilizing unconventional modalities as a part of their healing program, and many more are at least contemplating the use of such modalities. (See Chapter 3, Toward a General Theory of Psychic Healing.) Although the selection of specific healing modalities is based on the needs of the patient seeking health and the healing commitment of the team, certain basic components are uniformly present. These include nutrition and dietary counseling, and the use of physical exercise and self-regulatory regimes. Of equal importance are programs designed to help the person seeking health to achieve better understanding and management of emotional factors and the use of spiritual resources in the regaining of health. As an integral part of such treatment programs, appropriate use is made of the dynamic and therapeutic forces inherent in group work. All the preceeding are basic components of wholistic healing programs regardless of the specific healing modalities selected.

3. The Active Participation of the Person Seeking Health in the Healing Process

Central to wholistic healing is a focus on engaging the consciousness of the individual seeking health to help him or her to become an active participant in the healing process. This means the optimum utilization of the person's motivational structure, values, and aspirations in the service of health. In so far as possible, the person needs to be presented with *choices* about the courses of action leading to health, so that decisions for health are made on the basis of the person's *own decisions* rather than the imposition of prescriptions and proscriptions issued by authority. "Health professionals should provide resources and information to help persons make informed choices regarding their health. . . . A medical system that fosters dependency and undermines an individual person's confidence is clearly counterproductive to the ideal of individual freedom."[12]

It is necessary to recognize that traditional treatment models are firmly entrenched and, during the many years people have had to learn the role of "patient," these models have become deeply established. To many, assuming the role of patient means entering an essentially passive state of being, with the physician and the chemotherapy or elective surgery assigned the responsibility for making the patient well. For these and other complex reasons, some persons may not be in sympathy with a number of the components and aims of wholistic healing. Wholistic healing programs, on the other hand, emphasize and place reliance on the person's *own* responsibility, initiative, and full involvement in the regaining of health. In this connection, the thinking of physician Leonard Duhl, a professor of public health at the University of California, Berkeley, is of interest. He points out that health may not always be homeostasis and balance; "it is also an attempt to get ready for a new state and development. . . . Concern for health, therefore, is concern for utilization of the transition period of crisis stress, to redirect individual (self-healing) energy . . . the process toward health—the act of creating our own aliveness—that act is health."[13]

Over the past years, it has become clear that stress-induced illness is responsible for an increasing number of hospital admissions. This trend is only in its beginnings, and in the foreseeable future, admissions due to stress-induced illness can be expected to further increase. Although different people have varying stress factors, most stress is traceable to various combinations of vocational, familial, or social problems. Furthermore, a person is extremely likely to return to the identical stress-inducing environment after treatment. As a crucial part of the maximum active involvement in the healing process, such a person needs to be particularly encouraged to become aware of the sources of stress that have contributed to his or her condition. Even more important, he or she needs to be encouraged to initiate change designed to minimize stress or to learn ways (such as relaxation, massage, meditation, biofeedback techniques) to more adequately cope with stress.

4. The Healing Environment

Wholistic healing means the creation of a total healing environment including both the climate of interpersonal relationships and the physical environment. Most people suffering from illness are particularly sensitive to the emotional currents and undertones both in and among members of the healing team with whom they come into contact. As previously mentioned, the caring/loving and supportive emotional climate provided by the team plays an important role in the creation of a healing climate.

There is a growing recognition of this fact. For example, significant segments of the nursing profession are now placing less emphasis on the administrative and technical functions of nursing and are more concerned with the emotional/nurturance and understanding the nurse has to offer. Psychotherapists have also shown an increasing interest in the wholistic approach. Hospitals are beginning to use the principles of color therapy in their environment and are making available "loan art" for the patient. As previously stated, color and design, aesthetic objects, and self-selected printed messages and posters remain largely neglected in their use as supportive adjuncts to the healing program.[14] In short, wholistic healing is concerned with the creation of a total environment that facilitates total health—both the environment specifically designed to facilitate the healing process and the larger environment of the society and the world in which we live.

Wholistic Healing: Emergence of a Movement

The following short history of the wholistic healing movement is based on records to which the writers had access. It is already clear, however, that although a great deal of groundwork and research was done, this initial effort to compile a short record of the movement can make no claim to be comprehensive. More information, particularly pertaining to the early evolution of the movement, is needed. The authors would welcome any help with this task from readers so that a more comprehensive history can be included in a subsequent edition of this volume. (Chapter 2, Wholistic Healing: Historic Base and Short History.)

Contemporary antecedents of the wholistic healing movement are to be found in the fields of sociology, biology, anthropology, medicine, chemistry, philosophy, religion, physics, nutrition, and other disciplines. For numerous decades, organizations and responsible individuals engaged in these disciplines have been concerned with many of the concepts that lie at the core of the wholistic healing movement. Prominent among the organizations, some of whose aims and purposes parallel those of the wholistic healing movement, are the American College of Preventive Medicine, the Academy of Psychosomatic Medicine, and the American Psychosomatic Society.

Some of the organizations more recently formed to actively promote a number of the principles, concepts, and approaches to wholistic healing are the International College of Psychosomatic Medicine (1970), Association for Transpersonal Psychology (1972), The American Metapsychiatric Association (1974), The Center for the Healing Arts (1975), and the Health Network of the Association for Humanistic Psychology (1976). These and other organizations of similar as well as varied activities and interests are listed in Appendix B, Directory of Organizations.

At annual invitational meetings such as the May Lectures, initiated in London in May, 1974, and Council Grove, cosponsored by Menninger Foundation and the Association for Transpersonal Psychology, relatively small groups of well-known scientists, clinicians, and researchers gather to explore new and pioneering concepts related to medicine and health. During the early seventies, two organizations, the Hawaii Health Net and the Academy of Parapsychology and Medicine, launched programs that can be called the precursors of the wholistic health movement.

The Hawaii Health Net officially began in August, 1972, with a conference coordinated by Nancy Strode and Walter Strode, M.D., "Toward the Future of Health," held at the East-West Center, Hawaii. Futurist-economist Robert Theobald was the keynote speaker. His message emphasized that the institutionalization of formal organizations reduces their flexibility, and that professional specialization of human roles locks people into mental sets foreclosing new possibilities. To help rectify this situation, an open communications network, the Hawaii Health Net was formed.

The Health Net is a body of people from various disciplines interconnected through a communications network; conferences, meetings, and other activities promote that communication. Additional conferences sponsored by the Hawaii Health Net included the three-day "Toward the Future of Health and Whole Man," held in May, 1973, at Hawaii Loa College, and "Healthing Hawaii: New Experiences in Health as Human Wholeness," held in January, 1975. In August, 1974, a symposium entitled "Health on a Small Planet," one of a series of environmental symposia at Expo '74, was held in Spokane, Washington. This symposium added new dimensions of experiences, ideas, and people to the Hawaii Health Net and led to the establishment and spin-off of a Northwest Net with headquarters in Spokane.

According to physician Walter Strode, one of the originators of the Hawaii Health Net,

> . . .we must realize that we are searching for *promotive health* and not merely better health care, and this requires reconceptualization. . . . we have come to realize that new approaches to health as human wholeness follow from changes in our consciousness. As we ourselves

change, systems will change. . . . *Health as human wholeness*, then,
is both *what we aspire to and what we seek to live from*. The Network
provides us with a means for expressing the metaphor of human
wholeness operationally. . . . At the center of the Net's life-style is the
experience of human community, a core of persons-in-relationship.
This core provides a base of security or stability from which to move
into the new and unknown areas, provides the encouragement to bring
the unknown into creative dialogue with the known so that the Net can
always be in the process of 'becoming.'[15] [Emphasis added.]

The Academy of Parapsychology and Medicine, composed of physicians, allied health professionals, and others interested in a scientific
approach to frontier areas of healing, sponsored a four-day symposium
on "The Dimensions of Healing." This conference was held at Stanford University September 30 through October 3, 1972, and again in
October in Los Angeles, this time cosponsored by the University of
California at Los Angeles. Over 1300 professionals were introduced to
biofeedback, acupuncture, spiritual healing, and other modalities.
The academy sponsored a similar three-day conference featuring frontiers of science and medicine in October, 1975, in Phoenix, Arizona.
Also of interest is the February, 1976, publication of Volume 1,
Number 1 of the *Journal of Holistic Health*.[16]

It is clear now that this series of conferences, which heralded a
growing surge of interest by health professionals in new modalities of
healing, were by no means restricted to the West Coast. Similar meetings, on a somewhat smaller scale, were held in other parts of the
country from the early through the mid-1970s.

Two such events were "Holistic Patient Care and the Role of Body
Energies: Ninth Annual Symposium" sponsored by A.R.E. Clinic, Inc.
and The Edgar Cayce Foundation in cooperation with Atlantic University in Phoenix, Arizona, in January 1976; and the seventh annual
"ESP Body/Mind/Spirit Healing Workshop," sponsored by ESP Research Associates Foundation, held in St. Louis, Missouri, in June,
1976. At the 1972 and 1973 annual meetings of the American Psychiatric Association in Dallas, its Task Force on Transcultural Psychiatry
presented panel-symposia on psychic phenomena. Stanley Dean,
M.D., organized the 1974 panel in Detroit; it attracted an audience of
six hundred and fifty lay and professional people—the largest panel
attendance in APA history.

On the West Coast, the University of California played a central role in the genesis of the wholistic health movement. The University of California, through the School of Medicine, Extension Division and various health divisions, offers opportunities for both professionals and the general public to join together for weekend programs or brief workshops. The first pertinent programs included Healing I and II, consisting of lectures on wholistic healing held jointly by the Los Angeles and Santa Cruz university campuses in March and April, 1975. The meetings attracted approximately seven hundred and one thousand people respectively, including many professionals from throughout the state. Other presentations have included "Birth and Rebirth," held in September, 1975, in Santa Cruz, cosponsored by Gladman Memorial Hospital, Oakland; "Sound, Movement and the Healing Arts," in August 1976, at San Diego; "Ways of Healing: Ancient and Modern," in January, 1976, at San Francisco, in cooperation with the Institute for the Study of Human Knowledge; and "The All-American Medicine Show," held in September, 1976, at Santa Cruz. Ten-week courses, limited to fifty professionals, have also been offered at the University of California's Los Angeles, San Diego, Santa Cruz, and San Francisco campuses on such topics as "Acupuncture for the Management of Musculo-skeletal Pain," "Autogenic Training and Biofeedback," "Yoga: Clinical Applications and Techniques," "The Laying-on-of-Hands," and "Shiatsu: Acupuncture Without Needles."

In Northern California, the East West Academy of Healing Arts, under the direction of Dr. Effie Poy Chow, actively assumed the responsibility and coordination of the wholistic health movement, including the application for and obtaining of state and national grants for education and research, sponsoring of conferences and workshops, and communication of wholistic healing concepts to local, state, and national governmental leaders. Several conferences have been co-sponsored by the University of San Francisco, San Francisco State University, the Department of Public Health, the City and County of San Francisco, the Western Interstate Commission on Higher Education, and the Public Health Services of the Department of Health, Education and Welfare. The conferences, all held at the University of San Francisco, included "Holistic Approaches to Health Care," in June, 1975; "Holistic Health II and Healing Energies," in November, 1975; "Holistic Health III: Cultural Healing Systems: Rituals and Practices," in June, 1976; and Holistic Health IV: Stress and Tension:

Cancer/Death and Dying," in September, 1976. Short-term training programs held included "Acupressure," "Therapeutic Touch," and "Iridology."

In May, 1974, the International Cooperation Council, a coordinating body formed in 1965 composed of educational, scientific, cultural, and religious organizations, sponsored a well-attended symposium, "Healing the Whole Person I," in Los Angeles for the general public, also drawing many interested professionals in the health field. Further stimulation and exchange of ideas in wholistic healing was afforded a large audience of professionals and the general public at the two-day conference "Healing the Whole Person II," held in Los Angeles in May, 1975. Sponsoring this sequel to the 1974 symposium was the International Cooperation Council in cooperation with the Healing Council for the Whole Person, Los Angeles.

Close on the heels of this highly successful conference directed toward the general public, physicians and other allied health personnel were invited to San Diego, California, for the "Physician of the Future" symposium. Held in June, 1975, under the auspices of the Mandala Society affiliate and International Cooperation Council, this seminal conference was directed by David Harris of the Mandala Society, San Diego. Harris, the founder of the Association for Holistic Health, has played a leading role in the establishment of the wholistic health movement in southern California.

A most significant convergence of energies followed the "Physician of the Future" conference, which was attended by over 900 persons, including approximately three hundred physicians. Numerous smaller meetings of interested professionals have been held subsequently in San Francisco, Los Angeles, and San Diego to facilitate wholistic healing in a multiplicity of directions. As a result of these meetings, wholistic concepts have begun to be integrated into already existing organizations and institutions. There have been efforts to accumulate curricula for programs directed toward the allied health professions, as well as efforts toward establishing wholistic healing centers in many other sections of the United States as well as in California.

The Association for Holistic Health was incorporated in 1976 in San Diego to unite organizations and individuals creating wholistic health centers and education and research programs integrating body, mind, and spirit. A weekend symposium, "The Healing Center of the Future Conference," held in San Diego in September, 1976, was attended by over 2,300 participants. Sponsored by the Association for Holistic Health and the Mandala Society in cooperation with the University of California, San Diego School of Medicine, the purpose of the conference and subsequent week-long workshops was to "create a solid bridge between traditional medicine and the innovative healing arts." The 1977 San Diego conference was entitled "Experiencing the Medical Model of the Future," and the 1978 conference theme was "Holistic Health: A Top National Priority."

A number of conferences and meetings on wholistic healing sponsored by professional organizations are in the planning stages or have recently been held in Western, Midwestern, and Eastern states as the spread of this movement grows. For example, in June, 1976, the Western Region meeting of the American Public Health Association held in San Francisco featured a one-day symposium on wholistic health under the leadership of Richard Svihus, M.D.

It is evident that the wholistic healing movement is only in its beginnings. By 1978, meetings and conferences on new modalities of healing and wholistic health had been conducted in many parts of the country, and there were reports from numerous states about the establishment of wholistic healing centers.

In May of 1978, some 225 physicians from the United States and Canada met in Denver to form the American Holistic Medical Association. This was the "birth" in the medical profession of the wholistic medicine movement and its principles. One of the editors participated in the spirit of love and harmony in which the principles, by-laws, and purposes of the organization were founded. This organization provides programs in medical schools, research, education and support materials for both professionals and consumers interested in a wholistic medical practice. (See List of Organizations.)

An indication of the nationwide interest in new healing modalities was furnished in May, 1976 when the pharmaceutical firm of Hoffman-La Roche offered physicians three fifteen–minute tapes of a panel discussion entitled "The Natural Process of Healing." The panel of five physicians and one psychologist was drawn, for the most part, from faculties of medical schools. They discussed such topics as how faith healing techniques (like the laying on of hands and prayer vigils) have speeded up healing of wounds, relieved arthritis, cured infants suffering from colic, and caused regression of cancer. On the tape, one of the members of the panel, Lawrence Le Shan, Ph.D., who is also a contributor to this volume and who has trained many physicians in his psychic healing seminars pointed out, "The psychic healer is a specialist in mobilizing the patient's own resources." *It is significant that more than 27,000 United States physicians and psychiatrists (seven thousand of the latter), or a total of 7.1% of all U.S. medical doctors, wrote to request these tapes.* This is a clear indication of the nation-wide interest in both new modalities of healing and the wholistic healing movement, which is closely associated with these modalities. This response would also appear to suggest that many physicians in traditional medical practice who currently look at the wholistic ap-proach as an adjunct to their work are at a point of readiness to consider it as an alternative. The wholistic healing movement has entered the initial phases of a development that can be expected to accelerate rapidly in the years to come, with profound effects on the health care system.

Conclusion

Wholistic healing is a discipline of the healing process that helps a person deal with each of the dimensions of disharmony and disease in the body—the mental/emotional, physical, social, and spiritual dimen-sions. It is a process that does not force itself upon the being of the person; it is a harmonious process in and of itself. It is one that the person needs to cooperate with totally in order to achieve the desired goal of healing. Therefore it may take a change in consciousness of the person to achieve major facilitation of the healing process. To achieve this, a total environment approach is needed, such as is currently being pioneered by some of the wholistic healing centers. These cen-ters, as they exist now, are primarily learning centers and are serving as a proving ground for the movement.

Much remains to be learned and discovered through research. The research concepts of wholistic healing form a body of science and study that seeks to encompass and elucidate the unknown factors affecting the total health and energy of the human being, including both internal factors and those in an individual's interrelationships with others, with society, and with the environment. Research needs to be organized in such a manner as to build a large data base of relevant orthodox medical and scientific information as a point of reference. This data base can be expanded so that one is able to examine the presently undefined energies as well as the disciplines that at this point are not as yet encompassed by the body of the scientific community. Also, more research needs to be undertaken of the kind conducted by Dr. Kenneth R. Pelletier and colleagues of the Langley Porter Neuropsychiatric Institute in San Francisco. This group is studying the responses and characteristics of exceptionally healthy people.

Finally, wholistic healing is concerned with prevention, preventive programs, and the objectives of preventive medicine. We are therefore in accord with the point of view of physician Theodore Cooper, Assistant Secretary of Health of the U.S. Department of Health, Education and Welfare. "For one thing, *medicine will have to give more than lip service to its responsibilities in the broadening field of prevention.* In order to contribute to improving the quality of life, medicine will have to shift from its traditional passive role—providing care when the patient asks for it—to one of active involvement in seeking to address conditions in society that give rise to the very health problems that medicine is expected to solve."[17] (Emphasis added.) The whole field of prevention, despite and perhaps because of the research difficulties that it poses, remains one of the most promising and challenging fields for intensive research and study.

The research aims of wholistic healing are to expand the scientific field of knowledge and thereby expand the healing potential in the human being. It is our hope that this book will challenge the multiple disciplines to unify themselves into a wholistic concept in order to bring about an improvement in the health and harmony of the individual, the family, the community, and the world.

Notes

1. Jan C. Smuts, *Holism and Evolution* (New York: The Viking Press, 1961): 99.

2. Roy W. Menninger, "Psychiatry 1976: Time for a Holistic Medicine," *Annals of Internal Medicine* 84 (1976): 603–4.

3. Franz Alexander, *Psychosomatic Medicine: Its Principles and Applications* (New York: W. W. Norton, 1950).

4. Flanders Dunbar, *Mind and Body: Psychosomatic Medicine* (New York: Random House, 1955).
5. Howard R. Lewis and Martha E. Lewis, *Psychosomatics: How Your Emotions Can Damage Your Health* (New York: The Viking Press, 1972).
6. Flanders Dunbar, op. cit., pp. 281, 284.
7. C. Alberto Seguin, *Introduction to Psychosomatic Medicine* (New York: International Universities Press, Inc., 1970): 281.
8. Herbert A. Otto, "The Human Potentialities Movement—An Overview," *The Journal of Creative Behavior* 8 (1974): 258.
9. George Leonard, "The Holistic Health Revolution," *The New West* 1 (10 May 1976): 40–49.
10. Theodore Cooper, "A New Perception of Medicine's Role," *The Western Journal of Medicine* 125(1976): 2.
11. Kenneth R. Pelletier, "Mind as a Healer and Mind as a Slayer," *Lifelong Learning* (September–October 1975): 1–3.
12. David S. Sobel, "Limiting Assumptions," *The Western Journal of Medicine* 125 (1976): 15–16.
13. Leonard J. Duhl, "Health, Whole, Holy, Healing," *Gesar* (quarterly publication of the Nyingma Institute) 3, no. 3 (1976): 15–16.
14. Dr. Otto is in the process of assembling a set of wholistic healing posters for use by individuals and in healing programs.
15. Carol Strode, Nancy Strode, and Walter Strode, "The Hawaii Health Net Story," *Futures Research Working Paper Six* (Honolulu: Hawaii Research Center for Futures Study, 1975).
16. *The Journal of Holistic Health*, ed. Leonard Pellettiri, P.O. Box 23231, San Diego, CA 92123.
17. Theodore Cooper, op. cit., p. 2.

2

Harold Stone

Wholistic Healing: Historic Base and Short History

THE RUINS OF THE ancient Greek village of Epidauros lie in a beautiful valley only a few hours from Athens. The surroundings are a lush green, and there is a quietness that pervades the atmosphere, even in today's whirl of tour buses, guides, and snapping cameras. The entrance into the actual ruins brings with it yet a greater quietness and centering. There one sees the remains of a hotel where guests once stayed. There is the gymnasium which was the center of physical activity, but which also served as the auditorium where appeared lecturers and teachers from all over Greece. There is the temple to Asklepios himself, the god of healing. Here is where the ill person who came to Epidauros slept during the incubation rituals that were connected with the healing rites. There is the temple to Aphrodite and the mysterious Tholos with its spiral cut into the earth leading towards the center of the sacred precinct. Above, on a hill overlooking the whole valley, is the theater. Here one can sit on the top step and hear a voice from the stage speak in a normal voice. Most of the major gods and goddesses of the Greek pantheon were represented live in dramatic form.

A Living Mythology

Why should this very personal experience of Greek ruins be of any consequence now to those of us who are concerned with the issue of wholistic healing? To answer this question, we must have some understanding of the significance of these gods and goddesses for our own beings.

We are very complex psycho-social-physiological organisms, we human beings. We have a body, and we have a spirit. We have emotions, and we have a mind. We have a capacity for order and structure, for experience and ecstasy. We have a capacity for love and sensuality and a capacity for chastity and bodily negation. The Greeks took these basic human propensities and made out of them gods and goddesses. That is why mythology is of such consequence to us today. It gives us a picture of the basic qualities of man in projected form.

Apollo, then, is a representation of the basic capacity in us to bring order to our world. Dionysius has to do with that basic capacity in us for experience and ecstasy. Aphrodite expresses the basic human capacity for love and sexuality, and Artemis for chastity. Asklepios himself represents our innate healing capabilities. This is, of course, one of the very basic ideas of wholistic healing—that there is a dormant healing capacity within us and that the job of the health professional is to help to activate that healing potential.

What we find then at a place like Epidauros are the remains of what once was a center for wholistic healing. There were certainly aspects missing that we today would include. However, the basic ideology was there. The ancients recognized that healing required the development of these various capacities, or, to put it another way, healing required the participation of many of our different selves. That is why so many of the gods and goddesses were represented.

The origins of Greek medicine were in Thessaly at mount Pelion. Here was the home of Cheiron, the mystic centaur, with his knowledge of plants and herbs and all the forms of healing that we today would call esoteric. It was in this environment that Asklepios had his mythical birth and breeding. The god Herakles and many ancient heroes who developed healing functions were also pupils of Cheiron and learned the precepts rare that enabled them "disease and mental pain to 'suage."[1]

Early Healing Framework

The earliest forms of healing of which we have any traces whatsoever were of two kinds: direct intervention and indirect intervention.

Indirect intervention involved the employment of a wide variety of methods directed by divine communication through oracles, dreams, visions, or omens, and mediated by a priest. Direct intervention included the laying on of hands, the use of sacred relics, coming into contact with the image of a god, and contact with the priest or a sacred animal.[2]

We see, then, that the origins of medicine were in the hands of the priests and that there was no separation between psyche and soma, between the treatment of the mind and of the body. Illness was related to an imbalance, and healing would take place through the activation of the gods or goddesses, experienced in both outer and inner form.

One of the basic tenets of wholistic healing is that any treatment program is directed towards the whole person. Whatever the illness, no matter how organic or psychic it may appear to be, it is no longer possible to separate the mind from the body from the emotions from the spirit from the social nexus of the problem.

That is why there is such freedom and excitement in our considerations regarding healing. Any problem that we meet may have consequences in any of the above-mentioned areas, and more and more we realize the ever widening areas of knowledge and experience that can be brought to bear in dealing with the thing we call illness.

We have established, then, that the origins of medicine were, in fact, wholistic. This means specifically that the mind-body dichotomy did not exist. It means also that priest-healers saw themselves as agents for putting the healee in contact with the transpersonal forces that were the basis of the healing. This very important idea is critical to the thinking of wholistic healing. Our role is to help the patient connect to his or her own healing capabilities, and to discover his or her own inner authority, which will help to make the appropriate choices regarding healing.

I would like to give a little more background regarding the actual way that some of these early healing rites operated. By the late seventh or early sixth century B.C., Asklepios had emigrated to Epidauros, where he was worshipped along with Apollo Maleates. The patient would come to the temple at Epidauros and meet with the priest. Initially, there would be a fast or at least a very rigorous diet. The patient was garbed in white and was given a place to be and to sleep on the portico of the temple itself. Offerings were made on the altar, and the priest would offer a prayer to the god. An example is the prayer that follows, composed by Aristeides:

O ye children of Apollo/who in time past have stilled the waves of sorrow for many people, lighting up a lamp of safety before those who travel by sea and land, be pleased, in your great condescension, though ye be equal in glory with your elder brethren the Dioskouri, and your lot in immortal youth be as theirs, to accept this prayer, which in sleep and vision ye have inspired. Order it aright, I pray you, according to your loving-kindness to men. Preserve me from sickness; and imbue my body with such a measure of health as may suffice it for the obeying of the spirit, that I may pass my days unhindered and in quietness.[3]

After the prayer, there was a time of silence, the patients were asked to be afraid of nothing, not to whisper, and to go to sleep. During the night, priests would sometimes return with assistants dressed in the garb of other gods and goddesses related to Asklepios, and often accompanied by dogs and snakes. At these times, the priests would apply ointments to the afflicted parts of the body.[4]

In this heightened atmosphere of imagination and power, many cures did take place. Very frequently, patients reported healing dreams in which the god appeared and gave remedy for the illness; there were also situations in which the illness was gone the next day. How often this was a dream and how often it was related more directly to the activity of the priest is difficult to say.

We know from our own work in psychotherapy that the experience of this transpersonal energy in a dream or meditation may have a very healing effect, sometimes amazingly dramatic, on illness. For example, I once worked with a woman who had suffered from migraine headaches for over twenty years. We had spent a considerable time together with many changes taking place, but the migraines remained untouched. Then came the following dream, a modern healing dream, after which the migraines disappeared completely.

I am cleaning out my medicine cabinet, throwing away all my old headache medicines. My old girlfriend is with me. I find an ancient bottle with some liquid in it, and inside the liquid is a small snake. On the bottle is a label that gives the date that the snake was bottled. It was 1385 A.D. I know that I must let the snake out of the bottle. I am afraid. I finally go outside and open the bottle and let the snake out. It immediately grows larger and goes running off into nature.

This is not the place to enter into a discussion of the particular meaning and significance of this dream. It would take us too far afield.

I wish only to illustrate that the activation of healing energies can manifest themselves in many ways. Dreams that occur synchronously with the disappearance of symptoms are not uncommon, and they are current expressions of what we have been describing in these early incubation rituals.

There were, of course, patients who did not get well. They were told that they were impious or disobedient. This seems, of course, quite unfair, but it is not unlike the therapist who tells a patient who is not doing well that he or she is resisting, rather than consider the possibility that another approach or therapist might be more effective.

I have spent considerable time on these early forms because they are the origins of wholistic healing. The cleavage between scientific and theurgic medicine began to appear as early as the fifth century B.C. An early Kniddian author of Asklepiadai writes:

> To offer up prayers is no doubt becoming and good, but while praying to the Gods, a man ought also to use his own exertions.[5]

It does not seem like bad advice. The problem for us is that the exertions of mankind became more and more focused and soon began to leave out any healing system or remedy that did not conform to what has come to be called scientific medicine.

Contemporary Medicine

I would like now to leave our historical roots and move to the more recent history of wholistic healing. I do not intend to do a survey of who is doing what and who has written what. The field itself is so new that this book essentially represents its history. What I would like to do is to place wholistic healing in the context of scientific medicine to show the more recent evolutionary process.

In the first place, traditional medical practice is oriented towards symptomatology. There is a symptom that develops, an illness that must be gotten rid of. Disease, symptomatology, is bad and is to be eliminated. Complex systems of diagnostic treatment have evolved with this aim in mind. Such medical practice is described as the target approach. The idea here is that there is a specific target to be hit: preferably the elimination of the disease and, if this is impossible, the removal of the symptoms. The physician is the authority on the elimination of the disease and, in general, the patient remains rather passive during the entire procedure.

Health as Wholeness

When psychiatry came into being in the late nineteenth century, a very similar symptom-oriented approach was used. Neuroses were a form of illness that had to be eradicated. The analytic therapies began, however, to develop a different emphasis in their approach to emotional problems. There began to develop a health, rather than an illness orientation. The neurosis was not just something to be gotten rid of, according to Jung. The neurosis developed because of a psychic imbalance, and if the patient accepted the challenge, the neurosis gave him or her the opportunity to develop a different consciousness. This kind of thinking is basic to wholistic healing. Illness, no matter what kind, is no longer seen simply as something to be eradicated. It is seen in the context of a person's life space, and it is valued as being a possibility for moving someone into a very different kind of consciousness. Illness is seen here as an imbalance in the energy spheres of our emotional, rational, spiritual, physical, and social selves. Healing is concerned with the individual balancing of these energies. So it appears that the revolution that took place in psychotherapeutic thinking with the advent of the health-oriented therapies, now extends to healing generally.

Doctor-Patient Relationships

The second area in which psychotherapy was important in the evolution of wholistic healing was that of the doctor-patient relationship. The word *therapist* is derived from the Greek word *therapon*, which means "a comrade in a common struggle." Therapists who are generally associated with a humanistic tradition have realized this comradeship for a long time. There is no basic emotional life problem that our patients deal with that is not in some way ours. There is a commonality to the struggle all of us have in living life.

This idea of the "comrade in the common struggle" is difficult to comprehend in medicine. If a young man goes skiing in the Sierras and breaks his leg early Saturday morning, what possible common denominator can there be between his orthopedic physician in Los Angeles and himself? After all, the physician's leg is not broken. In fact, the orthopedist doesn't even ski. They are not comrades in a common struggle until the physician discovers that this man left L.A. at 6:30 P.M. on Friday and broke his leg early the next morning. On further questioning, the physician discovers that the patient could have gotten off early but was afraid to ask his employer, with whom he has a conflict, as he does with all authority figures. The physician struggles with authority, too, feeling like an adult in private practice and like an insecure child when with the main professor at the teaching hospital once a week. The treatment of the leg has now become more complicated, more human, and the young man with the broken leg and the orthopedic surgeon who can be made to feel like a child have the real opportunity of becoming "comrades in a common struggle." The problem is greater than the broken bone. The broken bone has become a manifestation of a deep common concern. This attitude towards illness, now a basic tenet of wholistic healing, has its origins in the health-oriented philosophies of the early analytic and later humanistic traditions.

The malpractice crisis that sweeps the country today has many roots. One of the central themes of this problem comes, I believe, from the split that has taken place between physician and patient as medicine has become increasingly technological and patients are treated medically as though their psyches did not exist. Comrades in a common struggle do not sue one another. Patients who have parts of their bodies administered to by authorities who take responsibility for healing them do tend to sue. I realize that I am simplifying a complex issue, but I do believe that these considerations are central to the problem.

There is still a third place where the psychotherapeutic tradition has fed into wholistic healing generally, and that is in relationship to the responsibility for healing. One of the major problems of traditional treatment of any kind is the abdication of responsibility on the part of the patient in regard to choices that the patient needs to make. The longer the health professional remains in a position of authority and power, the more the patient remains a son or daughter to that authority. We recognize, of course, the necessity of technical skill in the healing arts. We are talking now about patients being trained by health professionals to make choices that keep the responsibility for healing in their own hands. This means also recognizing where patients may have participated in the development of their own illnesses. Nowhere is this more dramatically seen than in the work being done with cancer, because the recognition by the patient of where he or she has participated in the development of illness becomes an essential ingredient of the overall treatment process.

Traditional scientific medicine has not totally neglected the patient's responsibility in the development of physiological illnesses. Certain symptom systems, e.g. ulcers, are generally regarded as being both organic and psychological in nature, and as such, are studied in the field of psychosomatic medicine.

The last major feeder element in wholistic thinking is the area of transpersonal psychology. Wholistic healing includes the spiritual area in its consideration since it views spirit as part of the basic human condition. The work of Jung was pioneering in this area, and his work on the archetypes and the transpersonal self led into the work of Assagioli and the psychosynthesis movement leading eventually into the meditative disciplines and their attempt to tap into transpersonal elements. These systems are critical to wholistic healing because each of them developed methods for tapping into these energies. These methods, with many variations, have become part of the methodology of wholistic medicine. This is particularly true of the use of visual imagery in its many forms.

This transpersonal psychology can be seen as originating in the philosophical systems of Plato and Kant, who saw us as the inheritors of basic ideas and image systems that interacted with environment in the course of our evolution. Jung picked up and developed the Platonic and Kantian thinking further. He added the concept of the Self as a personality construct that transcended the ego and that incorporated the objective psyche, the world of the transpersonal self. Our entry into this world was through dreams and active imagination, a form of visual imagery that, with variations, has become a central method in many healing methods.

The central issue for us, as I have mentioned previously, is that the activation of, and experience of, these transpersonal forces often exerts a remarkable effect on people's psychology that is accompanied commonly by serious and prolonged symptoms being changed and sometimes eliminated. Aside from the general positive effects of relaxation, this is why so much emphasis is being placed on meditative practices. They are seen as being an entrée into the world of the transpersonal self.

Psychotherapists often tend to think in terms of disowned selves. We grow up in a culture and develop along the lines of particular selves that are stressed in our family and culture. Other aspects of our being may be seen as alien. The integration of personality is connected to the owning of these disowned selves. We have discovered that most approaches to growth and change and therapy generally tend to help us own what has been disowned. These ideas are very basic to therapists, and they represent another important feeder element that psychotherapy has brought to wholistic healing. In the course of our scientific evolution, we have disowned many of the mysteries of man. Goethe says in one of his poems:

> *He whose vision*
> *does not encompass man's 3000 years*
> *lives forever*
> *within the day's dark frontiers.*

Wholistic Healing is open to all of these mysteries. It is not a question of either/or. There is no reason to polarize traditional and wholistic medicine. We simply live in a historical time when it becomes necessary for more and more people to bridge the worlds of rational and irrational, of spirit and body, of personal and transpersonal, of traditional and nontraditional. Wholistic healing is an idea that at its very heart is healing because its core is the bridging and reconciling of these and other opposites.

Entering into the world of wholistic healing is like opening Pandora's box. One suddenly becomes interested in everything that might have anything to do with healing, no matter how remote the connection might be. It is difficult to identify oneself as the ultimate authority or "knower"—an easy identification for many people in the healing arts—because one is constantly discovering more and more that is not known. This book is a beautiful expression of this fact.

Notes

1. Walter Addison Jayne, *The Healing Gods of Ancient Civilisation* (New Hyde Park, N.Y.: University Books, 1962): 226.

2. Walter Addison Jayne, *op. cit.*, p. 229.

3. Walter Pater, *Marius the Epicurean* 1: 39, as cited in Walter Addison Jayne, *op. cit.*, p. 279.

4. Lewis R. Farrell, *Cult of the Greek States* 3 (Oxford: Clarendon Press, 1896): 10.

5. Hippokrates, *de Insomnis*, sec. 4: 87, as cited in Walter Addison Jayne, *op. cit.*, p. 277.

3

Lawrence L. LeShan

Toward a General Theory
of Psychic Healing*

IN ATTEMPTING to understand the problems posed by the existence of
the paranormal, we must probe into the nature of reality as we know it
today. It is part of the faith of science that all phenomena that exist
must exist under the category of natural law, and that none exist under
the categories of magic or miracle. In following that faith and attempting to understand the paranormal in normal terms, it became necessary
to change the question usually asked about this class of phenomena.
Instead of asking "How do the 'sensitives' *do* it? How do they attain the
paranormal information?"—questions that had not yielded results after
long and careful work by serious men—I asked a new question: "What is
going on between the sensitive and the rest of reality at the moment
the paranormal event occurs?"

This question was put to some of the leading sensitives of our time in
direct discussion and through a study of their written material. It
became clear that at the moment they were acquiring the paranormal
experience they viewed the cosmos as if it were constructed in a special
way. I termed this way the "clairvoyant reality" and contrasted it with
the way we view the nature of reality in our everyday commonsense
life, which I termed the "sensory reality."

The clairvoyant reality is a coherent, organized picture of the way
the world works. It is a complete metaphysical system. It implies that

* From *The Medium, The Mystic, and the Physicist* by Lawrence LeShan.
Copyright © 1974 by Lawrence LeShan. An Esalen Book. Reprinted by permission of
Viking Press.

when one is using it, certain events (such as telepathy, clairvoyance, and precognition) are normal and explainable. Certain other events (such as being able to will or take action toward a goal) are paranormal in this system.

I then realized that two other groups of individuals had arrived at similar conclusions. The mystics and the Einsteinian physicists both agreed with the clairvoyant that there are two valid ways of perceiving reality, and on what these two ways were. Except for tricks of language and a few comparatively minor disagreements, all were completely agreed on the nature and existence of the clairvoyant reality. It proved impossible to differentiate statements describing it that were written by mystics from those written by physicists.

In order to test this theory, I attempted to use it to learn how to accomplish one of the functions long described as paranormal, and to teach it to others. If the theory predicted that this paranormal function occurred in a certain psychological situation, and I organized that situation and found that the paranormal function occurred, then it would be a pretty good test of the theory. Psychic healing was chosen for this test, and by following the theory and its implications it became possible for me to learn to be a psychic healer and to teach it to others.

My first question was, Does the phenomenon of psychic healing really exist? With what we know today about hysterical symptoms and hysterical suppression of symptoms, do the phenomena described as "psychic healing" exist apart from these? Prior to my work in parapsychology, I had spent fifteen years working full time on a project in psychosomatic medicine, and so was aware at least of the scope of the problems involved.

A survey of the literature in this field made it plain that the phenomenon of psychic healing *did* exist. There was enough solid experimental work and enough careful evaluation of reported claims to make this clear. After I discarded the 95 percent of the claims that could have been due to hysterical change, suggestion, bad experimental design, poor memory, and plain chicanery, a solid residue remained. In these, the "healer" usually went through certain behaviors inside of his head, and the "healee" showed positive biological changes which were not to be expected at that time in terms of the usual course of his condition.

The "explanation," or theories of explanations, were another matter entirely. Generally speaking these seemed to be divided into three classes.

The largest group of healers described their work as "prayer" and believed that success was due to the intervention of God. A second group believed the healing was done by "spirits" after they had set up a special linkage between the spirits and the patient. The third group believed that they were transmitters or originators of some special form of "energy" that had healing effects.

With the group that involved God in the healing process I could find no quarrel. I could not, nor did I wish to, disagree with this explanation. Nevertheless, science must go further than this. We are concerned with the "how" of things: "How" does God work? The poet-philosopher Petrarch devised the rationale of science within a religious framework when he described the world as the "theater of God," the "Teatrum Dei," and said man could admire God by understanding His handiwork. Within this framework, I would work in harmony with those who used God as an explanatory force.

A serious difficulty with the use of the concept of God is that, with it, one can do little either to further one's understanding of a process or to increase his efficiency at it. To improve one's healing ability he can learn to pray better, but that is about all. For a scientific approach and a scientific society, more was needed.

The second group used "spirits" as an explanation. I have no particular opinion, one way or another, on the existence of discarnate entities who intervene in human affairs. Even after hundreds of hours spent conversing with mediums in trance during which the medium claimed to be someone who was dead, I still see no scientific way to determine if these spirits are (1) what they claim to be; (2) a multiple personality split-off; or (3) something else. At present we do not seem to have a way to test any of these hypotheses. . . .

In addition, "spirits" are notably difficult to work with scientifically. If you do not get results today, it is because the "spirits" were not in the mood! In any case, with the "spirit" explanation, I had to concentrate on "how" the spirits do it, how they can heal. I could not prove or disprove the spiritistic answer, but I could go on from there and study the "how" of the healing process, whether spirits existed or not.

The third group explained the healing on the basis of an "energy" which they either originated or transmitted. Certainly this sounded more promising scientifically than the other explanations. However, since no one has been able to define this energy further than by giving it a name presently acceptable to science, nor to find any of its characteristics, it did not seem very useful.

Furthermore, there is a very real problem about the use of a concept such as "energy" if it is accepted into one's thinking too early in the process of exploration. Such a concept has implications; it shapes our thinking in ways we are often unaware of. Energy does "work," for example. Is "work" done in the psychic healing process? Tempting as it is to answer "yes," one had better be careful about it. The Christian Science healers (and they often accomplish very serious results) would certainly not agree with this. In addition, energy "flows" or "travels" between "two things." Are there "two things" in the psychic healing process? If so, it would mean that we find our explanatory system in the sensory reality and not in the clairvoyant reality.

I could point out other implications of the use of a concept like "energy" that worried me, but these should do to show why I was so cautious about accepting it as an explanatory system early in the game. Rather than seeking the understanding of healing in the explanations of the healers, it seemed plain that another approach was needed.

I assembled a list of individuals who could be described as "serious psychic healers." These included all the individuals who I felt reasonably certain *did* accomplish results in this area, who worked consistently in it, and about whom there was either autobiographical or good biographical material. It consisted primarily of Olga and Ambrose Worrall, Harry Edwards, Rebecca Beard, Agnes Sanford, Edgar Jackson, the Christian Science group, Parahamsa Yogananda, Stewart Grayson, and Kathryn Kuhlman. A variety of other healers, ranging from Padre Pio to Mrs. Salmon and Sai Baba, were also studied in this way through the material which was available on them.

This group all described behaviors that they felt were related to the healing effect. When I listed these behaviors, I found that they fell into two classes. The first class were "idiosyncratic behaviors," that is, behaviors engaged in by one or a few of the healers. The second class consisted of "commonality behaviors," behaviors engaged in by all of the healers. The assumption was made that it was this second class of activities that was relevant to the healing effect.

At this point in time I had a set of behaviors, a series of activities, that all the serious healers engaged in when they were trying to heal someone. This series had been teased out of the larger mass of activities they described as related to the healing. I could reasonably assume that I had come as close as I could at the moment to the "pure method," to the activities really related to the healing process, and I could discard the other, idiosyncratic behaviors as culturally or personally conditioned and nonessential. Exactly what were these activities? How could I describe them?

I found that, from the viewpoint of the experience of the healer (what he believed and observed himself to be doing), they fell into two classes. From an experiential viewpoint, there seemed to be two separate types of healing here. In a brilliant flash of genius I named these "Type 1" and "Type 2"!

The healers themselves had not made this differentiation as far as I could tell. Some used both, slipping back and forth without apparently noticing that the two phenomena were qualitatively different. Some used only one of them. To my best knowledge, this was the first time they had been separately delineated in detail.

Type 1 seemed to me to be the most important type. Many healers, such as Edgar Jackson and the Christian Science group, used it exclusively.

In Type 1 healing, the healer goes into an altered state of consciousness in which he views himself and the healee as one entity. There is no attempt to "do anything" to the healee (in Harry Edwards's words, "All sense of 'performance' should be abandoned"), but simply to meet him, to be one with him, to unite with him. Ambrose Worrall put this simply and clearly: "I followed a technique I have of 'tuning in,' to become, in a metaphysical sense, one with the patient." Edgar Jackson defined intercessory prayers (prayers for a patient's recovery) as "a subject-object bridge." And Edwards wrote that in psychic healing the healer ". . . then draws 'close' to the patient, so that 'both' are 'one.' "

These are clear statements. Jackson put the entire matter in a larger frame of reference:

> Prayer as a specialized state of consciousness moves beyond the usual considerations of real or unreal, conscious or unconscious, organic or inorganic, subjective or objective to a place where he is dealing with the totality of being at one and the same time in a way that produces sensitivity to the whole.

What we have here began to become clear. The healer views the healee in the clairvoyant reality at a level close to that in which all is one. However, he is focused by love, by caring, by *caritas*, on the healee: this is an essential factor. In Agnes Sanford's words, "Only love can generate the healing fire." Ambrose and Olga Worrall have said,

a "miraculous healing" in the course of which it regressed and cleared up. Carrel (a very highly trained and reliable observer) reported that the cancer followed the usual, well-known course a cancer follows when it regresses. These include specific courses of development in the formation of scar tissue fibers, changes in blood distribution, etc. This cancer, said Carrel, followed this progression, but many many times faster than he had ever seen or heard of it happening before.

I began to see the light on a possible way of explaining the biological changes. None of us do anything as well as we potentially can. We can all learn to read faster, jump higher, discriminate colors more precisely, reason more accurately, and so on through practically any abilities you can name. One of these abilities is the ability to heal ourselves, our ability at self-repair and self-recuperation. This too usually operates far below potential.

What appeared to happen in Type 1 healing was that because he was momentarily in an "ideal organismic situation," the healee's self-repair and self-recuperative systems began to operate at a level closer than usual to their potential. Type 1 psychic healing was not a "doing something" to the healee, but a meeting and uniting with him on a profound level, a uniting that permitted something new to happen. The reason, then, behind Shaw's comment on the lack of wooden legs at Lourdes is that the regrowth of a severed limb is beyond the ability of the body's self-repair systems. The rapid remission of a cancer is not.

Henry Miller had once written something that was in a curious way very similar to the way I had begun to see this:

> The great physicians have always spoken of Nature as being the great Healer. This is only partially true. Nature alone can do nothing.
> Nature can cure only when man recognizes his place in the world, which is not in Nature, as with the animal, but in the human kingdom, the link between the natural and divine.

When man is "at home" in both realities, when he is fulfilling himself as an "amphibian," living in both—in Miller's terms of the "natural and the divine"—the healing of many wounds can occur. The healer does not "do" or "give" something to the healee; instead he helps him come home to the All, to the One, to the way of "unity" with the universe, and in this "meeting" the healee becomes more complete and this in itself is healing. I was reminded here of Arthur Koestler's words: "There is no sharp dividing line between self-repair and self-realization."

This fit very well with one of the analogies used in Christian Science to "explain" this type of healing. Christian Scientists point out that a rubber ball retains its usual shape of roundness (here the analogy for "health") so long as there is no pressure to deform it (here the analogy for "illness"). As soon as the pressure is released, it springs back to roundness. The pressure, they say, is being cut off from God, is the lack of the knowledge that one is a part of God, or, in our terms, the All. When this "pressure" is "released" through the healer setting up a metaphysical system where the healee is included in the All, brought "home" to it, the healee's body responds by a tendency to repair itself and work toward health.

A basic theory had emerged for Type 1 healing. Now would come the crucial test of the theory: a test that involved learning to meet and unite with another person (and training others to do this) according to the theory, and see if it provided positive physical changes. But I have gotten ahead of myself. Type 2 healing remains to be described, since the analysis of both methods was done at the same time.

Experientially, Type 2 is quite different from Type 1. The healer perceives a pattern of activity between his palms when his hands are "turned on" and facing each other. Some healers perceive this as a "flow of energy," some as a sphere of activity. The hands are so placed—one on each side of the healee's pathological area—so that this "flow of energy" is perceived to "pass through" the troubled area. This is usually conceived of by the healer as "healing energy" which "cures" or "treats" the sick area. In a large percentage of cases (I would estimate about 50 percent in my own experience) healees who do not know the literature and do not know the expected response perceive a good deal of "heat" in the area. Frequently there are surprised comments like "It feels like diathermy!" "It's like an electric blanket!" "Where is all that heat coming from?" A smaller percentage of naïve subjects (about 10 percent in my experience) report a sensation of a great deal of "activity" in the area. A very few report a sensation of "cold." These sensations are almost invariably felt only in an area in which there is a real physical problem. One can "turn on" one's hands to any degree and it is still almost unheard of to get a perceptual response from the healee when the hands are held on each side of a healthy area.

In Type 2 the healer *tries* to heal; he wants to and attempts to do so through the "healing flow." In both Type 1 and Type 2 he must (at least at the moment) care completely, but a fundamental difference is that in Type 1 he *unites* with the healee; in Type 2 he tries to cure him. Harry Edwards, writing of Type 2, explained his attitude:

> When the author is engaged in this work, only one thing exists and that is his hands through which the healing power flows. The healer's whole being is concentrated on his fingers—nothing else seems to exist. The desired result is the only thing that is his concern.

Some healers see themselves as the *originators* of this healing power; others see themselves as the *transmitters* of it. Frank Loehr has called them the "God Withiners" and the "God Beyonders," respectively. In either case, the procedure and the experience are essentially the same.

This much I learned from reading the works of the serious healers, but I could not understand what was going on. Even now I do not have the faintest idea what Type 2 is all about or how it "works." And it frequently does "work," that is, produces positive biological changes in the healee. I know how to "do it," to "turn on" my hands and teach others how to "turn on" theirs. It seems perfectly reasonable to me that we may be dealing with some kind of "energy." It also seems reasonable to me that Type 2 may be a sort of "cop out" on Type 1 in which healer and healee say, in effect: "We are both too frightened of all this closeness and uniting that is a part of psychic healing. Let's pretend with each other that all that is happening is a flow of energy is coming out of the hands and treating the problem. That way we will both be more comfortable." It also seems reasonable to me that the most fruitful explanation of Type 2 healing may be quite different from either of the above two hypotheses.

At a complete loss for a theory about Type 2, the time had come to test the theory of Type 1. Following the theory, the test I set up was to train myself to go into the state of consciousness indicated and see if—as the theory predicted—positive biological changes would occur in the healee's body. If this worked, the next step would be to try to train others to do this. The others would be individuals like myself who had never done this type of healing before, and who were not accustomed to having paranormal experiences of any sort. If the theory pointed out that certain activities had certain results and that when these activities were carried out the results occurred, it would at least prove the theory to be a fruitful one.

I had therefore to teach myself to go into an altered state of consciousness of a particular type. For at least a moment, I had to *know* that the cosmos was run on field-theory lines, that All is One, and to do this somehow "centered" about the uniting of another person and myself in the clairvoyant reality. The next question was *how* to do this.

The writings of the various mystical traditions are a vast resource of training techniques for problems of this sort. I experimented with a wide variety of these techniques, trying with each one to understand its purpose, to relate that purpose to my goal and then to my particular personality organization.

Any way of dividing up these techniques into classes is bound to be faulty. Not only is there a great deal of overlap, but all techniques have as one of their goals a tuning and training of the personality similar to the way an athlete tunes and trains his physical structure. However, bearing this in mind, some general classifications can be made. One of these is a division into meditation techniques, rhythm techniques (as the Dervish dances, the chanting of Mantras, and the Hassidic body movements), and assault-on-the-ego-techniques (such as fasting, the use of hallucinogenic agents such as LSD, and various methods of the *Via Ascetica*, the way of the ascetic). It was clear from what I knew about myself—and found out further in experimenting—that the meditation techniques were closest to my own easiest path.

These meditation techniques are all partially ways of learning to discipline the mind, to make it learn to do what you want it to do. No one who works at one of them for five minutes is left in the slightest doubt that his mind is as undisciplined as—in St. Teresa's phrase—"an unbroken horse. . . ."

One way of classifying meditation techniques is the threefold division into what has been called in the East the Inner Way, the Middle Way, and the Outer Way. In the Inner Way, one concentrates on the spontaneously arising contents of one's own mind, upon the images and feelings that arise. In the Middle Way one strives for stillness of the mind; one withdraws from both internal and external perceptions. It has been called the Way of Emptiness. In the Outer Way one concentrates and meditates on an externally given perception; one relinquishes spontaneity and disciplines the mind to stay with this perception until it blends with oneself. One contemplates one thing, following the statement of William Blake: "If the gates of perception were cleansed, all things would appear as they are, infinite."

These divisions are not clear-cut, and various meditation techniques cut across these arbitrary lines. A Zen Koan, for example, is both a meditation technique of the Outer Way and an assault-on-the-ego technique, in that what is being meditated upon cannot be dealt with by the ego operating in its usual manner. The Theraveda techniques in which one concentrates on a spontaneously generated rhythm of one's own (as the rise and fall of the chest in breathing) are a combination of rhythm and meditation techniques.

Another way of classifying mystical training technique is major avenues of approach: the body (as in Hatha Yoga), the feelings and intuition (perhaps the most widely used avenue; examples include Bhakti Yoga, the way of Meher Baba, and the monastic practicing his prayers, devotions, and deepening his ability to love), or the route of the intellect. From what I understood of myself, and of American culture generally, it seemed that the way of the intellect would be best and fastest for my purposes. In the East this is known as the Narodhi Samadhi. In the West it was the approach followed by the Habad school of Hasidism. It starts with an intellectual understanding of the structure of the two ways of being at home in reality, which I have described earlier as the sensory reality and the clairvoyant reality. From this point, one trains himself to perceive and "be" more and more in the clairvoyant reality through various (primarily meditation) techniques. For myself, I had thus chosen the meditation approach, the Outer Way, and the intellectual Samadhi.

The Outer Way (the Way of Forms or Way of Absorption) has been more commonly used in the West than the other two paths. In the West it is often called contemplation and we hear of the lives of the contemplatives, as the Christian followers of this path were called. In the East it has been called "one-pointing," or the Buddhist "bare attention." The clearest book on this subject I know of is Evelyn Underhill's *Practical Mysticism*, from which I learned much.

Using contemplation as a central exercise, I gradually devised a series of techniques which it seemed would, if practiced enough, lead me to the state of consciousness that appeared to be associated with the positive biological changes that occurred in successful psychic healing. It took me about a year and a half of experimentation and practice until I felt I could achieve this state.

At the end of this time I felt ready to try. If the theory was right and what was being stimulated was the individual's own self-repair systems, I did not see how I could do any damage. If the theory was invalid, nothing would happen. It seemed ethically legitimate to try it.

Once again—as when I discovered that physicists also believed in the clairvoyant reality—I found myself surprised at what occurred and surprised at my surprise. This time I was surprised that positive biological changes *did* occur to healees when I was able to go into the special altered state of consciousness. So deep are the prejudices ingrained in us about the nature of reality being that of the sensory reality that I—in spite of all the intellectual understanding and the intensive training program I had put myself through—still somewhere felt that it could *not* work, that it was all fantasy and that "reality *was* reality." I was surprised at positive results and surprised that I was surprised.

The results of the "healing encounters" I now began to have fell into five classes:

1. I went into the altered state of consciousness and nothing happened so far as the healee was concerned.
2. I went into the altered state and positive biological changes occurred in the healee's body.
3. I went into the altered state and positive psychological changes occurred in the patient.
4. I went into the altered state of consciousness and there were telepathic exchanges between the patient and myself.
5. I was unable to go into the altered state of consciousness.

There were all possible combinations also between numbers 2, 3, and 4. Further, again to my surprise, there was no particular relationship between these that I have been able to discover. A patient might consciously observe nothing psychological during the session and still have positive physical changes. He might observe a very strong "calming," "relaxing," or "tranquilizing" effect with or without telepathic exchanges and with or without physical effects. The presence of one of these three factors appears at this time to have nothing much to do with the presence or absence of others.

In order to show the different types of results, I will describe some healing encounters which give a fairly accurate overall picture.

The general procedure followed in the healing encounters was simple. After enough general conversation so that we knew each other a little and felt reasonably relaxed together, I would ask the healee to simply get comfortable physically and to let his mind do as it pleased—not to cooperate in any particular way or to "try" to do anything, but to let happen whatever happened. I would then find myself a comfortable standing position (for no particular reason except that I concentrate more easily standing), close my eyes, and conceptualize this particular healee being in both realities at the same time. I would attempt to reach a point of being in which I would *know* that he not only existed as a separate individual inside his skin and limited by it, but that he also—and in an equally "true" and "real" manner— existed to the furthest reaches of the cosmos in space and time. When I *knew* for a moment that this was true and that I also coexisted with him in this manner—when, in fact, I had attained the clairvoyant reality— the healing work was done. Generally, I tried for two or three such moments in each encounter to "make sure," although this is probably more a statement about my own insecurity than it is about anything else.

Often I would use various types of symbols to help myself reach this point of knowing. For example, I might use the symbol of two trees on opposite sides of a hill with the tops visible to each other. From one viewpoint, they looked like two separate trees, but inside the hill, the two root masses met and were one. The two trees were really one and inseparable. Further, their roots affected the earth and the earth the rocks until I could know that in the whole planet and cosmos there was nothing that was not affected by them and affecting them. This sort of symbolization, different in each case, as the healee and I are different in each healing encounter, would often be useful in helping me reach the clairvoyant reality with the healee and myself centered in it. With practice, the situation often arose where no symbols were needed, where I could move immediately to the point of complete *knowledge* of both realities at once. Each healing encounter was different; symbols which would be useful in one would be empty and sterile in the next.

There is certainly something that the healee can do to increase the probability of a positive response to the healing. At present, however, I do not know what this is. In spite of experimentation (still continuing) on having the healee relax, meditate, or do half a dozen other things, I do not know at this time what the best activity (if, indeed, there is one best way for everyone) is for him to do. Curiously, belief in the efficacy of healing of this kind does not seem to be a factor. Our results seem to be as good with skeptics as they are with believers.

Sometimes, if the Type 1 healing described above goes well, I feel the palms of my hands begin to tingle and realize that I "want" also to do a Type 2 ("laying on of hands") healing with this person. When I have this impulse, I follow it, but never force it or try to do a Type 2 when it does not "feel" right to do so after a strong Type 1 encounter with the healee. The whole procedure rarely takes less than ten minutes or more than fifteen. There comes a certain point when it "feels" complete; there is the sense that whatever could be done has been done. It is then time to stop.

Frequently, I will go through this procedure and have a feeling of having been deeply into it, and as far as the healee is concerned all that has happened is that he relaxed for fifteen minutes in a comfortable chair. So far—in spite of a belief that in science the failures need study exactly as much, if not sometimes more than the successes—I have been able to find no clues as to why this happens with many healees, nor any ideas as to how to predict in advance which healees will respond in this way. The factors are certainly there, but so far I have not been able to analyze them.

With some healees, there is a positive physical response apparently associated with the healing encounter. Although coincidence has a long long arm and some of these cases are certainly "false positives" (that is, the positive physical response occurred for some other, unknown reason and the relationship in time to the healing encounter was coincidence), the successes have been frequent enough and impressive enough to persuade me that this research is worth continuing.

A woman, well known to me, 75 years old, had had a painful arthritis and swelling of both hands for over a year. Although she could hold and use a pencil, or a knife and fork, it was impossible for her to bring her fingers closer than one inch from her palm. Attempts to do so, or pressure from outside the fingers, brought severe pain. Persuaded by members of her family to let me try psychic healing, she agreed and said she was not "against it," but did not believe in it. She asked what she should do during the time I was working. I replied that she should read a newspaper and she did so.

I started with a Type 1 approach and in the course of about ten minutes felt that I had achieved the filling of consciousness with the field-theory viewpoint several times. I then moved into a Type 2 with her left hand only. It seemed to me that this was a strong Type 2, as I had the perception of a good deal of energy between my palms, which were on both sides of her left hand.

After about five minutes of the Type 2 I felt that the experience was over and stopped. We chatted a moment and she told me she had felt nothing unusual. I asked the other members of her family to come back in (they had gone into the next room when I started the healing). Her husband asked her if there had been any effect. She replied, "No, it's just the same as it was," and to demonstrate this "flapped" the fingers of both hands. To everyone's surprise—certainly including hers and mine—they swung easily to the palm and out again. She now had full and painless movement in the fingers.

This has not changed in the full year since the healing encounter. She had been taking Prednisone (a Cortisone preparation) for three days before the healing, but up to one minute before the healing encounter, it had no apparent effect.

The following healing encounters occurred quite early in the work before I had set up the basic rule of *never* doing a Type 2 without a strong Type 1 first. By and large, Type 2 results (when done alone) tend to be transient; Type 1 results strongly tend to be permanent.

A woman known to me, aged thirty-six years, had intermittent, very large "cold sores" for over twenty years. Two or three times a year she would get one on her lip and it would take approximately thirty days to heal. She and her family knew the phenomena thoroughly and what to expect each time.

I held one hand on each side of her face, not touching the affected area, for about twenty minutes in a strong Type 2 healing. Afterwards she reported that during the twenty minutes she had been conscious of several periods of heat, and one of "tingling" in the lip area. About one half hour later she left my office to drive home (a drive of about an hour); en route she felt suddenly a strong "tingling" in the lip area, she looked at it in the rear-view mirror, and in her words, "I nearly had an accident, I was so surprised. I pulled off the road and sat for ten minutes watching the new skin regrow. The dead skin in the center did not seem to change, but new skin slowly grew over the whole raw pink area." When she arrived home, her son and her husband both reacted in surprise to the complete unexpected change and almost complete healing of the cold sore.

The next day it had returned about one-third the size it had been when she arrived in my office the day before, and disappeared over the next week.

A woman, aged thirty-eight years, had an overstretched cartilage of the knee. Her physician had termed it a "loose joint" and told her that if she was very careful and did not put any weight on it while it was in a bent position, it would recover in a year to eighteen months, or if she immobilized it in a cast, in four to six months. The knee joint was quite swollen, had no strength to bear weight when moving from a full bent (90-degree angle) position to a straight position, although once straightened she could walk on it, and was constantly painful. She came into the end of one of the training seminars I was holding and all ten people present did a Type 1 healing with her. She said afterwards that she felt very relaxed, calm, and "loved" during the ten-minute session. For me at least, it was a very strong Type 1 with full focus established several times. This was in the early afternoon. By that evening the swelling was reduced and the pain had lessened. On awaking the next morning there was no more sensation of pain in the area, its full strength had returned, and the swelling—according to her physician—was about half of what it had been. This lasted for several months, and the swelling gradually diminished to normal. In the following eighteen months, there has been no recurrence.

This case concerns a fifteen-year-old boy who broke his back on a trampoline. A letter dictated by his father, a surgeon, on November 1, 1971, and written by his mother, reads in part that the "period of detraumatization is over, and we must face the fact that 'medically' Chris is where he will be forever. That means: No feeling below the chest. Some feeling on the backs of the hands and the thumb and first finger. Movement of the lesser flexor muscles in the arm so that he has limited movement and strength in his arms—with supportive braces he may be able to use his arms to a limited degree. Indomitable inner strength and a smile that still knocks you dead."

On November 7, a group made up of students who had been at one of the healing seminars and were now working at an advanced workshop did a distance healing with Christopher. We had a letter about him and a picture, and the group—none of whom had ever met Christopher—were deeply involved. Chris, however, did not know of our existence or that anyone was going to do a psychic healing with him. He was in Denver and we were in Greenwich, Connecticut. An earlier healing had been held Friday evening, but it was on Sunday between 11:55 and 12:15 in the day that the group really "turned on" in a very strong long-distance, Type 1 healing. In the early afternoon (2–3 P.M.?) Denver time, Christopher suddenly called out that he could "feel" his legs. It soon became apparent that he could not only feel pressure sensations, but "could even tell which of his toes was being touched at any given time." The father said (to the woman who had written the letter to us, a close family friend) "that there is no explanation for this since the period of detraumatization was well over and no hope was held for any further improvement or restoration in Chris's physical condition."

However, all results must be evaluated cautiously. The most dramatic single result I had occurred when a man I knew asked me to do a distance healing for an extremely painful condition requiring immediate and intensive surgery. I promised to do the healing that night, and the next morning when he awoke a "miraculous cure" had occurred. The medical specialist was astounded, and offered to send me pre and post healing X-rays and to sponsor publication in a scientific journal. It would have been the psychic healing case of the century except for one small detail. In the press of overwork, I had forgotten to do the healing! If I had only remembered, it would have been a famous demonstration of what can be accomplished by this method.

Coincidence has a long long arm and the unexpected *does* often happen. All reports of medical improvement by psychic healing (or by any other therapeutic technique) must be interpreted with this in mind. It is also true, however, that a technique must be evaluated in terms of its results, and not in terms of a previously held theory. If the application of a theory produces results in the predicted direction, its fruitfulness has been demonstrated and previously held theories which imply that these results could not occur must be abandoned or modified.

The third group of cases reported psychological effects only and no positive effects. Almost invariably (and there were no negative or disturbing psychological effects) these were reported in terms like "I felt very calm and relaxed," "It was as if I were tranquilized," "I felt so peaceful," "It was as if a great wave of warm love came over me." Although this comprises a considerable group of healees, and is a definite and consistent phenomenon, in a pure research sense these cases must be regarded as failures, since no physical changes were observed. There is a difference between results of an experiment from which one learns something new (it is hoped one learns something from *all* results) and results that conform to one's predictions.

In the fourth group of cases there were strong indications of telepathy exchanges between the patient and myself during the healing encounter. To put this more accurately, I should state that there was a movement of images and information *within* the Gestalt that had been formed and that included the two of us.

A woman well known to me, aged twenty-eight, had an area of psoriasis on the abdomen which had shown no signs of clearing up over a five-week period, in spite of various prescribed topical treatments. A Type 1 session was divided into two ten-minute periods with a ten-minute rest period in between. In the first period I visualized her as a part of the "All," and connected to it through white bands (the love she felt and had felt for others during her life) and by black bands (her perceptions of others and events). (She is a writer with a very sharp, perceptive eye.) During the rest period she reported first having had the sensation of waves of heat pouring over her and then a pattern of alternating lighter and darker waves of light intensity. I told her nothing of what I had been conceptualizing. During the second period, I was able to conceptualize her very strongly and one-pointedly in the same way and began to merge the bands of black and white into grays—symbolizing her relationships as "loveknowledge" (in Maslow's sense) rather than love *and* knowledge separately.

At the end of the session she was obviously deeply moved, and just wanted to sit quietly and not talk for a few minutes. Then, after drinking some water, she said that it had seemed to her as if she was surrounded by black and white clouds fanning out from her like the spokes of a wheel. They presently began to revolve around her, going faster and faster until the spokes of black and the spokes of white began to merge and blur. She then said to herself "They are outside of me. I'm inside. What would happen if I let them in?" She let them in, and after the session said that they were still inside and outside and she felt that they always would be. On questioning, she would not say that it had been a "good" or "bad" experience (although she now felt very good), but that it had been an "ecstatic" experience and that she now felt "as if I had just made love." She was deeply moved by the experience and we talked in generalities for a half hour.

This is a person I know quite well and have much respect and affection for. The next day she reported that there had been—during the night—a period of intense itching of the psoriasis and a sense that her entire abdomen was "breaking out" with it. In the morning the area was—to her inspection—unchanged. She said that she had since the session "a deep feeling of calm and competence."

And another relevant example: An exceptional healing session with a woman of sixty-five with multiple myeloma. I had met her a few times fifteen years ago. Through a mutual friend she knew of this work. I saw her at her house. A *very* strong Type 1 session. During it, the main symbol system I used was to visualize "A thousand Ilses," each a moment younger than the previous one, each holding the next youngest in her arms and (a word I have not used before) "approving" of her. From the future, older Ilses also formed a line following the same procedure. A gap was in the future part of the line, and I placed myself in it. At this point, the Gestalt solidified very strongly, went from black and white into full and rich color (unusual for me) and really filled the total field of my consciousness. To my surprise, the imagery took on a life of its own and one of the younger girls—in middle adolescence—left it and with a wicker basket over her arm went into a brightly lit field gathering flowers near some trees. This seemed only good, so I let it happen and simply lived with and participated in the picture for some time.

Afterward I asked Ilse what her experience had been. She replied that three things had happened. First, she felt a great deal of pleasant heat throughout her entire body and now felt very good and relaxed. Secondly, she had two strong images. The first concerned an incident at twelve that she felt had changed her entire life. In the town in Northern Germany where she had been raised there were two kinds of pretty girls: those with black hair, blue eyes, and white skin like her sister's, and those with blond hair, fair skin, and blue eyes. "And there I was with mud-colored hair, slate gray skin, and these washed out pale blue eyes." When the nurses dressed up her sisters, they "did not even bother to put a bow in my hair, it was hopeless." One day her mother had gone downtown and she went to her mother's room for something. She caught sight of herself in her mother's full-length mirror. "I realized that I was not pretty, but that I *approved* of myself. Since then I have always *approved* of myself and it has made a great difference in my life." (The word "approve" was both times spoken with real emphasis.)

The second image was of herself, as a young girl "gathering flowers in a bright, sunlit field with trees. I was putting them into a wicker basket on my arm."

After the session it was apparent from both our feelings that there was a deep and warm relationship. We sat talking as two people who have had a long, caring relationship for some time. When I left, she spontaneously kissed me on the cheek, which, for a person of her personality and background as I understand it, was a highly atypical action.

In the fifth group, I was simply unable to go into the altered state of consciousness with the patient healee.

There are experientially two separate phenomena here. In the first, the patient actively does not want the healing. This is a clear experience that one of my students in psychic healing has described as "feeling as if you were running into a rubber wall." Often a person has been "persuaded" by family or friends to try this type of healing and does not want to. The feeling that results when the healer tries is unmistakable; it just cannot be done. Put bluntly, it is impossible to "unite" with someone who does not want to unite with you.

The second class of those with whom I could not go into the altered state of consciousness is not so easy to define. Sometimes it was probably due to a fatigue state or distraction of my own that I could not transcend. At other times, it may have been due to something in the healee or to the "mix" our two personalities formed. We know so little about the best (and worst) healer-healee pairings that at this stage all we can do is be aware of our ignorance and our wish to overcome it. The experience in these cases was simply that I could not move into the world of the One; the symbols I used remained empty and just images, the world of the many remained the world I was in.

As it became clear that the first stage of testing the hypothesis of "how" psychic healing worked checked out, the time for the second stage drew closer. This was to determine if it could be taught to others. In the past, the ability to "do" psychic healing had always been regarded as "a gift of grace" or due to a special personality organization. Although I had never done any psychic healing before, it was possible that I had the special personality organization (or "gift of grace") and the reason I had never done it was because I had never tried to. From this viewpoint, the theory and self-training might be irrelevant to the results. I might, for all I knew, have been a "natural" healer and had this ability activated by my interest. The only way to test this was to see if the theory could be used to train others. If it worked there, if following the procedures indicated by the theory could lead others to the ability, I could be reasonably sure that the theory was valid and had not worked the first time merely by coincidence.

The first training seminar was held in September, 1970. I let it be known at the annual convention of the Association for Humanistic Psychology that I was interested in holding such a training seminar. With ten participants (mostly psychologists and others who were interested in the human potential movement), I went off to a private Florida estate which had been offered by Margaret Adams, the owner. The three and a half days scheduled was a very short time, but most of the participants learned to do Type 1 healing. Later seminars were scheduled for five days, and although the pace was still terribly exhausting, it proved possible to teach the majority of participants how to go into both Type 1 and Type 2 states during this time.

Participants were selected for the seminars on the basis of several qualifications. A strong ego structure was needed, as the exercises used are often quite powerful types of meditation, and the time available is too short to allow for members going on "trips" with them. Second, a good ethical approach to life is, from my point of view, important. And third, I selected the kind of people I felt I would like to be associated with in a new field. In the first five seminars I generally also ruled out people who had had a number of psychic experiences or who had ever been involved in psychic healing. The reason for this was that I was less interested in training those already in this area than I was in trying to see if individuals who had never been so involved could be trained. It is important to note, however, that the very act of applying for a seminar in itself was a selection system. Academic or formal qualifications were not considered as standards for acceptance, as I believe that they mean very little. I tend to agree with a patient of mine who once observed that she knew a lot of Ph.D.s and M.D.s who were educated far beyond their intelligence!

The procedure at all the seminars was structurally similar. First came a theoretical discussion of the concept of the sensory reality and the clairvoyant reality. (All students were asked to read my monograph on the subject *before* we started so we did not start from scratch.) A series of exercises composed the bulk of the seminar. These were designed to accomplish three purposes:

1. To strengthen the structure of the ego—a sort of personality calisthenics.
2. To loosen the individual's usual concepts of dealing with space, time, the location of the self, etc., and to make him emotionally aware that there were alternative valid ways of conceptualizing in these areas.
3. To move in a step-by-step progression until one arrived at the altered state of consciousness theoretically associated with psychic healing.

At the end of this series, the group did Type 1 healing on each other and had a good deal of practice at this. On the last day, a small group of individuals with medically described physical problems would come in, one at a time, and the group would hold healing encounters with them. At one point or another, depending on the fatigue level of the group, a short series of exercises leading to Type 2 healing would be held.

Five days is a very short time for this procedure, but it proved feasible. The pace was exhausting, three sessions a day with each session ending when the group was too tired to go on. The pace was so intense and the pressure so heavy that it was necessary to hold the sessions in a residential setting and in a non-urban atmosphere so that the contact with nature could refresh the participants. At present, I and some of the advanced students who received training in teaching the seminar are experimenting with other forms of structure, such as several intensive weekends in a row.

Overall, this general format proved successful. As I learned more and more how to put the exercise series together and how to pace the progress, and as I learned from the contribution of those involved, the seminars improved, and more and more of the participants learned how to go into the altered states. At the seminar in September, 1971, all the students became quite proficient at this, continued to practice it after the seminar and—working together—became an amazingly strong healing circle. It was this group that, at a three-day follow-up advanced seminar, was involved in the case of the boy with the broken back described above.

It was clear from these results that if one followed the implications of the theory, a training method for psychic healing could be devised. If one then went through the training, it was possible for most people to become fairly effective at psychic healing, and further practice improved this ability. This seemed the most important type of test I could devise of the validity (or fruitfulness) of the theory. Other tests of the more usual "experimental" type have been devised, . . . but the healing approach seems to me to be the most critical test of the general theory of the paranormal implied in the concept of the clairvoyant and sensory realities.

There is still, of course, a tremendous amount we need to learn about psychic healing. We do not know its limits or in what types of physical problems it is most effective. We do not know its implications for emotional problems, or how it can best be integrated with standard medical and psychotherapeutic procedures. We know little about how to select the best candidates for training, or how to set up the best healer-healee pairings. We need to know much more about training, about the comparative effectiveness of group and individual healing, and about how to form healing groups. We have no adequate theory for Type 2 healing, and we have only impressions about the comparative effectiveness of the two types or if, indeed, they are more than experientially different. We have no idea how to predict which healing encounters will be associated with positive biological changes and which will not. We are very much at the beginning of this work.

References

Bergin, C. R. "The Effects of Psychotherapy: Negative Results Revisited. *Journal of Counseling Psychology* 10 (1963): 244–55.

Cannon, W. B. "Voodoo Death." *American Anthropologist* 44 (1942): 169–81.

Carkhuff, R. R., and Truax, D. B. Training in Counseling and Psychotherapy: an Evaluation of an Integrated Didactic and Experimental Approach. *Journal of Consulting Psychologists*, 29 (1965): 333–36.

Chance, P. Parapsychology is an Idea Whose Time Has Come. *Psychology Today* 7 (October 1973): 105–20.

Egbert, L. D.; Battit, G. E.; Welch, C. E.; and Bartlett, M. K. Reduction of Postoperative Pain by Encouragement and Instruction of Patients. *New England Journal of Medicine* 270 (1964): 825–27.

Frank, J. D. *Persuasion and Healing*. Baltimore: Johns Hopkins Press, 1961.

Frank, J. D.; Nash, E. H.; Stone, A. R.; and Imber, S. D. Immediate and Long-term Symptomatic Course of Psychiatric Outpatients. *American Journal of Psychiatry* 120 (1963): 429–39.

Friedman, H. J. "Patient-Expectancy and Symptom Reduction." *Archives of General Psychiatry* 8 (1963): 61–67.

Gliedman, L. H.; Nash, E. H.; Stone, A. R.; Imber, S. D.; and Frank, J. D. "Reduction of Symptoms by Pharmacologically Inert Substances and by Short-Term Psychotherapy." *Archives of Neurology and Psychiatry* 79 (1958): 345–51.

Medical World News. "Finger-Tip Halos of Kirlian Photography." October 26, 1973, 43–46.

Rogers, C. R. "The Characteristics of a Helping Relationship." *Personnel and Guidance Journal* 37 (1958): 6–16.

Schofield, W. *Psychotherapy: the Purchase of Friendship*. Englewood Cliffs, N.J.: Prentice-Hall, 1964.

Torrey, E. F. *The Mind Game: Witchdoctors and Psychiatrists*. New York: Emerson Hall, 1972.

Truax, C. B., and Carkhuff, R. R. *Toward Effective Counseling and Psychotherapy*. Chicago: Aldine, 1967.

Uhlenhuth, E. H., and Duncan, D. B. "Subjective Change with Medical Student Therapists: Course of Relief in Psychoneurotic Outpatients. *Archives of General Psychiatry* 18 (1968): 428–38.

4
Walter S. Strode

An Emerging Medicine:
Creating the New Paradigm*

The Scientific Method

MANY OF MY COLLEAGUES may be disturbed by the contents of this paper, and understandably so. As a physician, I have been disturbed by these ideas for several years. They do not fit the model of medical practice in which I was trained 25 years ago. They threaten the professional and economic base on which I stand and which has undergirded my concept of reality. The majority of physicians whom I know and with whom I share responsibility for the care of patients are products of Western, rational scientific thought. The medicine we practice results from application of the logical scientific method to the understanding and treatment of disease. For several years, I have found myself in the uncomfortable position of believing in at least two seemingly contradictory value systems. It would have been much easier to shift quickly from one to the other, and perhaps I should have done so, if it had been possible. But I have chosen not to, for reasons which are still unclear to me. I think they involve a persistent identification with old friends, a certain wistful nostalgia for the recent past, a fear of the hazy outlines of the future, of the new realities of an emerging paradigm— and a hope that it may be possible to combine the best of both worlds.

In order to make clear the problems with which medicine, and

* Reprinted with permission from the *Straub Clinic Proceedings* (April–June 1975) vol. 41, no. 2.

indeed all of society today, are trying to deal, it may be helpful to describe the more important elements of the old paradigm—the patterns which shape medicine today. A hundred years of practice based on the concepts of Galileo, Newton, Koch, and Pasteur, to mention only a few, have resulted for us in a generally agreed-on view of reality. And this is understandable, particularly when we see how much mileage we have obtained from a certain way of looking at problems and of producing solutions. The scientific method really works—we all know this. We almost automatically reject "non-scientific" views, at least in the field of medicine. To do other than this is to invite the scorn of fellow practitioners, as well as to encourage the possibility of medicolegal problems for the physician.

Scientific, logical thinking is based on the concepts that man can be and is an observer, apart from the process he studies; that there are fixed laws governing the functioning of the universe which are there to be discovered; and that ultimately there is only one reality to all of life. It has been only since Einstein[1] and Heisenberg[2] that we have begun to have the first uneasy glimmerings that these concepts are subject to challenge. They, in essence, represent basic themes which humans have constructed to help them understand the workings of their complex universe. "Reality" is not ultimate—there are many realities. Recent writings of Carlos Castaneda[3-6] bring us to this disturbing conclusion.

Present Patterns in Medicine

This paper partly reflects my experience in an exciting new program—The May Lectures. Some of the concepts for a "new medicine" are emerging from programs of this kind. The May Lectures program is very new; there have been only two conferences so far. The first took place in London in May 1974, the second in Airlie, Virginia (near Washington), in April of this year. The program has developed with the primary initiative and energy of Rick Carlson, a brilliant young lawyer with a particular concern for and several years' experience in the health care field. The major focus of the program has been to bring together a relatively small group of well-known scientists and researchers who are exploring new and profoundly different ideas related to medicine and health. Some of the presenters have been

Elmer Green (biofeedback research at Menninger Clinic), John Platt (mental health research at the University of Michigan), Willis Harman (director of the Center for the Study of Social Policy at Stanford Research Institute), Werner Erhardt (of *est*), Andrea Pujarich (author and physician exploring psychic phenomena), and Roslyn Lindheim (professor of environmental design at UC, Berkeley). Also participating are professionals in the Program in Humanistic Medicine in San Francisco, Gay Luce (codirector of the Senior Actualization and Growth Exploration program in Berkeley), and others. More "traditional" physicians in practice and in government have been added to the mix, along with health policy planners. Out of several days of interaction have emerged new understandings of where we are going today in medicine and, hopefully, where we want to go. Total participation in each program has been limited to 60 to 75 persons. I describe the May Lectures program as only one of many signs indicating profound "scientific" interest in alternative medical futures—there are others.

John Platt lists some of the signals of the revolution in health care which we are now encountering:

1. The rapidly growing mass of drug resistant infectious diseases.
2. The escalation of significant iatrogenic diseases.
3. Problems of aging, which are calling for community-oriented research.
4. A focus on patients' rights, as exemplified by the issues of abortion, informed consent, death and dying, and human experimentation.
5. The appearance of a growing number of "radical young doctors" whose goals in medicine differ from those of other physicians.
6. A large contingent of so-called "public doctors"—physicians who have never had private patients.
7. A growing concern for health problems of the underdeveloped countries.
8. The self-help medicine movement.
9. "A new sense of justice," where the highest priority in society requires us to do the best for those worst off.

What are the characteristics of today's medicine? Rick Carlson[7] recounts five that we can see as typifying everyday practice for most of us:

- mechanistic
- interventionistic
- inside the body
- tool intensive
- accepting of science

Notwithstanding the facts that probably all physicians are aware of mind-body relationships in health and disease, and that most of us have concerns for more than the narrow specialty we practice, the way the health care system actually operates today forces one to accept these five descriptions as relatively accurate. We physicians *do* understand the body as a complex machine, and we *do* usually treat symptoms and disease by intervening either surgically or medically within the patient's body, and we *do* diagnose and treat primarily through the use of tools (technology), and the whole system *is* certainly science-based. Is it possible that this set of characteristics might not be appropriate for the future? Could it be that this paradigm might be replaced by one more effective for an emerging new reality?

A Medical Critique

Most criticism of the health care system today is directed at what we can call the operational level: not enough doctors and paraprofessionals, poor distribution, skyrocketing costs. Oddly enough, there is also a major concern for quality of care, but very little focus on the prior question of effectiveness. Although it is admittedly difficult to measure output of medical care (we need more than mortality and morbidity yardsticks), surely we need to know how effective our efforts are at the same time as knowing how good they are.

An evaluation of our health care system needs to proceed from a different point—at the conceptual level—and this significantly alters our usual discussions. Approaching the problem on this level we see a different and more basic set of issues.

Fragmentation of Persons

Although specialization has seemed to be the best way for medical practitioners to handle the flood of new information, knowledge, and techniques of the last 50 years, inevitably it has led to our knowing more and more about less and less. We have tended to lose our concern for the whole human being at a time when a holistic understanding of health is crucial. The trend back toward family practitioners and primary care is not nearly adequate to reverse this direction.

Iatrogenesis

All of us would agree, I am sure, that if we could not help a patient we would not want to do him or her any harm ("primum non nocere"). Our current diagnostic and therapeutic attempts certainly are far more effective than those of our fathers, but the undesired bad effects of these same techniques have escalated incredibly. We are probably all familiar with the often-quoted statement that 15% of encounters with the health care system result in iatrogenic illness. I was skeptical of this figure, but a recent six-month survey by our medical records department revealed that even in our own hospital experience the figure was 11%. It's true that many of these cases are not serious and are either correctable or self-limited. However, a good number do result in serious morbidity or mortality.

Disease-Orientation

Despite our concern for health, no one can reasonably disagree that, as physicians, our primary attention remains on disease. Those who are more humanistically inclined might assert that we are illness-oriented, illness representing the disease plus the person who is ill. But this is not the same as a concern for *health*. The American public continues to feel that health equates with medicine, and that good medical insurance coverage will guarantee good health. This is probably the basic assumption underlying the specter of national health insurance, which will surely lock the United States into a relatively nonchanging medical model for the foreseeable future. Health is more than the absence of disease, more than therapy or prevention, no matter how effective and modern.

Loss of Control

Although physicians still exercise most of the power, with consumer groups and the drug industry also pressing hard, for the most part our health care system is out of control. Who really determines the basic direction of medical trends? Physicians? Patients? Medical schools? Government planners? Probably none of these. Perhaps more than anything else the direction of medicine follows the often unplanned and unco-ordinated outputs of research, of technology in general. Certainly, one wonders if important concerns for ethics, for social and political benefits, and for justice have a discernible effect on the direction we are going.

Futuristics

Three years ago when I reduced to 60% the time I devote to medical practice, my wife and I entered wholeheartedly into the study of "the future" as a new discipline. I brought with me all of the enthusiasm and beliefs my training and experience as a physician could have provided anyone. Those who knew me then would probably agree that I had accumulated the usual criteria of "success." The scientific method was really working for me then, and it obviously still works a lot of the time. But I am much more critical of it now, and much more willing to look for new explanations, new ideas, new patterns. I used to be happy with my ability as a well-trained technician to intervene in the body of a patient in an attempt to change a part or improve a dysfunctional process. My concept of disease then was based on the idea that something *outside* the body had an unfortunate effect *on* the body, producing symptoms of disease. I saw that my job was to discover the cause, eradicate it if possible, and reduce the symptoms if cure was impossible. In a very real way, I was applying man's conquest of Nature to the human body's problems.

As we study thoughtfully the field of futuristics, especially as it applies to medicine, it becomes alarmingly clear that extrapolation of the medical (scientific) model may not solve all of our medical problems. In fact, it seems likely that the harmful effects of the medical model could be responsible for its eventual failure. The major health problems of the present and foreseeable future are not those which can be solved by application of the present medical model alone. The way we can prevent this "failure of success" is by being receptive to ideas, concepts, theories, and practices that lie well outside of what we comfortably accept as logical scientific thinking.

This does not necessarily require a rejection of the past, or even of the present—and fortunately so, as this rejection would probably be a major stumbling block to change, since it would glaringly indicate that we have been wasting our lives following false ideas.

Intelligent creation of alternative futures requires the keeping of what is of value from the past and the elimination of what is not going to work in the future. The new paradigm requires new patterns, and these are inhibited by the presence of old patterns, even when we see that the old patterns aren't working too well anymore. So it is difficult, frightening, and threatening. But it is the real challenge of being human. . . .

If the dinosaur had been aware of the inappropriate relationship between himself and his environment, he might have been able to alter one or the other, or the pattern itself. But, unlike humans, he was unaware, and that marked his end. Humans should be able to do better.

Some Suggestions

A new concept of medicine, a new idea of what constitutes health, a fresh understanding of science, and a different view of humans in society seem called for at this time. Pragmatically, this is the case because the concepts we've been living with have become less and less appropriate. But beyond pragmatism, growth toward increasing complexity and differentiation are what characterize human development. Eternal search for better, more effective ways seems to be part of what being human is. New patterns are constantly being created; but, with a lack of perspective, humans are often satisfied with lesser cures, smaller repairs. The systemic vision necessary for survival requires our developing a holistic view of mankind, and a holistic view of ourselves is what our new pattern in medicine must include.

Physicians are characteristically so caught up with the all-consuming job of caring for sick people that we do not usually have the time or extra energy required to step away from what we are doing, to see it in a larger perspective. But for those of us who can do this, there are visible many individuals and groups exploring the elements of a new paradigm. In the last two years I have been part of at least ten such explorations, usually in the form of conferences, workshops, seminars, courses, and the like. All of us should be aware of these new directions and should contribute to them, so that our intelligence and our experience can also inform the new patterns.

Elements of a New Paradigm

Programs such as the May Lectures, the Kennedy Center for Bioethics in Washington, the Hastings Center in the state of New York, the recent EXPO-sponsored "Health on a Small Planet" program in Spokane, the Program for Humanistic Medicine in San Francisco, to mention several, are indicative of the underlying concern many of us have about the basic assumptions of scientific Western medicine. In various ways, most of these efforts are challenging traditional beliefs all of us have held about the effects of what we are trained to do.

Basic social change is in order—a real paradigm shift is occurring. Of course, changing techniques, improving mortality rates, finding new causes for disease, lowering cost of care, evenly distributing available resources are all good things, and it would be hard for us to stop pursuing these goals. Interestingly enough, however, Ivan Illich in *Medical Nemesis*[8] makes a very strong case for *not* doing these kinds of things. He feels that the changes required are so profound and basic that lesser improvements will serve only to perpetuate the present inappropriate and rigid system. Although some readers might agree with him, it seems to me less than human to bypass process for the sake of ultimate product.

As the recent May Lectures program came to an end, most of the participants had no difficulty agreeing on critical assessments of modern medicine. Building a new paradigm, however, requires more than criticism. It requires creativity, imagination, and an open-mindedness to new ideas—especially ideas that may seem opposed to comfortable and secure concepts of long-standing. Most of all, we must be willing to assume, even if we are threatened, that old ways of doing things may be inappropriate and ineffective. If self-interest is our real motivation—and I think it is—then we must be willing to look anew at where our real self-interest as physicians and as human beings lies.

Several basic questions emerge which seem to highlight the elements of a new paradigm for an emerging medicine:

The Question of Wholeness

Can we see that health is not the absence of disease, not prevention, not exclusively body-orientation at all? Health has really to do with human wholeness, and this wholeness is concerned systemically with the mind, body, and spirit of individuals. It is also concerned with humans as part of a greater universal whole. "Healthing" has something to do with helping each of us optimize our potentials for becoming whole persons.

The Question of Dependency

All of us realize that we are involved with a medical care system that greatly promotes dependency of patients on doctors, on hospitals, on medication, and on technology. Patients tend to become passive recipients of therapy, rather than active participants in a healing and healthing process. The burgeoning of self-help and share-care movements today emphasizes that persons need to and can be responsible for their own conditions, their own healths.

The Question of Field Effects

Disturbing as it is to many of us who are uneasy with esoteric ideas, we are beginning to realize that humans are linked in energy fields that are profoundly important to our healths. Oriental theories based on "chi," such as those associated with acupuncture and herbal medicine, point toward concepts that are not incompatible with Western medicine. Many of us summarily reject, as unscientific, healing practices whose explanations are conceptually at odds with our beliefs. The problem really lies in ourselves, in our unwillingness to hurdle the language barriers and the constructs of others, when the basic understandings are really not too different from our own. We do not have a monopoly on the "truth."

The Question of Limits

In the same way that we have begun to scrutinize ecologically the long-standing ideal of growth, particularly as measured in terms of gross national product, we need to examine just how far our present technologically-oriented medicine can take us. The Club of Rome report[9] has started a series of conferences and discussions that point out the finite limits to growth of which this planet is capable. In the same vein, because of iatrogenesis, because of impersonalization, because of the emergence of stress diseases, because of system size and momentum, because of new "facts" and theories that transgress old concepts, there are clearly limits to medicine that we must identify and respect.

The Question of Reality

Basic to this entire argument is whether we are willing or even able as individuals and as a profession to agree that the universe possesses multiple realities, as Pearce[10] suggests. Specifically, for example, can we deal constructively with the power of the mind? If we are able to accept the existence of paranormal phenomena such as psychosomatic illness, voluntary control of autonomic functions through biofeedback training, clairvoyance, telepathy, telekinesis, and extrasensory perception, even though we do not presently understand them, perhaps new modes of healing will be allowed to surface. Many native healers seem to possess abilities that go beyond mere showmanship, beyond delusion and hysteria. The work of Lyall Watson[11] clearly shows this. Being open to such possibilities seems to be the only way we will ever hope to understand and utilize them.

A New Medicine?

As with all futuristic endeavors, one is tempted (and even urged by others) to peer into the crystal ball, examine the Tarot cards, cast the I Ching, and sketch for willing listeners a picture of the future. "What will medical practice look like in the year 2000?" All physicians are familiar with the hazards of predicting length of life in a patient discovered to have a fatal illness. Yet much pressure is exerted on us for such kinds of soothsaying. How much more difficult it is to foretell the shape of a new system of medicine, especially if we might no longer be the purveyors of truth in such a system. I recall hearing of a person who refused to have any truck with futurists, but who admitted that he would like to know where he was to die—because, if he knew that, he would never go near the place. I am willing only to offer general suggestions.

We might begin to do all we can to encourage individual responsibility in our patients. This can take the form of "demystification" of medicine by providing as much understandable information as we can to our patients, so that they will actually share as much as possible in all decisions regarding their healths and their illnesses. Share-care can readily become a reality in all of medicine and can lead in many areas to the promotion of self-help groups of all kinds.

We might take the initiative in establishing interdisciplinary meetings and discussions with all fellow-healers—including osteopaths, chiropractors, naturopaths, homeopaths, psychic healers, herbalists, and nutritionists. In the last two or three years, I have found that we have much to offer each other if we are given such opportunities in nonthreatening and accepting situations.

We might begin to allocate resources increasingly to holistic and humanistic efforts of all kinds in health care. This could mean reducing resource allocation to technological research and development. Attempts at technology assessment in medicine are profoundly needed and should certainly include citizen participation on equal terms with physicians and researchers.

We might, as a profession and as a country, seriously encourage research into the areas of the paranormal, into energy field implications, and into eastern medicine and primitive folk medicine in general. The primary goal here should not be discovering new tools and techniques for professionals to use on people. Rather, we need to develop a systemic and holistic picture of humans in their total environment, so that we can see clearly the interdependent effects of manipulation of any part of the system. . . .

Basically, we need to realize that medical care supplies only a small fraction of a people's health. The self-interest of all of us, physicians and nonphysicians alike, forces us to accept that we must truly be resources for people, rather than insist that people be resources for us.

It has been said that a new world is only a new mind. Geneticist Theodosius Dobzhansky believes: "Man and man alone knows that the world evolves and that he evolves with it. By changing what he knows about the world, man changes the world he knows; and by changing the world in which he lives, man changes himself."[12]

Are we willing to share in the creation of a new medicine that will fit our changing world?

Notes

1. Clark, R. W.: *Einstein, the Life and Times.* New York, World Publishing Co., 1971.
2. Heisenberg, G.: Uncertainty Principle or Principle of Determinancy, Encyclopedia Americana, Vol. 27, 1975, pp. 355–356.
3. Castaneda, C. *A Separate Reality.* New York: Simon & Schuster, 1971.
4. —————. *Journey to Ixtlan.* New York: Simon & Schuster, 1973.
5. —————. *Teachings of Don Juan: A Yaqui Way of Knowledge.* New York: Simon & Schuster, 1974.
6. —————. *Tales of Power.* New York: Simon & Schuster, 1974.
7. Carlson, R. *The End of Medicine.* New York: Wiley-Interscience, 1975.
8. Illich, I. *Medical Nemesis.* London: Calder & Boyars, Ltd., 1975.
9. Meadows, D. *Limits to Growth.* New York: Universe Books, Corp., 1972. ment of New York: Universe Books, Corp., 1972.
10. Pearce, J. C. *The Crack in the Cosmic Egg.* New York: Simon & Schuster, 1971.
11. Watson, L. *Supernature.* London: Hodder & Stoughton, 1973.
12. Dobzhansky, T. *In* "Human Imagination in the Age of Space" by William R. Cozart. *Motive*, March/April, 1967.

Part II

Evolving the Framework of Wholistic Healing

5

James W. Knight and Herbert A. Otto

Utilizing the Psychic or Natural Healer and Other Modalities in Medical Practice: Some Guidelines

SINCE THE BEGINNINGS of organized medicine, physicians in many parts of the world have sometimes collaborated with psychic or natural healers during their medical practice. There is a similar history of physicians using other modalities ranging from herbology to various forms of massage, physiotherapy, and systems of body manipulation. In the vast preponderance of such instances, collaboration between physician and healer and the physician's use of other modalities were conducted in the hope that colleagues and the public would not take undue notice of this activity.

Today, due to the growing interest in parapsychology and paranormal phenomena, the increasing recognition of the vast powers and potentials inherent in the human being, and the thrust of the wholistic healing movement, a new climate of tolerance, openness, and inquiry has emerged. This new climate of tolerance and, to some extent, acceptance is noticeable at scientific meetings and gatherings in various parts of the world. For example, approximately ten years ago tests of natural or psychic healers were beginning to be conducted in the USSR to separate effective healers from charlatans with the eventual objective of using those with proper talents and capacities in healing teams or as a part of the health care establishments.[1] It is the purpose of this chapter to provide some guidelines for the physician interested in providing a wholistic base for his or her healing practice.

Identification and Selection of a Healer

The first question that confronts the physician interested in using a psychic or natural healer in his or her practice is How and where do I find such a person? (It should be clear that references in this chapter to a psychic or natural healer also refer to the utilization of a so-called psychic diagnostician, i.e., a person who has the ability to arrive at an accurate diagnosis of a person's health problem using paranormal or unconventional means or approaches. In a similar manner, a natural or psychic healer is a person who may use intuitive, clairvoyant, or telepathic capacities of sensing or knowing, and who is utilizing a part of his or her total energy system to affect healing or to bring greater harmony to the energy system or psyche of the person seeking healing.)

The initial step toward the location of a healer is *to get word out, on as broad a base as possible, of the physician's interest in the area of psychic or natural healing.* It has been our experience that establishing such lines of communication usually brings results. The informal communication network in most communities functions both quickly and adequately. By talking to such key persons as ministers, teachers, and counselors, information and leads are often forthcoming shortly. Patients can also be an excellent source of information and, in many instances, hear about the activities of a psychic healer in the community before the physician does. (Since most patients fear ridicule and perceive the psychic healer to be in competition with the physician, they are naturally reluctant to share this type of information.)

Once a psychic healer has been located, the next step is to get some preliminary approximation or assessment of the healer's capabilities and techniques. This is preferably done by contacting persons who have received treatment from the healer, in order to arrive at some determination of outcomes. Many persons who seek out a healer have first consulted community physicians before seeking other help, and their medical records can be helpful in checking results. However, it is always best to seek first-hand accounts and to personally speak to the patient who has been treated by a healer. This also gives the physician the opportunity to clarify understanding of the healer's modus operandi—i.e., to determine the specific procedures utilized during a healing session. These may include such means as touching the person seeking a healing, dialogue, or prayer.

The next step involves determining if the healer is interested in working jointly with a physician as a part of a healing team (or a wholistic healing center). If there is such an interest, it would be well for the physician and healer to have a series of talks to clarify attitudes and beliefs and to establish the philosophical base from which each operates. The two should attempt to determine each person's belief system about how healing takes place. Closely related to this is a mutual exploration of attitudes toward wholistic healing and wholistic health care. (In this connection and prior to such an exploration, the physician may suggest that the healer read Chapter 1 of this volume, Wholistic Healing: Basic Principles and Concepts.)

An underlying aim in this whole process, of course, is to establish whether personal compatibility can exist between physician and healer: whether they are able to work with each other, respect and like each other, enjoy working together, and share a sufficient community of interest.

Finally, throughout this process of getting to know each other, the physician should work toward a mutual determination of whether the general abilities and attitudes of the healer are such that he or she can fit into a wholistic healing program. In this connection, the following questions need to be explored: What are the healer's attitudes toward the keeping of medical records in relation to his or her activities? Can the healer work in an environment that may initially be critical? What is the healer's viewpoint toward research? Once such matters have been clarified, a firm foundation exists so that physician and healer together can move toward an explication of staff and healing-team relationships.

Staff and Healing Team Relationships

Review of the section Wholistic Functioning of the Healing Team in Chapter 1 would be of value at this point. A series of meetings with all members of the healing team (including the office staff) needs to be scheduled to build good team relationships. Obtaining the services of a competent outside consultant to lead this initial phase of team building is often the best and most productive course.

During this initial period of creating the team, it can be of considerable value to go through one of the structural group experiences designed to build close interpersonal relationships. The Depth Unfoldment Experience, or D.U.E., developed by one of the writers is of particular value in this connection and has been widely used in the United States and abroad for over a decade.[2] It is the purpose of the D.U.E. to build a caring group climate distinguished by open communication, empathy, and understanding. Focus on these goals is an important aspect of team building and maintenance. During the initial period of team building it is also important to explore blocks that may stand in the way of proper team functioning. These may include past grievances and resultant feelings of resentment of team members toward each other or toward persons in authority within the team, and similar matters. Clarification of each person's role and function within the team needs also to be undertaken in the recognition that this is an ongoing process throughout the life span of the team. Emphasis always needs to be on conveying that any contribution or sharing by team members is welcome and to be encouraged. After the team has been formed, members still need to be encouraged to contribute any ideas or suggestions that would improve the functioning of the wholistic healing team or center. Team sessions often yield many suggestions of considerable value. *Implementation* of suggestions the team considers most valuable is directly correlated with team morale and more productive and creative team functioning.

It is best to conduct team building utilizing the democratic leadership principle, rotating leadership responsibility on a voluntary basis among group members. Throughout both team building and team maintenance, emphasis is on working toward a harmony of purpose and goals. In this connection, it is of the utmost importance to develop the type of team climate in which members feel free to share their personal problems with each other and to seek positive directions and guidance. Not only does what happens at home and in private life affect the quality of work, but the team's ability to welcome and accept the sharing of personal problems is experienced as deeply nourishing, caring, and supportive by members.

The Patient and the Healer

If the healer is generally known to be a part of the health care team, referrals to him or her must be made with full advance knowledge and consent of the patient. Some brief description, verbal or in writing, of the capabilities of the psychic, diagnostic, or healer should be provided to the patient, as well as a list of goals or objectives to be obtained. For example, the senior author of this chapter often makes referrals something like the following:

> In taking care of your medical problem over the past few months, I have noticed there is another deeper underlying problem that we have not touched. I have sensed, through my communication with you, that you are open to other modalities of healing. There is a psychic healer whom I refer patients to. I am convinced the healer may be able to help you to open yourself up to find the cause of the problem and bring about a healing process.
>
> The extent of the relationship that you develop with the healer is dependent on your own ability to cooperate in the healing process. The psychic healer helps you to develop an altered state of consciousness and works with your energy system. The healer can also give you an awareness of the level of disease or disharmony present in your body, mind, or spirit. The healer will then use healing energy to remove the blocks and bring all parts of you a positive, creative program of thought and activity to take with you when you leave.

If the healer is functioning outside the healing team, his or her function should be described similarly. But in addition, it is important to obtain a signed release for exchange of information between the physician and healer and vice versa.

The relationship between healer and patient is very delicate and is built on mutual respect and trust. This leads the healer to a sensitivity that enables him or her to identify the person's beingness of mind, emotions, physical body, and spirit. Identification of the obstructive process (disease) is then possible. Patient and healer can then work in harmony to bring about a healing that changes the client's consciousness, thereby altering the course of the life process and improving the state of health. At no time should the healer be allowed to force his or her will onto the patient; the healer always needs to obtain the patient's consent on either a verbal or a nonverbal level. The healer must recognize the right and responsibility of the patient to manage both the energy and the substance of his or her life processes, in the awareness that the healer can be a vessel of energy and consciousness to awaken and energize the patient. It is not the function of the healer to exercise power over the patient. The healing is done in a spirit of love, not condescension, awakening the capacities and powers within the patient and helping him or her to take charge of life on all levels of his or her being. The attitude encapsulated in the foregoing passages also needs to be that of the entire healing team.

Administrative and Related Matters

Records of all healing activities and services need to be as objective as possible so that they may become a part of a data base. Such a data base can later be validated in relationship to other more allopathic medical data. A system for follow-up study needs to be developed in order to further expand the validation process. This system may point up other needs not immediately apparent while also furnishing services to patients.

Public relations can play an important role in the physician's use of a natural or psychic healer in his or her practice or the establishment of a wholistic healing center. The healer needs to be brought to the community's attention through the development of a step-by-step educational program or through informal means. This may be done in the wholistic healing center as a part of the education program or in an outreach program such as a series of public meetings. For example, the physician may sponsor, or find an organization such as a church or education institution to sponsor, a series of talks on such subjects as parapsychology, new modalities of healing, and biofeedback, using local or out-of-town speakers. In conjunction with such a series, the physician may wish to make a brief opening or closing talk, or have the speaker make reference to the theory and practice of utilizing natural and psychic healers and the wholistic healing movement. Another possibility would be to end such a series of lectures with a presentation on "The Wholistic Health Movement: Some New Dimensions in Healing." It is particularly important at such times to issue special invitations to the professional community and to have a question-and-answer period at the end of each presentation so that uncertainties and misunderstandings can be resolved.

More informally, the healer also may be presented to the physician's colleagues who are open to this type of involvement. This can be done so as not to bring embarrassment to either party and on a high level of professionalism. The medical community needs careful reassurance that the healer's role is complementary to and in harmony with the overall medical diagnostic and treatment program. It should be made clear that the healer's role is not designed to take the place of the medical treatment program.

The economic and legal base for the utilization of a healer in medical practice is a subject of concern and needs clarification. To accomplish this, however, certain long-range goals have to be reached. There is a need to establish clear-cut guidelines for evaluating the qualifications of the healer. Such guidelines could lead to a licensing program so that natural and psychic healers could be utilized as paramedical aides working under medical supervision. If this were accomplished, insurance carriers and governmental programs might ultimately move toward including the healer in a fee schedule for service.

As it is now, the healer cannot charge for services and must depend on a donation that is subtly or frankly suggested by someone other than the healer—i.e., the physician. The senior writer of this chapter has found this to work quite well on a limited basis. The desirability of the open acceptance and inclusion of a healer as part of a wholistic healing team cannot be overemphasized. It allows a much needed greater depth of coverage than health care systems can now provide with their overworked, overscheduled physicians.

The Use of Other Modalities in Healing and Medical Practice

The use of considerable range of other modalities in the wholistic healing practice is long past due. The particular modality or modalities selected as a part of the treatment are, of course, dependent on the needs of the patient. It is important to consult and plan with the patient in regard to the use of other modalities as a part of the treatment program. A considerable number of them are available. Among these are the Intensive Journal,[3] Autogenic Training,[4,5] biofeedback,[6,7,8] various forms of body awareness and massage,[9,10,11] physical fitness programs such as yoga,[12,13] Tai Chi,[14,15] swimming, plus regular physical exercise programs suited for a specific disease and the limitations it imposes.[16,17]

The writers believe that nutritional education, and counseling with patients and their families, are modalities of particular importance. Use of these modalities is of special value in relation to many medical problems, including respiratory disease, high blood pressure, coronary artery diseases, and many types of cancer. [18,19]

A counseling program utilized as an integral part of wholistic healing can help establish a clear picture of primal and contributing causes that may lie within the patient, his family, or others as well as in his vocational environment. A counseling program can also help a patient to become fully committed to a course of corrective and healing action after he or she has been helped to acquire an awareness of the factors leading to the disease. [20,21] In short, a counseling program can effectively deal with the psychosomatic or functional problems that, in the opinion of many physicians, constitute between sixty and seventy percent of their general practice.

Finally, as part of the counseling procedures, an on-going program of psychological in-depth interviewing and testing could be developed to examine and reveal to a greater depth to the physician and patient the causes contributing to a disease process. [22] Such a program could also reveal a tendency toward a certain disease before it had made major inroads. The thrust of such a program would be basically preventive for, with further psychological counseling and utilization of some of the modalities discussed previously, the person may not become a full-fledged patient.

Physician and Healer Collaboration and the Use of Other Modalities: An Opportunity for Research and Further Study

The wholistically oriented physician is faced with a singular number of opportunities for research and further study. The decision to pursue these opportunities does depend on intellectual curiosity and desire to understand the functioning and causes of healing—that is, the framework that produces certain outcomes.

A number of excellent volumes on the basics of medical research for the practicing physician are currently available. First and foremost, however, all study and research begin with adequate record keeping including, if possible, written (or tape-recorded and transcribed) statements by the person seeking health as to what transpired during treatment plus the outcomes that were noted. Any corroborative observations or statements by the wholistic healing team members are of course of value and need to be included in the records. Many physicians use dated Polaroid photographs as a record of the patient's condition before, during, and after the treatment process.

Follow-up interviews six months and a year after treatment are of great value. Again, written statements of changes observed need to be obtained from the person who received treatment. Finally, by inviting skeptical yet interested colleagues to participate in the studies and the assessment of records, the work can acquire increased validity, and valuable allies may be gained.

As previously mentioned, computer data base collection programs to process medical, biofeedback, laboratory, and other data are of singular value in conducting research involving other modalities and authenticating validation programs.

From the long-range perspective, the economics of research present a difficult problem. The writers would like to suggest that physicians set aside a certain amount of their fees for research. A portion of this amount would be contributed to a recognized community research program and a portion would go to a more regional or national research project or center. Results from such research would then be made available to the physician at regular intervals.

In Conclusion

The utilization of a psychic or natural healer plus the use of a wide range of other modalities by the physician constitute a progressive and very challenging step into the future. It will take a lot of doing as well as a lot of dreaming to reach the goals of wholistic healing: to give the patient the responsibility and tools of power to achieve control of his or her whole being, using the spirit, mind, emotions, and physical body in health; and to harmonize with the healing team and others to bring about a more healthy community and world in which to love, play, and work and to be happy.

Notes

1. Shiela Ostrander and Lynn Schroeder, *Psychic Discoveries behind the Iron Curtain* (Englewood Cliffs, N.J.: Prentice-Hall, 1971).

2. Herbert A. Otto, *Group Methods to Actualize Human Potential* (Los Angeles, Calif.: Holistic Press, 1975): 30–42.

3. Ira Progoff, *At a Journal Workshop* (New York: Dialogue House, 1975).

4. J. H. Schultz and W. Luthe, *Autogenic Methods*, Autogenic Therapy, vol. 1 (New York: Grune & Stratton, 1969).

5. Karl R. Rosa, *You and AT* (New York: E. P. Dutton, 1973).

6. Neal E. Miller et al., *Biofeedback & Self-Control*, Aldine Annual on the Regulation of Bodily Processes and Consciousness (Chicago: Aldine, 1974, 1975).

7. Articles of current research in the field of biofeedback may be found in the published quarterly of the Biofeedback Research Society, *Biofeedback and Self-Regulation* (New York: Plenum).

8. Barbara B. Brown, *Stress and the Art of Biofeedback* (New York: Harper and Row, 1977).

9. Alexander Lowen, *Bioenergetics* (New York: Penguin, 1975).

10. Wilfred Barlow, *The Alexander Technique* (New York: Alfred A. Knopf, 1973).

11. George Downing, *The Massage Book* (Berkeley: Bookworks, 1972).

12. Indra Devi, *Yoga for Americans* (Englewood Cliffs, N.J.: Prentice-Hall, 1959).

13. *Breath, Sleep, The Heart, and Life: The Revolutionary Health Yoga of Pundit Acharya* (Lower Lake, Calif.: Dawn Horse, 1975).

14. Justin F. Stone, *T'ai Chi Chih!* (Albuquerque: Sun, 1974).

15. Li Po and Ananda, *Wave Hands Like Clouds* (New York: Harpers Magazine Press, 1967).

16. Mike Spino, *Beyond Jogging* (Millbrae, Calif.: Celestial Arts, 1976).

17. Kenneth H. Cooper, *Aerobics* (New York: M. Evans, 1968).

18. A Nutritional Evaluation Profile, Form F-1, may be obtained from Dietronics, P.O. Box 44244, Dallas, TX 75234.

19. Another computerized nutritional survey is available through the Wellness Resource Center, Mill Valley, Calif.

20. Refer to Joseph LaDou, M.D., et al., "Health Hazard Appraisal in Patient Counseling," *The Western Journal of Medicine* 122 (February, 1975): 177–80.

21. The Wellness Resource Center, Mill Valley, Calif., offers a package of materials for professionals interested in wholistic diagnosis.
22. For a discussion of the Holmes-Rahe Scale, used by one of the authors of this article, see "Life Crises and Disease Onset" by Richard H. Rahe, M.D. and Thomas H. Holmes, M.D., available from the Department of Psychiatry and Behavioral Sciences, University of Washington School of Medicine, Seattle, WA 98195.

Bibliography

Bailey, Alice A. *A Treatise on the Seven Rays*. Esoteric Healing. Vol. 4 London: Lucis Press, 1972.

Hall, Manly P. *Healing: The Divine Art*. Los Angeles: Philosophical Research Society, 1971.

Hammond, Sally. *We Are All Healers*. New York: Harper and Row, 1973.

Kinnear, Willis, ed., *Spiritual Healing*, Los Angeles: Science of Mind Publications, 1973.

Loomis, Evarts G., M.D. and Paulson, Sig J. *Healing for Everyone*. New York: Hawthorn Books, 1975.

Nolen, William A., M.D. *Healing: A Doctor in Search of a Miracle*. New York: Random House, 1974.

Ponder, Catherine. *The Dynamic Laws of Healing*. Santa Monica, Calif.: DeVorss, 1966.

Shealy, Norman C., M.D. *Occult Medicine Can Save Your Life*. New York: Dial, 1975.

Tournier, Paul. *The Healing of Persons*. New York: Harper and Row, 1965.

Vitvan. *Teachings for the New Age: Healing Technic*. Baker, Nevada: School of the Natural Order, 1946.

6

Evarts G. Loomis

The Wholistic Health and Growth Center Concept: The Background and History of the Meadowlark Experience

TWENTY-FIVE HUNDRED years ago, pilgrims came from far and wide to the remote healing sanctuary of Epidauros in the hills of northern Greece. As they entered the grounds of the sanctuary of Asklepios, the mythical god of healing, they read these words:

> *Pure must be he who enters the fragrant temple;*
> *Purity means to think nothing but holy thoughts.*

Perusing transcripts describing the well-preserved tablets with their accounts of the healings scarcely matched today, one is immediately struck with the vital importance of the need for the seeker to find within himself a pure and harmonious state that is conducive to a return to health and wholeness. The contemporary Plato describes the lack of this consciousness among many of the city doctors of Athens: "You ought not to attempt to cure the eyes without the head, or the head without the body, so neither ought you to attempt to cure the body without the soul—and this is the reason why the cure of so many diseases is unknown to the physicians of Hellas, because they are ignorant of the whole which ought also to be studied; for the part can never be well unless the whole is well."[1] What have we learned in the ensuing twenty-five hundred years? Perhaps nothing is more fundamental in our search to discover the new medicine than this profound understanding that renewed health comes from within the heart of man.

The Center, the Period of Visualization

I trust you will be patient with me if I attempt to reveal something of the expansion of the wholistic concept within my own consciousness. Many years of study, visualization, and meditation are, I believe, of prime importance for those who would become involved in this type of work. The roots of the healing center must reach deeply into the consciousness of the founder and leader, or the project is likely to miscarry, and funds secured to obtain property are likely to vanish into thin air. Secondly, an eagerness to get the show on the road can easily lead to serious mistakes in the securing of staff, with similar results.

I am now very thankful that my early attempts to secure funds were unsuccessful, for I am well aware of what would have happened had I succeeded. I made many mistakes in the choosing of staff in the early years of our Meadowlark project, which greatly held back the forward movement of the project. I can see so clearly now that my intellectual picture of the future Meadowlark was far ahead of my heart-felt knowing. Therefore, anxiety and staff problems were prevalent, polluting the atmosphere that is the very basis of all healing.

Some of the books that have been formative in picturing the concept for me have included P. D. Ouspensky's *Tertium Organum*, R. Bucke's *Cosmic Consciousness*, William James's *Varieties of Religious Experience*, The Gospel of Sri Ramakrishna, the writings of Vivekananda, Alexis Carrel's *Man the Unknown*, Lecomte du Nouy's *Human Destiny*, Sinnott's *The Biology of the Spirit*. Donald H. Andrew's *The Symphony of Life*, the writings of Phinneas Quinby (the physician who cured Mary Baker Eddy), Thomas Sugrue's *There Is a River* (the story of the healings of Edgar Cayce) and all the writings of Albert Schweitzer, whose life decided me on a career in medicine.

May I just briefly review other areas of growth potential in my own consciousness that seemed to have a place in readying me for my particular role in this area. About thirty-five years ago, while working as a medical officer at the Grenfell hospital in northern Newfoundland, the phrase "medicine of the whole man" came to me out of the blue, and I have been stuck with it ever since. In addition to the hospital work, there were many trips on the ocean in a one-cylinder motorboat or in a dispensary ship as we visited the fishing villages up and down the coast. These and long treks across the snow-covered barrens in winter on a dog sled gave much time for contemplation and the opportunity to be aware of one's relationship to the vast, vibrant closeness of Nature. In this type of isolated practice, one has a great opportunity to build up a sense of self-confidence, for frequently you are the last resort for your patients. You either do the medical, surgical, and psychiatric work called for, or it doesn't get done. As the old saying goes, Man's extremity is God's opportunity.

I recall the case of a young woman with epilepsy who in spite of full doses of anticonvulsant medications was having one seizure after another. We talked about her life and her frustrations and usually ended up with a prayer, sometimes audible and at other times silent, she being a Roman Catholic and I a Quaker. At any rate, her seizures became less, and when last heard from a year later, she had had only one seizure in a year and was on no medication.

Then there were two years in China doing medical relief work for the Friend's Ambulance Unit. Each morning, our international staff met together as a group, placing our problems in silent meditation. The results were many lessons in the positive results of applied faith.

Nineteen forty-six found me back with my family in California, and a few years later I was searching for the location for the realization of a long-anticipated center for practicing medicine of the whole man. In the hills overlooking the Mojave Desert we found an 80-acre ranch that seemed just right, but there seemed to be no way to raise the necessary $50,000. Then we found a 300-acre ranch that we considered and even went so far as to place it in escrow. Evidently we weren't supposed to have it, as it was taken away from us by a legal trick that astounded our real estate agent, who never could figure out what happened. Finally, our search ended in Hemet, and here everything began to click. Here we found a beautiful 600-acre ranch that had just gone on the market for an amazingly low figure, and further, there was a marvelous feeling about the place that seemed to pervade its very atmosphere. Later events made it evident the earlier locations would have been wrong. Two air force bases and much smog have come into the area of our first choice, and to cap it off, after we moved to Hemet, pictured on the front page of the *Los Angeles Times* was the other ranch, which had burned to the ground.

The Staff

We are entering a new age in which one might hope quality will again find its rightful spot, considerably replacing quantity, as expressed in high salaries and multiple advanced degrees. However, since we are in a period of transition today, we cannot altogether overlook the latter. Many, many mistakes have been made by taking on staff members who turned out to be sicker than some of the guests. Incidentally, we don't have any patients. They are all guests, inasmuch as we have yet to find the person who is really well in the sense that is under consideration. Of cardinal importance in a center such as Meadowlark is the ability of a staff member to demonstrate empathy and to have no need to point a finger of criticism toward a guest or another staff member. The prevalent atmosphere of love and acceptance would seem to be where healing really starts, and it should be felt the moment a new guest enters the grounds.

While at present we can accommodate eighteen guests at a time, we feel the ideal health community should not exceed twenty-five. Beyond this number, the feeling of interrelatedness and family atmosphere seems to be lost.

Currently, the Meadowlark staff consists of thirteen full-time employees and ten part-time workers. There are an administrator-manager, two psychological counselors, and three hostesses who are trained listeners and have had special experience in psychosynthesis, Intensive Journal, or other techniques. There are four cooks, a housekeeper, a receptionist, a secretary, a polarity therapist, groundsmen, and maintenance men. Volunteers are on call for special mailing, library work, electronic repairs, or other projects.

All new staff members must complete a one-to-three-month probation period before becoming full staff members. Salaries are small and frequently paid partly in board and lodging. Consequently, dedication must be great. The satisfaction of seeing guests come through seemingly impossible situations into new and unexpected dimensions of life more than pays for the lack of financial security. This type of living is a great impetus in stretching one's understanding of the meaning of living in faith.

Guest Selection

At this point it might be appropriate to consider what type of guests are invited to share in this experience of renewed health and growth. First, they must be ambulatory and quite able to take care of their daily needs. While we do have an R.N. on the staff and living nearby, she does not have time to do special duty for any one guest.

The newly arrived must personally have made the choice to come and not be there at the insistence of some family member or friend. In the latter case, few meaningful results are likely. We suggest that people living in Southern California come to open house, which is held every Sunday afternoon, to meet some of the staff and possibly have an interview with the doctor. We want to be very sure the prospective guest wants to get well and is ready to take on the responsibility of his or her healing, with the assistance of our doctor and staff. If, from telephone communication or letter, we think there is any question of psychosis or an alcohol or drug problem, we want an interview with the patient or even a psychiatric consultation as to the appropriateness of the guest's coming. We have found it most important not to have more than one or possibly two guests who may have any real degree of depression in residence at the same time, as their negative mood can affect the whole atmosphere most unfavorably.

The Meadowlark Experience

Arrival time at Meadowlark is Sunday afternoon. People come from all over the country and Canada; some drive, others are met at nearby airports. After arrival, they are assigned to their rooms and then asked to come to the main house for tea, where they are met by members of the staff and some of the other guests who are staying over. At this time, the nurse and I meet them personally and have a chance to discuss with them what they would like to gain through the Meadowlark experience. If there are medical needs, we review any medical records that have been brought with them and plan what laboratory work and what type of examination will be needed. Following dinner Sunday evening, there is an orientation period with a staff member to acquaint the newcomers with the program for the coming week. To further enhance the family atmosphere, only first names are used for both guests and staff members, and the title "doctor" is purposely omitted except off the grounds at the medical office.

The day's program starts each morning with the notes of our cook's flute or a rising bell at 7:00 A.M., followed by meditation in the chapel for those who care to attend. The early birds may want to get up even earlier for an early morning walk or a plunge in the pool or to jog around the track. Some of our guests will have come for the experience of a directed fast, one of Nature's oldest healing methods. They will meet with me regularly each morning at 7:15 as a group. There may be the problem of overweight or the need for detoxification from tranquilizers, cortisone, coffee or tobacco; chronic illness of almost any kind; or a hunger for the spiritual experience so uniquely afforded by this method. During this time the body's energy reserves can be given free rein with no need to be used for the digestive process and attending to daily business or routines. It is thrilling to see the effects of fasting on arthritis, diabetes and hypoglycemic states, chronic headaches, high blood pressure, colitis, and other medical problems that are ordinarily quite resistant to help, or where drug dependency has developed. Following water fasting, supplemented with herb teas or juice, we may take some guests through a medical ecology program, much as described by allergist Theron Randolph and psychiatrist William Philpott.[2]

It is becoming increasingly evident that much illness is associated with the overuse of certain foods in the diet, especially milk, wheat and corn products, or coffee and tea. When these are used beyond the body's ability to provide the necessary enzymes, vitamins and minerals for their conversion into energy, typical addiction problems follow with a myriad of symptomatic manifestations. It is important to point out at this stage that fasting and starvation are in no way synonymous. With a little experience, the physician will become familiar with the signs that indicate the stopping point for fasting.

After the daily individual evaluation of each faster by nurse and physician, there is a discussion of the process and symptomology, and a consideration of dreams the fasters have been asked to record. During periods of cleansing, many dreams have something to do with cleansing—for example, a visit to the laundromat. The fast's appropriate length is determined individually according to each guest's needs and progress. Going off the fast is a most important and critical period. Day by day the diet is expanded until the regular diet is once more appropriate, possibly with the omission of certain foods that have been found deleterious for the individual, should he have gone through the food-testing program. Perhaps the most significant aspect of the fast is the accompanying clearing of the mind and personal insight into life's problems. These are further enhanced each morning by instruction and the practice of meditation.

At eight o'clock, guests and some staff members join together for breakfast, which consists of Swiss Muesli (fresh fruits in season, cut up, with raw oatmeal soaked in pineapple juice overnight, seeds, and homemade yogurt), followed by eggs or cooked cereal and fresh home-made whole-grain bread or muffins. The cereal and muffins are made of flour that was stone-ground just previous to baking. Pero and herb tea take the place of coffee. And so the new nutrition program commences.

At ten o'clock three days a week, there are classes in body balance followed by an experience in "heart to hand" art. This class begins with a group of relaxing exercises to unwind the tensions that tighten up the spine and limbs and cause so much disease, and include a period of autogenic training to quiet the mind and prepare it for the expression in color or clay. The teacher may suggest, "Just draw what you are feeling. You don't have to be an artist, just let the colors flow onto the paper." At times there is a musical background, or there may be silence. Afterwards, the drawings or molded pieces of clay are observed by the group at large to see what has emerged. Much direction and clarification of problems mysteriously comes to the fore, followed, in later classes, by answers. One morning a week I have the fun of personally leading the class in movement and music. This is an experience in moving out of some of the rigidity of everyday routines and attempting to take on the rhythm of our mate or employers. The music is varied to suit the feelings of the group and to help the body to refind its own natural tempo and begin to flow with everyday life situations without tension. Many guests have told me they used to dance or sing but haven't been able to for some years since some tragic event in their life. It is a thrilling experience to see them begin to move once more and find again their ability to dance, sing, or play the piano.

Lunch is at 12:30. Let us take time out to talk about the exceedingly important role of nutrition, which has too long been neglected by the medical profession. Early in our work in establishing the center, as more and more of the medical failures sought us out as a last resort, I discovered that I must study nutrition. At this time, the theme of hypoglycemia was just beginning to attract public notice. As one guest after another had a glucose tolerance test, it became evident that the problem of glucose metabolism was involved in a high percentage of these failures. For the past ten to fifteen years, no refined sugar or flour has been served at our table. The meals are made up of about fifty to sixty percent raw vegetables and fruits, with meat or fish being served only twice a week. We grow as much of this raw food as possible on the ranch, using as best we can some of the principles set forth by Rudolf Steiner in his general concept of biodynamic gardening. The rest we obtain from farms we know avoid the use of artificial fertilizers and pesticides. We feel the quality of carbohydrates, proteins, fats, vitamins and minerals is more important than the quantity, as is illustrated by the eighty years of experience of the world-famous Bircher-Benner clinic in Switzerland. Too often, in totaling the grams, the biological activity of the food is not taken into consideration. Such activity may be absent due largely to high-temperature cooking, processing, or the addition of chemicals that have little or no place in the human economy. Everything in this universe is in a state of vibration, and the rate of frequency determines its state of vibrant life or relative death. Foods are no exception. It is a common experience that an apple just picked off the tree is not the same apple as one that has been on the kitchen table a week or more. We know that with aging the all-important Vitamin C content drops, but as yet we are not measuring the biological fields. I believe when we are able to do this, the whole field of nutrition will be revolutionized. Biochemist and nutritional food supplement manufacturer Dr. Anthony Pescetti assures me that foods cooked for any length of time at a temperature over 130 degrees F. are rapidly being destroyed. As we look at the human body, it should be obvious you can't make a silk purse out of a sow's ear. The increasing sales of hamburgers, french fries, cola drinks, potato chips, and imitation foods such as mass-produced ice cream have an important relationship to the declining health of our country and the rising incidence of arteriosclerotic degenerative diseases such as cancer and brain dysfunction in children and the aged.

Following the interactions and sharing of guests and staff at meals is a rest period with time for a swim or walk, and a time for relaxation before further encounter groups or individual sessions. These may take the form of a psychosynthesis experience or a group Intensive Journal session where there may be an opportunity for dialogue with some part of our being from which we have become alienated, such as the body. This latter might particularly be the case in the instance of deforming arthritis or obesity.

One of the most frequently employed techniques of psychosynthesis is the "waking dream." Following a period of guided relaxation, the therapist makes certain suggestions to the guest. Under the direction of the subconscious, these suggestions take the individual into the area of his or her blocking emotions or at times into a superconscious or mystical state of being—a source of great inspiration.

In conclusion, may I briefly relate case histories.

Betty, the thirty-three-year-old wife of a dentist, was finding it hard to get out of bed in the morning and face the world. She was having intense headaches, palpitations, hand tremors, and a feeling of pressure in the bladder area, which was a great inconvenience. She was found to have multiple allergic and endocrine metabolic problems, malnutrition, malabsorption, and maladaptive food problems. She was started on a water fast, followed by meals of single foods. It was discovered that milk was responsible for her stuffy sinuses, corn made her shaky and weak, bananas gave her a headache, and rice and strawberries produced all her bladder symptoms. Her treatment consisted of homeopathic and nutritional supports. Sulfur 200x (a homeopathic preparation) was used to help normalize her biological energy fields; adrenal cortex extract assisted her endocrine problem; and large doses of B complex, vitamin C, hydrochloric acid, and digestive enzymes helped meet her nutritional and metabolic needs; she was also given extra calcium and magnesium. In addition, she was provided the opportunity of looking at the conflicts between her own and her husband's needs, which were causing much marital conflict. Two months later, she was free of headaches and had no more bladder trouble, and her depression had lifted. A year later her marital life was vastly improved. She rotated foods in her diet to avoid too much of any one food in a given space of time, to avoid her previous symptoms, and she no longer needed adrenal cortex injections, except on rare occasions when she was under undue stress. She no longer needed to see her urologist for dilations of the urethra. If, however, she went off her diet, she experienced a return of her former symptoms.

Then there was Janet, aged thirty-one, who, following a divorce, started using alcohol, after which things went from bad to worse. At Meadowlark she went on a juice fast for four weeks. The first three

days were somewhat rough, with headaches and nausea. Let me share
with you in her own words:

> At last, I am! I am part and parcel of the eternal! Of the whole good
> of the universe. Now I feel, deep within, my worthwhileness, my
> ISNESS, my myness . . . that part of me which is unique and only me,
> and yet shares in every one of the me's around me. Nature is in me
> too—the skies, the rocks, the animals,—all is me—yet I am I. They are
> one—yet we are all a part—we are one. What does it feel like? It feels
> like nothing I have ever experienced before. It is at once sweeter,
> humbler, and yet more elevated and stronger than anything I once
> deemed precious in my life. It feels like the glowing color of gratitude.
> What a relief! A tremendous incredible relief. It means I don't have to
> prove my worthwhileness anymore, and that's impossible anyhow.
> What is IS. What great energy that took to measure up to what seemed
> acceptable to others! I am getting free. I don't have to have others'
> approval. No more arrows of self-condemnation. How I laugh now at
> those cartloads of books that I tried to ingest. It wasn't there. It was
> right here—in me all the time—residing with infinite patience and kind
> compassion—just waiting for me to slow down, step within my
> self—TUNE IN—FIND AND BE!

Finally may I share an example of the waking dream experience—a
dialogue with Edward P. "Can you visualize a mountain?" "Yes."
"Would you like to climb it?" "Yes. There is a good path, and it bears
around to the right, winding toward the top. There are many flowers
along the path and a rich loam beneath my feet. As I get higher, there
are fewer plants. It is interesting that I do not seem to tire, and the cool
fresh air seems to really invigorate me. I am nearing the top. I can see
off to great distances. Now I find myself immersed in a great white
light, and what's more, I am the Light. My body seems to fade away
and everything is one. There is no separation anymore."

After a bit, the descent is made back to the house setting where the
guest actually is. This type of experience (which has been somewhat
abbreviated) is always accompanied by profound changes within the
person and a new sense of values and outlook on life.

In conclusion, I hope I have been able to share with you the great
joy of participating as a physician in the inner life of fellow human
beings in their depth search for meaning, and the resulting exhilara-
tion that accompanies it as they discover new-found vistas of life,
which are the by-products of health at a new level.

Notes

1. Plato, *The Dialogues of Plato*, Britannica Great Books, vol. 7 (Chicago: Encyclopaedia Britannica, 1952) Charmides p. 3.
2. Philpott, William A., "The Value of Ecological Examination as an Aspect of the Differential Diagnosis of Chronic Physical and Chronic Emotional Reactions," *International Academy of Metabology Journal* 3, No. 1 (1974): 62.

Bibliography

Andrews, Donald Hatch. *The Symphony of Life*. Unity Village, Mo.: Unity, 1966.

Assagioli, Roberto. *Psychosynthesis*. New York: Viking, 1971.

Bircher, Ruth. *Fasting Your Way to Health: The Bircher-Benner Approach to Nutrition*. Translated and edited by Clair Loewenfeld. London: Faber and Faber, 1961.

Blaine, Judge Tom R. *Mental Health through Nutrition*. New York: Citadel, 1969.

Bucke, Richard. *Cosmic Consciousness*. New York: E. P. Dutton, 1901.

Cheraskin, E.; Ringsdorf, W. M.; and Clark, J. W. *Diet and Disease*. Emmaus, Pa.: Rodale, 1970.

Coulter, Harris L. *Homeopathic Medicine*. Falls Church, Va.: American Foundation of Homeopathy, 1972.

du Nouy, Lecomte. *Human Destiny*. New York: McKay, 1947.

Grenfell, Sir Wilfred. *Forty Years for Labrador*. Boston: Houghton Mifflin, 1919.

Hauscha, Rudolf. *The Nature of Substance*. London: Vincent Stuart, 1966.

Hawkins, David, and Pauling, Linus, eds. *Orthomolecular Psychiatry: Treatment of Schizophrenia*. San Francisco: W. H. Freeman, 1973.

James, Williams. *The Varieties of Religious Experience*. 1902. New York: Macmillan, 1961.

Karagulla, Shafica. *Breakthrough to Creativity*. Los Angeles: deVorss, 1967.

Loomis, Evarts G., and Paulson, Sig. *Healing for Everyone: Medicine of the Whole Person*. New York: Hawthorn, 1975.

Luce, Gay Gaer. *Body Time, Physiological Rhythms and Social Stress*. New York: Random House, Pantheon, 1971.

Ouspensky, P. D. *Tertium Organum*. New York: Knopf, 1920.

Pfeiffer, Carl C. *Mental and Elemental Nutrients*. New Caanan, Conn.: Kent Publishers, with Publications Committee of the Brain Bio Center, 1975.

Price, Weston A. *Nutrition and Physical Degeneration*. Santa Monica, Calif.: The Price-Pottenger Foundation, 1970.

Progoff, Ira. *At a Journal Workshop*. New York: Dialogue House Library, 1975.

Reiser, Oliver L. *Cosmic Humanism*. Cambridge, Mass.: Schenkman, 1966.

Schweitzer, Albert. *Out of My Life and Thought*. New York: Holt, 1949.

Shelton, Herbert M. *The Hygienic System of Fasting and Sunbathing*. Vol. 3. San Antonio, Tex.: Dr. Shelton's Health School, 1934.

Sinnott, Edmund. *The Biology of the Spirit*. Los Angeles: Science of Mind, 1973.

Sri Ramakrishna. *Sayings of Ramakrishna*. Mylapore, Madras: Liberty Press. Rev. ed., New York: Harper and Row, 1939.

Stromberg, Gustaf. *The Soul of the Universe*. New York: David McKay, 1940.

Sugrue, Thomas. *There Is a River: The Story of Edgar Cayce*. New York: Holt, 1942.

Tompkins, Peter, and Bird, Christopher. *The Secret Life of Plants*. New York: Harper and Row, 1972.

Tournier, Paul. *The Meaning of Persons*. New York: Harper and Row, 1957.

Vithoulkas, George. *Homeopathy, Medicine of the New Man*. New York: Avon, 1972.

Williams, Roger J. *Nutrition against Disease: Environmental Protection*. New York: Pitman, 1971.

7

John C. McCamy and James Presley

Nutrition and Wholistic Health*

NUTRITION can be as complicated as a maze. If you start studying every available book on the subject, you will encounter intricate biochemical and medical facts every few pages. Experts frequently clash, sometimes exchanging violent words. One authority insists on this, another on that. Who is right? What is one to do?

The Human Life Styling approach to nutrition can be summed up in three words: *Keep it simple.*

Accordingly, we have outlined a simple approach that is safe and can only benefit you. At the end of this chapter you will find a check list of ten prescriptions designed to cover the nutritional needs of most people. That, basically, is the nutritional program for Human Life Styling.

First, though, we will outline the predicate for that check list, by presenting a survey of certain nutritional principles that will help you understand why we think the simplified steps will improve your health.

You don't have to remember anything in this chapter but the check list at the end. Our purpose is only to explain to you, in as nontechnical language as we can, background material for the ten steps.

The important thing, after you've read this chapter, is to start *using* the check list.

* Reprinted from *Human Life Styling* by John C. McCamy, M.D., and James Presley. Copyright © 1975 by John C. McCamy, M.D., and James Presley. By permission of Harper & Row, Publishers. Nutrition is only a part of the total program of Human Life Styling developed by Dr. McCamy.

The best part of it is that you won't be asked to sacrifice yourself by "dieting." Instead of "giving up" things, you will be asked to substitute. Basically you will be substituting food for nonfood. By food, we mean fresh, whole foods without poisons or other additives. It is food that is as unprocessed as possible before it reaches the dining table. On the other hand, by nonfood we mean items in our diet that do not contribute fully to our nutritional needs. They may have been overmilled or overprocessed. They may have additives. They may be relatively empty of nutritional value, except for calories. They may be performing the same function in the body as drugs do.

Among a group of Dr. McCamy's patients, especially older ones first reporting in, he found that as much as 80 percent of their diets consisted of nonfood. All we are asking in this chapter is that you eat food, in order to do for your body what is natural and normal.

Simple? Yes. Easy? Not necessarily. For many, it may involve a radical change in life style.

You do not have to change overnight. Changes can be made slowly and in their relative order of importance. This will enable you to steadily lower your risks of falling victim to almost all illnesses, while at the same time instituting the program gradually. Instead of embarking on a crash program, you will be changing your entire life style. That takes time.

If you need the security of a cliché at this stage, remember: Rome wasn't built in a day. Give yourself time to change. But see that you do change, periodically showing progress. Keep a record. Write down your personal nutritional goals after you have finished this chapter. Check yourself weekly or monthly; better yet, have someone else check your progress for you, as a doctor would. Another person can be more objective about it than you may be.

Set yourself a time schedule, aiming toward an optimal diet in, say, six months—or a year. This is more likely to work in the long run. If you can pull off a personal revolution in less time, and keep the innovations as part of your permanent life style, then fine! But for most of us it is more effective to hew away slowly at a new regimen, modifying our life habits one at a time. . . .

For the next several pages we will be examining specific elements of nutrition in terms of resistance and susceptibility, as a prelude to the nutritional recommendations. We do not claim this is the definitive word on nutrition; instead we have attempted to classify the various facets in order of their relative importance.

We will begin with refined carbohydrates, which Dr. Weston A. Price has labeled "the white plague." Refined carbohydrates consist of sugar and white starch products. These overrefined nonfoods may be the leading cause of disease in this country today. Think back to early primitive man and his diet. Whatever he ate, we can be certain of one thing: he had no refined carbohydrates. Of these, sugar is the most pervasive.

Sugar

Sugar is a true susceptibility factor. It has no redeemable nutritional value; it is a pure carbohydrate devoid of other dietary factors. In plain words, it contributes calories—nothing else.

There are six major reasons why sugar should not be eaten. They apply to all refined carbohydrates, but especially to sugar because of its high concentration.

1. *Sugar, being a refined substance, is like a drug; it is absorbed too rapidly into the system.*

Our bodies were never meant to have such a staggering load of sucrose as you find in a cola, a ginger ale, ice cream or a piece of cake. Almost as soon as it hits the digestive tract, *whoosh!* it goes straight into the bloodstream. If it's drunk, it goes in faster than if it's in a solid form. This creates a sudden demand on the pancreas to supply insulin to control the sugar, possibly a hundred times more than the insulin output should be for such a brief period of time. There suddenly is more glucose than the body needs.

2. *This brutal overload of sugar upsets the entire endocrine balance.*

The endocrine system of the body consists of the ductless glands such as the pancreas, adrenals and pituitary. These are all interrelated. High insulin levels can depress thyroid and pituitary function. It may be a factor in early menopause. As the dumped sugar throws one gland out of kilter, the others become unbalanced. Eventually malfunctioning endocrine glands may affect the brain and, therefore, all other parts of the body.

3. *Sugar is deceptive because of its concentration, and this leads to overconsumption.*

British researchers T. L. Cleave and G. D. Campbell have labeled this as perhaps its leading danger. Citing the five-ounce-a-day average per person that is consumed in Great Britain, they emphasize that a person would have to eat two and a half pounds of sugar beet to supply that much sugar. Who would eat so many sugar beets every day? The concentrated nature of sugar leads readily to overconsumption. Cleave and Campbell build a convincing case that overconsumption of sugar (and refined starches) can lead to diabetes, obesity and coronary thrombosis. Dr. John Yudkin, another distinguished British scientist, thinks that in addition to these diseases, sugar may also be a factor in cancer, eye disorders, accelerated aging and other medical problems.

4. *Because it is overrefined, sugar is an incomplete carbohydrate.*

It has none of the protein and other food factors that accompany it in a natural food. This means sugar lacks the nutrients that are needed to metabolize it. If these nutrients aren't with the sugar at the time, they must come from the body's reserves. Thus, sugar may rob the body of vitamins B_1 (thiamine) and B_2 (riboflavin), niacin, vitamin B_6 (pyridoxine), magnesium, cobalt and other factors. Or, if the sugar doesn't metabolize completely, the body is left with waste products like lactic acid and pyruvic acid, which can become a factor in the degeneration of all the tissues and may lead to the development of arteriosclerosis.

5. *Sugar is an empty calorie.*

It contributes nothing of value to the diet. Zero. Actually it is worse than zero—a minus. You do not need it at all. It leads to obesity. An empty calorie is a sick calorie. It keeps you from eating food that is valuable. Good, whole food has all the nutritional factors in the proper combinations and provides the necessary calories, too. No soft drink, for instance, has any food value at all. Why waste money and health on empty calories?

6. *The fiber has been removed from sugar.*

Through the process of evolution, man in his natural state was accustomed to digesting foods with the fiber intact. His digestive tract requires coarse foods. The druglike sugar, lacking fiber, becomes the highly unnatural substance that figures in the five preceding objections. Its lack of fiber also figures in its role as a cause of tooth decay and gum disease. Children who are on high-sugar diets get tooth decay; those who eat large quantities of sugar cane (with fiber intact) do not have cavities.

In this country we consume an average of 120 pounds of sugar per person per year—adult and child. Many eat as much as 400 pounds per year. That's a national glut of sugar. (In 1900 the average was less than four pounds per year per person.) It causes no end of medical problems. Two ways it can affect health relate to its impact on blood sugar levels. It may overtrigger the insulin mechanism and cause hypoglycemia, or low blood sugar; or over a long period, perhaps twenty years, it finally breaks down the insulin-producing system, resulting in diabetes. Hypoglycemia is a major stress factor today. But since there are no lesions to be studied with a microscope, most doctors do not recognize it. Many doctors still advise patients to eat more sugar for hypoglycemia. This only starts the process over, as insulin overreacts. The patient has a ten-minute sugar high, followed by two miserable hours of fatigue.

Yudkin and others have related sugar consumption to coronary heart disease, demonstrating that it, rather than fat, is the primary villain. Sugar has been shown to raise the cholesterol and other lipid (fat) levels in the bloodstream. The study of Yemenite immigrants to Israel is merely one example out of many. In Yemen these people used hardly any sugar at all; when they first arrived in Israel they had little incidence of heart attack, arteriosclerosis or diabetes. After they had been in Israel for several years, however, and had greatly increased their consumption of sugar, the immigrants' statistics in all three of these diseases soared alarmingly.

The old home economics view that desserts every day make for balanced meals is absolutely wrong. Work done by the Southern Academy of Clinical Nutrition has placed refined sugar at the top of the list in relation to illness. It has no redeemable nutritional value.

Old-line nutritionists are sometimes caught in the trap of believing there is no difference between one carbohydrate and another. Asked "Do you think there's a difference between eating 100 grams of baked potato and 100 grams of a cola drink—they're both carbohydrates, right?" they may reply, "Yes, they do the same thing," being unaware not only of the absorption rates of the two but of differences in their nutrients. To give you some idea of the very complicated process that goes on in the body during digestion, note the chemical reactions that take place, as shown in Figure 7.1. The body must have the necessary nutrients for metabolism. The whole potato has it, the cola does not.

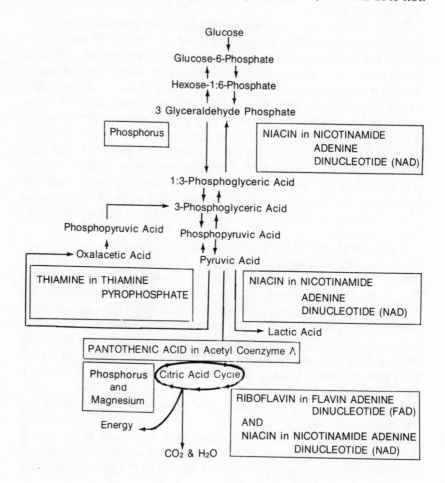

Just remember that digestion is a highly complex process by which cells change food into energy, requiring a complete supply of nutrients. Cofactors such as B vitamins, magnesium and cobalt are necessary at many points in the cellular cycle.

Many people have been aware of the dangers of white sugar for years, yet it is still widely believed that some form of sweetening is necessary. This view goes against the evolutionary history of man. You should shun not only white sugar, but also brown and light brown sugar. This includes every food product in which sugar is added, whether it be pastries, canned fruit, cookies, soda pop, packaged cereals or candy in its many forms. Sugar in these products is too rapidly absorbed for the human being to handle safely. What about honey as sweetener? Undoubtedly it is far better than refined sugar, but it, too, is a concentrated sweet. . . . By justifying sugar or a lot of honey to yourself, you open the door of logic to daily heavy loads of alcohol for all age levels. . . .

Most people's symptoms improve merely through the eliminating of sugar from their diets. Frequently just three days without it is enough to make a difference. But what do you replace sugar with? Food—fresh, whole fruits like apples, grapes, bananas and papaya. Fruit contains sugar, too, but in a natural state with all the factors needed to make it a healthy part of you.

White Starches

Other refined carbohydrates fall into the same category as sugar. The reason sugar is worse is that it is eight times more refined than white starch. That makes it eight times worse. But this does not lessen white starch's role in disease as a susceptibility factor. White flour, white bread and "snack foods" have been overmilled. Whole-grain fractions have been taken away to increase storage life—and profit. The results are white rice, white spaghetti, white macaroni, white soda crackers, potato chips and any other kind of starch that man has tampered with.

Classifying sugar and white starch together in their effects on the body, British scientists Cleave and Campbell have blamed these refined carbohydrates for causing one disease that takes many forms, including coronary thrombosis, diabetes, peptic ulcer and hemorrhoids. Briefly, their argument about peptic ulcer is that protein is a buffering agent for hydrochloric acid, which attacks the stomach lining. When carbohydrates are refined, the protein is removed totally or almost so. Fats, starches and sugars do not affect the acid; only protein does. With fiber removed from these products, they are chewed less, and thus less alkaline saliva accompanies them to the stomach. The acid that forms in the stomach is enhanced by the absence of natural buffering processes. After years of such a diet, an ulcer appears.

Ironically, ulcer patients are usually advised to avoid coarse foods, when it is the absence of coarse foods that caused the condition. Frequent feedings of refined foods are encouraged—though it is the loading of the stomach that causes hydrochloric acid to reappear. Cleave and Campbell advise, on the contrary, feeding of unrefined food only when hungry, a profound but logical departure from present-day practices.

What injures stomach membranes, insist Cleave and Campbell, is not coarse food but unbuffered hydrochloric acid.

They go on to explain how white starches cause varicose veins and hemorrhoids. First white starches, having lost their fiber in milling, lead to constipation as they fail to provide the bulk necessary to push waste through the bowels. The constipated mass in the colon exerts pressure on the arteries and veins at the back of the abdomen. This unnatural stress creates abnormalities that eventually become varicose veins or hemorrhoids. Coarser foods, such as unprocessed bran, on the other hand, keep the waste pushing through the bowels with regularity, thereby preventing constipation and its associated disorders. A comparison of American Negroes and tribal Africans, both of relatively similar racial stock, indicates that colon problems are common among American blacks, but rare with Africans; it is another instance of refined versus unrefined diets.

The solution to these problems is simple. It is no sacrifice to give up tasteless white dough. It is a pleasure for the palate to substitute whole, natural carbohydrates. Take a fresh potato. Bake or lightly boil or steam it, and eat the skin, too—that's the way to maximize its nutritional benefits. But if you peel it, overcook it and then mash it before consuming it, you might as well eat the plate instead.

A good way to change over from sugar and white starch is to gather the family in the kitchen and let them help you throw out all the junk:

the candy, cookies, chocolate-coated "goodies," white bread, Danish pastries, fruit drinks (not fresh juices) and white crackers. Bring in whole-grain breads, fresh fruit juices, wheat germ, unprocessed bran and whole-grain cereals. Learn to make bread. Substitute fresh meals for TV dinners. The older children may be disgruntled for a while, but remember this is an entire life style change. They may become the leaders. It is important that the whole family participate. You can't program your children to avoid junk if you eat it yourself.

Additives and Poisons

The average American eats from the storage shelf and in quick-food stands, where many foods, such as ice cream, may have scores of additives to soften, color and flavor. Delicatessen foods such as bologna and frankfurters contain nitrates, which have been classified as leading factors in colonic cancer.

Ideally, if you can do it, replace chemically preserved foodstuffs with food you grow yourself or buy from a farmer who uses no additives or sprays on his crops. Organic gardening is done without the use of commercial fertilizers and pesticides. If you can't do this, try to buy from a fresh fruit and vegetable stand. Check labels on everything you buy. Reject those that list among the ingredients BHA, BHT, artificial flavoring, artificial coloring, or other such terms that indicate petroleum derivatives and other chemical additives. . . .

Smoking

Smoking is included in this chapter on nutrition in order to simplify the program. Almost everyone knows the dangers of smoking by now. The Surgeon General long ago made it official. It is more than a matter of nicotine and tars. Smoking brings a very high heat into the sensitive tissues of the respiratory system. Furthermore, since growing tobacco plants are drenched with pesticides, the smoker is exposed to those poisons also.

The dangers of smoking aren't restricted to the smoker. Nonsmokers in the same room with a smoker are forced to breathe in the noxious gases caused by combustion processes, which may be more deadly than the original smoke sucked in by the smoker himself.

Smoking is completely incompatible with health. Along with the risks of cancer, bronchitis and emphysema, smoking depletes the body of its nutrients. It blocks oxygen transfer from the lungs into the blood, leading to imbalances in electrolytes and blood gas. There may be other losses, of which we aren't aware.

Dr. McCamy has found in his practice that most people will stop if the risks are clearly stated and the patient is advised (as we now advise you, as of this moment), "You *must* stop smoking for any level of acceptable health."

It is difficult to stop smoking. If you try cutting down, you might change at first to a pack a day of one of the filter-tip cigarettes, which taste so bad you'll wonder why you smoked in the first place. That could induce a positive attitude. Then after a month on a low tar cigarette you'll need to stop completely. Tapering down almost never works; too often people return to smoking too much. Nicotine tablets only help take away the slight nicotine effect, without reducing the need for doing something with your hands. Whatever you do, a period of nervousness can be expected until you get it under control.

Whenever possible, substitute. Carry twenty carrot or celery sticks in your pocket, and every time you want a cigarette take out a carrot stick and mouth it as you would a cigarette. It may sound silly, but try it. Just don't substitute foods that might be fattening.

Or take a brisk, brief walk instead of a cigarette. If you're at the office, take three slow, long, deep breaths, then walk to the water cooler and back. That's your cigarette. You may do this a hundred times the first day. A lot of walking and a lot of carrots, but after two or three weeks it'll drop down to ten or twenty times a day or much less. The carrots won't make you fatter, the walking will help you, and few people breathe deeply enough anyway. Think of it as substitution: *I'm going to do this instead of smoking. I'm doing something for my lungs. I'm improving the health of my mouth. I'm keeping my hands occupied. I'm helping my mind function better.*

The craving for a smoke may not be completely absent for years. This depends on the individual. If the problem is greater than you feel you can handle by yourself, seek out Smoke Watchers or any such group that may be available locally.

The entire Human Life Styling program will help smokers get off their habit. Aerobic exercises especially prove valuable. It's hard to run, walk or ride a bike if you're smoking. Exercise dramatizes the handicap; hard breathing makes you realize what has been happening to your lungs. We have found that the average smoker, after being on the total program for six months, just didn't want to smoke anymore.

Saturated Fats

There is almost no need in the human diet for saturated fats. In this nation we use tons of saturated fats in the form of chili, fried foods, hamburgers and hydrogenated foods.

When the cholesterol scare first came up about a decade ago, margarines became all the rage. That's great, we thought. It's better than butter and it will lower cholesterol! What we didn't know at the time was that the process starts with perfectly good corn or soy oil, which then is hydrogenated. Hydrogenation means that the hydrogen bonds in the fat are welded, producing a hard fat that is solid at room temperature—a saturated fat. It is harder than butter.

Since hydrogenated fats are the hardest and worst of all, they should be avoided wherever they appear in commercial margarine, peanut butter, mayonnaise or any other food. If you use these foods, make certain that the label confirms that they are unhydrogenated; usually you have to buy them at health food stores.

Beef fat is very hard at room temperature, while chicken and fish fat are markedly softer. Safflower and vegetable oils, on the other hand, are liquid at room temperature; they are unsaturated.

You need fat in your diet. The Southern Academy of Clinical Nutrition has proved that we need fat to live. It is a resistance factor. But we need more unsaturated fat. We need "fresh" fat, not the burnt or used kind one finds in short-order stands that deep-fry fish, chicken and potatoes. Avoid eating anything fried. The heating of fats, including unsaturated fats in frying produces carcinogens.

Ideally you would use only "fresh," unsaturated fat such as that in safflower oil, soy oil, saffron oil or corn oil, and these in salads rather than in cooking. Avoid *all* hydrogenated foods. If you're a heavy beef eater, alternate your beef meals with chicken and fish. Diet is recognized as basic to any treatment of high blood fats; all drugs for lowering cholesterol or triglycerides have some side effects. If you can't get unhydrogenated, unsaturated fats at your grocery store, demand it even if you have to scream at them. Or go to a health food store.

Inevitably the question arises as to whether or not to use whole milk. If you can obtain certified raw milk and it seems appropriate to drink it, go ahead. You might note, however, that about 30 percent of the population is allergic to milk to some degree and many people drink too much of it. If you have bowel problems, you might consider doing without milk, to see if that helps. There is a controversy in nutritional circles over milk. Dr. Melvin E. Page thinks no milk at all should be allowed in the diet; Adelle Davis recommends a high milk diet of around two quarts a day. We stand somewhere between these views. Whole milk contains saturated fat, but up to a glass a day of raw milk or some cheese may be acceptable if you have no adverse reaction.

Drugs

To simplify, we have classified as drugs: alcohol, coffee, tea and other caffeinated drinks, marijuana, sleeping pills, LSD, tranquilizers, diuretics or water pills, diet pills, "speed," aspirin and pain killers. All of these tamper with the body in some way and provide no nourishment. Any drug may have a side effect, ranging from suppression of the appetite to robbing the body of vital nutrients. The average American takes from three to five such mind-and-body altering drugs a day. Unless there's an urgent medical reason, it's best to shun them all.

Except in the case of very high blood pressure, the simple practice of restricting salt, increasing potassium and taking vitamin B_6 will eliminate the need for diuretics. Dr. John M. Ellis has proved that vitamin B_6 alone will relieve edema, or water retention, in most instances.

We consider it illogical to use diet pills. An appetite suppressant makes for an imbalance in the hypothalamic hunger mechanism, the weight-control mechanism and the bodily mechanisms regulating depression and awareness. . . . The way to lose weight is to methodically change your life style—for life. As you get more in tune with the rhythms of nature, you will not need drugs.

Alcohol, like sugar, is an unnecessary caloric. Ideally, no empty calories should be taken in. Different people handle alcohol in different ways. If you are in absolutely impeccable health, then it might be acceptable for you to have one drink a day, as long as it is not mixed with a soft drink or sugared liquid.

Coffee is an addictive drug. If you drink coffee and you don't believe this, then stop it totally tomorrow and see what headaches and depressions you will have until your body adjusts to living without it.

A high correlation with illness has been found in people who drink more than two cups of coffee a day. We've seen patients who were drinking ten, twelve, fifteen cups and wondering why they were nervous! There are probably millions of people in this country who drink more than ten cups of coffee every day. It is a susceptibility factor. Caffeine stimulates the sympathetic nervous system and the secretion of acid in the stomach; yet many patients with heartburn have never been advised to stop drinking coffee. They should have stopped at the first, tiniest sign of heartburn. Why wait until there's a bleeding ulcer?

Coffee also, for reasons not yet understood, has a fairly high ranking in the cancer profile. It could be in the processing, where sulfuric acid is used, or it could be the result of the fungi growing on the coffee beans after they have been stored too long. Or it may be the simple excess stomach acid irritation.

The high incidence of cancer correlates with heavy tea drinkers as well. Generally, what applies to coffee will fit tea also, though tea has less acid. All cola drinks and chocolate also contain caffeine.

Coffee, tea, cola and chocolate all perform the one disservice to the body that sugar does. Because they pull stored body sugar from the liver too quickly, they raise the blood sugar too high, then lower it. The best way to prevent this is to take an orange juice break in the morning instead of a coffee break. One study along these lines, conducted by Dr. McCamy, demonstrated that efficiency will go up 20 percent.

When you stop any of these caffeine drinks, you will suffer withdrawal symptoms, as you'd expect from a drug. These may include headaches, listlessness, general aches and nervousness—which gives you an insight into what this drug has been doing to you. The best way to stop is to taper down until you reach one cup a day. Hold the line there for two or three days. Then stop—or rather substitute. There are several coffee substitutes on the market, made in this country and in Europe. These, usually of grain or bran, are preferable to decaffeinated coffee, which after all has only the caffeine removed and retains some acid. Herbal teas are best of all, and there is a wide variety available. For chocolate substitute carob, which tastes better anyway. These are pluses. Decaffeinated coffee is a zero. Coffee, tea, cola and chocolate are minuses. Other aspects of the program will help you rid yourself of these crutches, . . . abnormal activities for the body.

Liquids

When the body is thirsty it needs one thing—water. People who quench their thirst with sweetened soft drinks are running a gamut of risks. By the time their thirst has been slaked, their blood sugar has been enormously raised, they have been alkalinized and they have swallowed a number of chemical additives. If thirsty, drink water.

Studies have shown that hard water is better for heart health. Many American cities today have polluted water supplies. For these reasons, spring water is preferable if you can get it, or distilled water.

Try to drink water at room temperature. Of the tribes of natural man studied for this book, none drank iced liquids. Even in the civilized world, Americans are the major consumers of iced drinks. It's abnormal for the human body. Those who drink an excess of cold liquids have more upper respiratory infections. What seems to happen is that cold liquids chill the cells in the throat and lower their resistance; the mucus supply drops immediately and bacterial invasion follows more readily.

On occasion you may wish to substitute small amounts of fresh fruit juice or vegetable juice without additives or sugar. Take the trouble to ensure that it is a genuine juice. Many juice drinks are artificial and may, like an orange drink, contain petroleum additives. Read the labels!

Protein

The literature on protein has become contradictory and confusing. Some nutritionists feel we need 80 grams of protein a day. Most people consume much less than that. Dr. McCamy has made one study indicating that upper- and middle-class women have deficient intakes. One reason for this is that foods we think of as protein are actually low in quality. Frankfurters, fat hamburgers and bologna are mainly fillers with little protein.

So the first step is to increase the quality of your protein. Eat simple foods: fresh fish, broiled; fresh baked turkey or chicken; some beef, pork or veal; eggs and some milk products. Haddock and cod are superior sources of protein. Have liver at least twice a week. Organ meats are of far higher quality protein than other cuts of meat, much better than steak and muscle meats.

Eliminate frankfurters, delicatessen meats and commercial chili. If you want to make your own stews or chili, use only fresh ingredients. Spices should be used only if you have no heartburn or bowel problems.

You will usually find that the best sources of protein are good providers of other essential nutrients as well. Eat eggs, milk, cheese, fish, chicken, beef (especially organ portions), soybeans, legumes and nuts, and you will not only ingest high-quality protein, you will also have calcium, iron, vitamin A and the B vitamins.

Some say that 80 grams of protein daily is far more than we need; others opt for a nonmeat diet. During a recent visit to Lausanne, Dr. McCamy reviewed work by Swiss and Scandinavian nutritionists that helped explain how a vegetarian could get along so well. Most of us in the United States apparently are in acid balance because of our carbohydrate and meat diets. When a person shifts his diet to more vegetables and fruit, this bodily condition changes to an alkaline balance. These Europeans' work shows that an alkaline balance ensures a much higher absorption of protein and generally better assimilation of food, and that more protein is held actively in the blood serum. The researchers found that the average person could get by on as little as 20 grams of protein daily, which is one-fourth of what some nutritionists say is necessary. We are not advocating such a change—although ecological reasons may make it necessary sometime in the future—but wish to indicate to you the range of opinions on this subject.

At the famed Bircher-Benner Klinic at Zurich, raw fruit and vegetables make up the bulk of the healthiest diet, for the sickest people. It appears that the sicker people often can't metabolize protein or fat efficiently.

Our suggestion: Improve the quality of protein and vary it by using both animal and vegetable sources together for an enhanced effect.

Meals and Freshness of Food

Americans by the millions have nothing but coffee for breakfast, grab a quick grilled lunch wolfed down with a cola drink or a beer, climaxed by a huge dinner at home. They follow up dinner with beer and potato chips and fall asleep in front of the television set. It is too much for their enzyme systems to handle at one time, and they sleep with half-digested proteins in their stomachs, a quite unhealthy practice. In the morning they are nauseated and wonder why they can't eat breakfast. Then the cycle begins again and they are tired all day.

They are not only eating the wrong things, they are putting an emphasis on the wrong meals. You need nutrients during the day when you are using energy, not after you've done your day's work. You need to take in body fuel early in the morning, so you'll have it when you need it. Most people will benefit by the policy of eating breakfast like a king, lunch like a prince and supper like a pauper. Certainly breakfast and lunch should be the larger meals.

A tossed salad and a soup can make a marvelous supper. Unless you expect to be up late, it should be sufficient. If you're in the habit of going out for dinner, why not change the routine? Go out for lunch. The same food is often served then as at dinner, and it may cost half as much earlier in the day.

For maximum utilization of your food, eat raw fruit or vegetables at every meal. The fresher food is, the better it works for you. A food grown on fertile soil, just picked, has all the enzymes and nutrients it will ever have. The longer it takes to reach your plate from the tree or vine, the more it loses in deteriorated enzymes and vitamins. This is also true of meat and fish; they have the highest food values when just slaughtered or caught.

Fruits and vegetables in some commercial markets have been stored for weeks or months before they are sold. Add to this the fact that many people go all week without eating one raw food. Such diets rank very high in cancer profiles. We need the enzymes, the roughage and all the nutrients that raw foods have—and that are usually missing in processed, canned and frozen foods.

The ideal way is to grow your own food organically, without pesticides or commercial fertilizers, and eat the food fresh, and preferably raw, as it comes from the garden. Cooling, packaging, heating, even slight heating, decrease its value. With fruit, fresh off the tree is best, from a fruit stand or from a farmer you know is next best, a market is third best, and frozen is fourth. Canned fruit should be ignored altogether. (Some diabetics, hypoglycemics and arthritics may have to restrict even some fresh fruits, like bananas, which are high in natural sugars, but for about 90 percent of us these are part of a good diet.) If you eat all fresh foods, with 50 percent raw and the rest cooked lightly or baked, you'll be making an excellent start toward better health. By using some frozen foods, while avoiding canned or packaged goods and eating nothing fried or burnt, you'll make commendable headway. At the very least, eat something fresh and raw once a day, and shun smoked or grilled foods.

The easiest way to remember this is to tie it in with your meals: Eat at least three raw foods every day.

If you have a clinical illness such as diverticulitis, you may be able to handle raw juices. Get a juicer and prepare raw juice for each meal.

If you have a tendency toward food binges, it's best to avoid snacks completely. Eat only at meals. Chew each bite *thoroughly*. This helps make digestion more complete, as the food is broken down and mixed with saliva. Don't eat while watching television or a movie: devote full attention to your meal. If you have no problem of overweight or of overeating, legitimate snacks of real food are acceptable. Popcorn without butter or salt is not bad. Fresh vegetables or fruit is better.

A good rule of thumb is to chew each bite at least ten times. Many foods will require more chewing to make them perfectly digestible.

Start off with a bowl of homemade soup tonight for supper. In the morning you'll wake up hungry. Then begin refueling your body right—normally and naturally.

Supplements

If you lived in a mountain valley, raised your crops and all food organically, worked hard manually and had relatively no stress, you probably wouldn't need vitamin and mineral supplements. But we are living an abnormal life style in a highly urbanized civilization with a complex technology that keeps us under unrelenting stress. Our requirements must take these factors into consideration.

Air pollution, as well as smoking, increases our need for vitamin E and other nutrients. A stressful situation, in which you feel tight inside all day, may require 3,000 or even 4,000 units of vitamin C, plus larger amounts of pantothenic acid and other B vitamins, for the adrenal glands to function properly. Jet lag, or the stressful experience of crossing time belts in a brief period of time, makes additional demands on our bodies; the precise needs haven't even been learned yet.

Even if you ate well, you still would have to contend with today's poor agricultural methods, geared only to quantity production. The vitamin C in a commercially grown orange may be only one-tenth of what it was thirty years ago, because of our depleted soils. Trace minerals aren't being replaced in the soil; fertilizers only add nitrogen, potassium and phosphorus. The same is true of almost all other commercially grown agricultural products.

Diet surveys among patients have indicated that few people in this country are getting even the minimum daily requirements (MDR) of all the nutrients. That's just enough to avoid deficiency disease, the borderline beyond which you are risking a clinical disease, such as scurvy, beriberi or pellagra. Radiant health will require much more than this borderline of the MDR. A normal person who feels fantastically well may need ten times the vitamin intake of the MDR.

Dr. Weston A. Price, in his epic study of nutrition and health all over the world, found that the best primitive diets have supplied at least *four* times the minimum requirements set by modern medicine.

Everyone probably needs a general vitamin-mineral supplement, from natural sources if possible, plus a formula designed to assist our adrenal glands in coping with today's urban stress. The stress complex should contain at least 5 to 10 milligrams of vitamin B_2 and B_6, 10 to 20 milligrams of pantothenic acid, and 100 to 500 milligrams of vitamin C. If sufficient vitamin E is not present in the general vitamin, 50 to 200 milligrams of vitamin E is advisable.

Remember, however, that every one of us has specific needs. Getting a hormone analysis of the body would be ideal. Certainly everyone can benefit from a computerized dietary survey. In the appendix of this book there is a list of nutritional organizations to which you may write to obtain the names of physicians who may be able to help you with this.

Your Nutritional Check List (For Everyone)

If you concentrate on the ten steps in Table 7.1, you will be able to increase the resistance factors and lower the susceptibility factors in your diet. Refer to this outline frequently as a memory refresher and to review your periodic progress.

Table 7.1

The Program   *Points*

1. *No* refined carbohydrates (sugar, sweets, white starches). There is no place for these in human nutrition. They are major factors in the causation of most illnesses.
   No sugar   10
   No white starch   5
2. No smoking. This has long been known to be a disease 10 factor. You must want to stop. Carry short carrot or celery sticks or nuts as substitutes. The whole program of diet, exercise and stress reduction will help.
3. Alcohol is an unnecessary caloric. Drink none unless in 5 *good* health and at your proper weight, then only one drink per day.
4. Use unsaturated fats. Safflower oil is best, corn oil is fair. 2 Do not use saturated fats such as meat or bacon fat, or margarine unless it is unhydrogenated safflower margarine. *Do not fry foods.*
5. Eat raw fruits or vegetables at every meal. Start the meal 5 with them. Buy foods as fresh as possible, from farmers or markets, and organically grown, if possible.
6. Have a large breakfast, like a king; a medium lunch, like a 2 prince; a small supper, like a pauper. Have a protein snack at 10 A.M., 3 P.M. and 9 P.M. if you need it; toasted soybeans are excellent. The body needs nutrients when it is using them.
7. No coffee, tea, colas, chocolate or other caffeinated beverages. 5 Herbal teas, decaffeinated coffee or coffee substitutes are possible alternatives.
8. Nutritional supplements. Most people need the minimum 5 below. Some people may need more, even when they are eating properly. Calcium and magnesium supplements may be needed if little milk is consumed. If you take extra vitamin C, it should be spread out over the day and taken with food. It is helpful to have extra reserves of vitamin C

before special demands on the body, as before running
exercises or before business meetings. Minimum requirements are:

   (a) A general vitamin, preferably from natural sources.
   (b) A stress complex formula, including equal portions
       of vitamin B_2 and B_6 (5 to 10 milligrams), pan-
       tothenic acid (10 to 20 milligrams) and vitamin C
       (100 to 500 milligrams).
   (c) Vitamin E, 50 to 200 milligrams, twice a day.
9. Increase the quality of protein. Liver is best, followed by   5
   chicken, fish, beef, legumes, nuts and dairy products.
   Combine vegetable- and animal-source protein at meals to
   include all and to enhance each type. Eat no junk meats
   such as bologna, frankfurters or salami.
10. Drink hard spring water, if available. Use no iced drinks.   2

(For those who wish to measure their progress numerically, an
optional point system is provided. Strive toward a weekly or monthly
total of 30 points. Set an ultimate goal of a perfect score—56 points.)

Besides nutrition, a full health program must include exercise and
movement, environmental factors, and work on one's emotional stress
reduction.

Sources

Dr. Weston A. Price's studies are extracted from his *Nutrition and Physical
Degeneration: A Comparison of Primitive and Modern Diets and Their Effects*
(Santa Monica, Calif.: Price-Pottenger Foundation, 1945). It would be difficult
to overpraise this excellent work. Anyone who is less than totally convinced of
the vital link between poor nutrition and degenerative disease is advised to read
it.

A study of diet and IQ in childhood is noted in "Effect on Intellect of Child's
Malnutrition Held Reversible," *Family Practice News* 3, no. 17, p. 3.

Documentation of nutrition's role generally and especially during pregnancy
can be found in Roger J. Williams, *Nutrition Against Disease: Environmental
Prevention* (New York: Pitman Publishing, 1971). Another well-documented
work is E. Cheraskin, W. M. Ringsdorf, Jr., and J. W. Clark, *Diet and Disease*
(Emmaus, Pa.: Rodale Books, 1968). Other worthwhile sources include Adelle
Davis's *Let's Eat Right to Keep Fit* and *Let's Cook It Right* (New York:

Harcourt Brace Jovanovich, 1970 and 1962); Catharyn Elwood, *Feel Like a Million!* (New York: Devin-Adair, 1956); Joe D. Nichols and James Presley, *"Please, Doctor, Do Something!"* (Atlanta, Tex.: Natural Food Associates, 1972); George Watson, *Nutrition and Your Mind: The Psychochemical Response* (New York: Harper & Row, 1972); Melvin E. Page, *Degeneration-Regeneration* (St. Petersburg Beach, Fla.: Nutritional Development, 1949); Frances Moore Lappe, *Diet for a Small Planet* (New York: Friends of the Earth/Ballantine Books, 1971); Linda Clark, *Stay Young Longer: How to Add Years of Enjoyment to Your Life* (New York: Devin-Adair, 1961; paperback, Pyramid Books, 1968). Of particular value to dentists is Abraham E. Nizel, *Nutrition in Preventive Dentistry: Science and Practice* (Philadelphia: W. B. Saunders, 1972).

Primarily, our concept of the section on refined carbohydrates is that of T. L. Cleave, G. D. Campbell and N. S. Painter, *Diabetes, Coronary Thrombosis, and the Saccharine Disease*, 2d ed. (Bristol, England: John Wright & Sons, 1969). John Yudkin, *Sweet and Dangerous* (New York: Peter H. Wyden, 1972) further builds the case against sugar. A recent report of the Yemenite immigrants is in Gil Sedan, "Israeli Scientist Proves the Case Against Sugar," *Let's Live*, August 1973, pp. 104 ff.

Several books about specific vitamins that have proved helpful include Linus Pauling, *Vitamin C and the Common Cold* (San Francisco: W. H. Freeman, 1970); Irwin Stone, *The Healing Factor: "Vitamin C" Against Disease* (New York: Grosset & Dunlap, 1972); John M. Ellis and James Presley, *Vitamin B_6: The Doctor's Report* (New York: Harper & Row, 1973); and Wilfred E. Shute with Harald J. Taub, *Vitamin E for Ailing and Healthy Hearts* (New York: Pyramid House, 1970). The Stone book explores a large number of diseases in which vitamin C may play a healing role. The Ellis-Presley book establishes a number of relationships between vitamin B_6 deficiency and disease disorders, including rheumatism and arthritis, hormonal imbalances of pregnancy, menopause and the birth control pill, heart disease and diabetes. A detailed clinical report on vitamin C therapy is Frederick R. Klenner, "Observations on the Dose and Administration of Ascorbic Acid When Employed Beyond the Range of a Vitamin in Human Pathology," *Journal of Applied Nutrition* 23, no. 3-4 (Winter 1971), pp. 61-68.

Of the wealth of valuable information that has come from the hearings of the Select Committee on Nutrition and Human Needs, United States Senate, chaired by Senator George McGovern, we might single out *To Save the Children: Nutritional Intervention Through Supplemental Feeding* (Washington, D.C.: U.S. Government Printing Office, 1974) and Part 7 of the hearings, on school nutrition programs (1973). The effects of prenatal and pediatric malnutrition are explored in "Malnutrition and Brain Development," *Roche Image of Medicine & Research*, undated; "Finds Multivitamins Help to Prevent Birth Defects," *Family Practice News*, October 1, 1973, p. 8; and "Carbohydrate Metabolism, Congenital Defects Linked" *Family Practice News*, November 1, 1973, p. 25; Tom Brewer's column in *Medical Tribune*, October 24, 1973; Myron Winick, "Nutrition and the Growing Fetus," *Obstetrics & Gynecology* 1972, pp. 47-49.

A detailed technical examination of blood fats can be found in Robert I. Levy et al., "Dietary and Drug Treatment of Primary Hyperlipoproteinemia," *Annals of Internal Medicine* 77, no. 2 (August 1972), pp. 267-94.

Proof of alcohol's impairment of cardiac function is given in L. Gould et al., "Cardiac Effects of Two Cocktails in Normal Man," *Chest* 63 (June 1973), pp. 943-47.

Malnutrition in the U.S. is reported in "Highlights from the Ten-State Nutrition Survey," *Nutrition Today*, July/August 1972, pp. 4-11.

A careful scholarly and perfectly damning examination of smoking, Alton Ochsner, "On the Bitter Truth About Tobacco," *Executive Health* 9, no. 12 (1973), documents the aging effect of smoking, as well as its relationship with heart disease and stroke, cancers and sudden death. "There is no such thing as a safe cigarette," this distinguished doctor concluded. Dangers to nonsmokers who breathe others' fumes are noted in "Personal Air Pollution," *MD* (March 1972), p. 82.

The improvement of cardiovascular symptoms through health lectures on nutrition is reported in Cheraskin and Ringsdorf, "Reported Cardiovascular Symptoms and Signs Before and After Dietary Counsel," *Alabama Journal of Medical Sciences* 9, no. 2 (April 1972), pp. 174-79.

Finally, one of the most comprehensive, regular sources of readable nutritional information is *Prevention*, the monthly magazine published by Rodale Press, Emmaus, Pennsylvania. It is, incidentally, well-named.

8

Herbert A. Otto

Toward a Wholistic Psychotherapy, Counseling, and Social Work Treatment Program

OVER THE PAST ten to fifteen years, the helping professions have slowly but markedly moved in the direction of developing a "total" or wholistic treatment program. This movement reflects an on-going evolutionary process involving most, if not all programs. It seems that as we add to our knowledge of how people can best be helped to regain health and function better, treatment programs tend to be increasingly comprehensive, "total," and wholistic. The writer's interest in the concept of a wholistic treatment program grew from private practice and particularly his work with nonpatient groups as a part of the Human Potentialities Research Project, the University of Utah. Based on this work, initial concepts and an approach were developed and subsequently published (in 1967, new edition in 1974) in a chapter entitled "Toward a Holistic Treatment Program," which appeared in Harold Greenwald's volume *Active Psychotherapy*.[1]

Since this initial formulation of a wholistic treatment concept in 1965/66, two major schools of psychotherapy-behaviorism and transactional analysis have made their appearance. Both schools represent a movement in the direction of the wholistic treatment program because, to some extent, they use methods and approaches that focus on and utilize the patient's life space outside the individual treatment session. On the basis of conversations with colleagues over an extended period of time, it is clear that, year by year, more and more members of the helping professions are using what can be called wholistic treatment modalities. These are divided into two general types: (1) those that focus on both the psyche and the soma, and (2) those that actively utilize aspects of the patient's interpersonal and physical environment outside of individual or group sessions as a part of the treatment program.

In spite of some progress, however, the movement toward a wholistic treatment program is still in its infancy. The superannuated Freudian model (with its emphasis on the past history of the person seeking help and its narrow focus on one-to-one [therapist/patient] verbal interaction restricted to the office) still dominates the helping professions. The vast majority of treatment programs continue to perpetuate the mind/body dualism by concentrating on the psyche and largely ignoring the soma while making little, if any, active use of the total environment of the person seeking help.

Nevertheless, at this time in the history of the helping professions, there is a greater readiness and thrust to develop a wholistic treatment program than has ever existed before. Briefly stated, the *wholistic treatment program is based on the health model perspective of the person and includes group and individual sessions while working with both the psyche and soma and actively utilizing all possible resources and vectors in the life space of the person seeking help.*

Due to the space limitations of this contribution, only a broad outline of the wholistic treatment program will be presented.

The wholistic treatment program consists of psychotherapy, counseling, and social work; treatment is generic and has seven basic components. They are: (1) the health model perspective of the person seeking treatment, (2) combined group and individual treatment, (3) body work, (4) optimum utilization of the life space in the treatment process, (5) working with the belief system, (6) use of the self-concept and self-image and human sexuality as major factors in treatment, and (7) the new eclecticism and the expanded therapeutic team. Each of these components will be briefly explored.

1. The Health Model Perspective of the Person Seeking Treatment

The wholistically oriented therapist clearly recognizes that, whatever the nature of the total symptom configuration presented by the person seeking treatment, the symptom is not only a (symbolic) way of asking for help, but also represents the person's best way of coping as a part of a process of reaching toward health. From this perspective, the basic thrust of the human organism is seen to be toward health, with symptom formation as a part of this process. Symptom formation is not only an expression of need, but it often provides clues to the underlying need structure of the person. If these needs are not adequately recognized or met, the symptom-formation process gains in strength as needs become more pressing and dominant.

In this way, the symptom formation creates a disturbance within the personality process. Progressively, symptom formation (the signaling for help) pervades or permeates the process of personality and becomes the dominant force. Just as a person may cry so intensively and loudly for help that his voice finally fails, the symptom signal can cause "organismic overload." In short, the intensification of the symptom-signaling system can lead to organismic dysfunctioning, exhaustion, and even death. Yet *the main function of the symptom system is to initiate movement toward health by seeking to elicit help and support from the total environment.*

From the wholistic perspective the process called personality remains essentially a mystery that we are far from understanding fully. In this connection, the human potentialities hypothesis is relevant: namely, that the average healthy human being functions at less than ten percent of capacity while being endowed with vast latent powers, capacities, and resources. From this perspective, the human being is also perceived as an energy system operating at a low level of capacity and affecting and being affected by the surrounding interpersonal and physical energy systems that are a part of the environment. Again, from this perspective, the hypothesis of *interpersonal energy transmission* as a process of helping a person's energy system to achieve increased harmony emerges as a valuable paradigm useful in the understanding of both treatment and healing.

The health or nonmedical model of the person, if it becomes an integral part of the therapist's belief structure, can have a marked effect on the treatment process. The person is no longer seen as "pathological" or "dominated by pathogenesis," but as an individual who is (strongly) reaching for health and asking for help.

Behavioral scientists and communication specialists have concluded that verbal communication occupies twenty-five percent or less of the communication spectrum. The therapist who functions from a health model of the personality is more likely, on a nonverbal level, to convey a message of hope to a person seeking help than the therapist who sees the patient as essentially dominated by pathology. The impact of subverbal or subliminal cues in therapy and human communication has not as yet received sufficient recognition. Suffice it to say, the sophisticated therapist is keenly aware that unspoken attitudes and feelings can and do have a profound impact. In this connection, it is clear that Attitude Regeneration Workshops are needed to help therapists and others assimilate the health model of the personality on both an emotional *and* a cognitive level. This could do much to facilitate both the treatment process and healing and is a necessary first step for the practitioner interested in the wholistic treatment approach.

2. Combined Group and Individual Treatment

In the years ahead, the helping professions can be expected to increasingly recognize the value of combined group and individual treatment. *The emphasis will shift to group treatment* with individual sessions scheduled at key points and as needed throughout the treatment program. It is indeed unfortunate that historic precedent (particularly the Freudian treatment model referred to previously) has established the weight of a tradition that focuses on the one-to-one (patient/therapist) session as the primary mode of treatment.

If a group is conducted by a well-trained and sensitive facilitator, however, group treatment has a number of distinct advantages over the traditional treatment pattern:

A. Manipulation of the therapist by the person seeking help is minimized, if not eliminated.

It has long been recognized by sophisticated therapists that the stronger the symptom formation (and signal for help), the greater the possibility of manipulation of the therapist. Therapist manipulation is today a very widespread and neglected issue—in part because it is an issue that affects the self-esteem of the therapist and in part because the use of supervision and/or consultation by therapists is not sufficiently widespread.

In a group treatment program, manipulation of the therapist is minimized because, in a well-functioning group, some participants are aware of this manipulation and either react to it in some manner or communicate their awareness. In a group, manipulation usually involves *multiple manipulation*—which greatly enhances the possibility of failure.

B. The function of "authority attitudes," or hostility toward authority, is more easily worked with and minimized in group treatment.

As a result of multiple experiences with authority figures, a lifetime's accumulation of attitudes and feelings toward persons in authority is brought to treatment by persons seeking help. Unless adequately worked through, this complex of feelings usually hinders treatment. In a group setting, as authority attitudes impinge on the treatment process, they can be more easily identified, accepted, and worked through *using the support of participants* with similar problems.

C. In a well-functioning group, the resources of participants are brought to bear on the treatment process and the participants are exposed to the multiple health vectors present in each other.

From the perspective of wholistic group treatment, *it is one of the primary functions of the therapist to recognize and bring to bear on the treatment process the participants' strengths, resources, and capacities.* In effect, group members both contribute to the creation of and participate in the therapeutic process. It would not be amiss to say that in a well-functioning group, participants become therapists to each other.

Finally, regardless of the emotional status of the person seeking help, areas and elements of healthy functioning are usually present. These can play a vital and often supportive role in treatment as participants interact with and are exposed to such health vectors.

A semantic differential is another factor that can prevent optimum interaction between therapist and participant. It has been my repeated observation that peer-to-peer communication is often vastly more effective in the course of the therapeutic process than therapist-to-participant communication. (This also applies to the participants' defensive maneuverings, which are often very effectively handled by peer group members.) Again, the therapist's skill to a large extent is reflected by his/her ability to nurture and sustain a climate where such therapeutic interventions or interactions between peers are maximized. In effect, participants in group treatment have a great deal to give to each other and, it should be added, to the therapist.

D. Treatment modalities that support the ego and enhance self-esteem and self-image are more effective in group settings.

Based on the writer's work with more than 800 groups over a sixteen-year period, focusing particularly on the use of ego-supportive group methods,[2] a number of observations and conclusions emerge. It is clear that the relationship matrix of the group is experienced as deeply nourishing and supportive, particularly in those groups where the creation of a deeply caring climate is seen as an important goal or objective by the facilitator or therapist. The experience of caring and being cared for (being accepted, understood, supported, and loved) differs *qualitatively* in a group as contrasted with one-to-one treatment. For optimum personality growth and progress in therapy, *the person seeking help needs to experience the quality of caring in both settings*. Over a decade of use of such methods as Strengths Acknowledgement,[3] the Your Strength Method,[4] the Primal Sensory Experience,[5] has repeatedly demonstrated the effectiveness of ego-supportive group modalities in self-esteem and self-image enhancement.

E. Group treatment offers significant economies to both participants and facilitator or therapist.

It is crystal clear that, if a therapist utilized most of his/her available treatment time to facilitate groups, a vastly increased number of persons seeking help will have an opportunity to work on their problem within a therapeutic setting. There are obvious economic advantages to both the persons seeking help and the therapist. Even more important, it is my impression (and a surprising number of colleagues concur) that combined group and individual treatment (with the emphasis on the former) in many instances appears to bring earlier therapeutic results.

If we consider the overall nature of the "mental health problem" i.e., the persons in need of treatment in the United States and other countries, it is evident that there is a pressing shortage of both skilled therapists and therapeutic time. One of the most effective ways to alleviate the shortage of treatment time is through a massive investment in the training of people-helpers to prepare them for work with groups. Federal and state incentives for such training need to be provided and the selection and training of paraprofessionals as group facilitators encouraged.

3. The Use of Body Work as an Integral Part of Treatment

An important aspect of the wholistic treatment program is the emphasis on treatment of the psyche and soma *simultaneously*. The sophisticated helping person, whatever his or her profession, today is aware that the psyche and soma are interrelated and that working with both aspects of the personality fosters optimum healing. There is also increasing recognition that the emotional status of the patient is usually reflected or expressed in body functioning and/or somatic symptoms. This recognition is based on the work of the early pioneers in psychosomatic medicine, such as Franz Alexander[6] and Flanders Dunbar,[7] in the late forties and early fifties. Since then, a considerable body of research has borne out these earlier findings. Today it is also evident that ego structure, self-image, and level of self-esteem are closely interrelated with muscle sheath, structural and total body functioning, and the body image.

A growing number of members of the helping professions recognize the need to work with both psyche and soma simultaneously. However, they have difficulty overcoming the early professional training that prohibits or restricts touch between patient and therapist. Although today many members of the helping professions use "supportive touching" during therapy, there has been a general reluctance to take the next step—i.e., the utilization of body work in treatment.

Training in body-work systems has become increasingly available over the years.[8] Nevertheless, as many of the writer's colleagues have pointed out, they do not have the time to take this (at times lengthy) training. One way out of this dilemma is to work out a referral arrangement with a qualified body-work systems practitioner. This makes simultaneous treatment of the psyche and soma possible. In most urban settings, a number of qualified body-work persons can be found; they are often willing to give demonstration of their work at professional meetings and similar gatherings.

Among the many body-work systems now available are those that focus primarily on muscle sheath and structural integration, such as bioenergetics;[9] Rolfing;[10] the Feldenkrais method;[11] and various forms of massage.[12] Pesso's psychomotor therapy is in a category by itself.[13] Finally, various Oriental body-work systems, such as acupressure and Shiatsu,[14] are also receiving attention. Autogenic Training,[15] which has been popular in Europe over the past two decades, is increasingly used in this country.

Finally, physical exercise programs including jogging, running, swimming and other sports can be effectively used as components of the wholistic treatment program.

An often neglected body-work modality is massage. In this connection, it is of interest that, while working with nonpatient couple groups in the early seventies, the writer found that "touch starvation" was a fairly widespread phenomenon.[16] Many couples discovered, much to their amazement, that, although their sex life was satisfactory, their need for skin contact (through stroking or massage) had not been met for prolonged periods. Based on this work and work with older persons, there was evidence that massage, given by a caring person, can have a marked positive effect on the self-image and the body image. Massage is suitable both for fostering relaxation and for purposes of toning and energizing and merits increased use by members of the helping professions.

4. Optimum Utilization of the Life Space in Treatment

The traditional model of therapy referred to previously, with its emphasis on the one-to-one treatment session in the office, has led to a tragic neglect of the life space of the person seeking help. This life space consists of the time between office sessions—i.e., the total interpersonal and physical environment. In the vast majority of instances, aspects of this life space can be used to support and foster therapeutic aims and goals. Among the helping professions, social work is perhaps most concerned about the therapeutic utilization of the life space. Unfortunately the profession of social work has not carried this concept far enough, and the current trend among social workers entering private practice is to revert to the traditional therapeutic model.

The utilization of life space as an integral part of the wholistic treatment program involves three dimensions: (1) the Action Program concept, (2) utilization of the interpersonal environment, and (3) utilization of the physical environment. The Action Program concept was developed as a part of the work of the Human Potentialities Research project, the University of Utah, before the advent of behavioral therapy and was first published in 1962.[17]

An Action Program

An Action Program involves a task (or action) decided upon *jointly* by the person seeking help and the therapist, which will strengthen the person, which is consonant with the aims and goals of treatment, and which (preferably) will be completed in the time between sessions. The nature of the Action Program of course varies with the individual's needs, the timing and progress of therapy, and many other factors. The use of Action Programs allows a dynamic extension of therapy into the life space of the person.

The Therapeutic Utilization of the Interpersonal Environment

The therapeutic utilization of the interpersonal environment of the person seeking help begins with his/her analysis of the total matrix of relationships, including relatives, friends, and acquaintances. Such an analysis usually proves to be highly perceptive and accurate. (Use of the Relationship Field Chart is helpful in this connection.[18]) Key questions to be explored are, Which of these relationships are strengthening and are supportive? and conversely, Which relationships undermine self-esteem or the self-image or are pathogenic? The aim here is, as a part of treatment, to encourage association with and to involve selected individuals in the relationship matrix who are identified as nourishing and supportive. Many therapists have discovered to their surprise that, for example, a simple telephone call to certain family members or other persons in the relationship matrix can mobilize considerable support or defuse destructive interaction.

The Physical Environment

The physical environment of the person seeking help can also be utilized to foster therapeutic aims and goals. The person asking for help can be encouraged to rearrange the furniture of one room in such a way as to foster more positive attitudes and feelings about the room. In this connection, it can be pointed out that this positive change in the physical environment will act as a reminder that he or she is engaged in a treatment program designed to bring personal growth and positive change. This utilizes positive reinforcement and is especially effective at certain points in the treatment program.

Also valuable is an analysis of the aesthetic dimensions of the living environment of the person seeking help. Key questions here are, What keepsakes, mementos, art, photographs and other objects trigger negative associations and feelings? and conversely, How can more positive aesthetic or symbolic objects be introduced into the living environment? This type of restructuring (again utilizing positive reinforcement) is especially effective in certain instances. It is not sufficiently recognized that objects in one's living environment trigger strong associations, memories, affective responses and attitudes in some people. The immediate environment thus continues to affect the emotional status. As one person put it, "When I got rid of that lamp I almost threw at my husband and made some other changes, it gave me a completely different feeling when I stepped in that room."

Finally, *diet* and *fasting* need to be included as an integral part of treatment programs. They are of special value in relation to the body-image and self-image and can be utilized in an ego supportive manner as well as contributing to raising the general level of health.

5. Working with the Belief System

It is an integral part of the wholistic treatment program to assess as well as to work with specific components of the *belief system* of the person seeking help. These components of the belief system include: (1) determining the person's understanding of the nature of the helping process (2) assessment of the lifestyle, including life goals (3) exploration of the meaning of existence to the person—including the spiritual resources, or religious belief system, as well as the area of values, (4) work in the area of facing death and dying.

Working with the belief system begins with an *assessment of the person's understanding of the helping process*. The objectives are (1) to determine the nature of the person's understanding of the helping process (2) to deepen and expand the person's awareness and understanding of the helping process (3) to demythologize the treatment process in order to help the person assume optimal responsibility for his or her healing. (Therapy is not something the therapist does to the patient.)

Some of the following questions are also explored: Is the person open to the possibility that the human energy system and the transfer of energy can play a role in healing? Is the person open to the possibility that knowledge or insights into his or her condition may be obtained through parapsychological or extrasensory means? If the answers to these questions are in the affirmative, there exists the possibility of utilizing the resources of a psychic healer as a part of the treatment program. It is recognized that, in most professional settings today, the readiness to utilize such a resource, even if available, does not exist. However, from the perspective of wholistic treatment, utilization of such a resource *is both desirable and necessary because the person seeking help can be expected to benefit.*

Lifestyle assessment includes past and current lifestyle (with emphasis on the latter) as well as the wished for or ideal lifestyle and life goals. *Exploration of the meaning of existence* includes encouraging the person to ask himself or herself such primal questions as What is the meaning of my existence? What am I here (in this world) for? *Exploration of the person's spiritual resources* or the nature of the religious belief system is also undertaken. Emphasis here is on determining the quality of faith, i.e., to obtain an understanding of the emotional commitment in this area. For example, in some persons religious beliefs are shallow and superficial and play a very minor role in life, while for others religious faith and values are on the level of a deep emotional commitment or spiritual resource. An assessment of the nature of the *value system* is also undertaken to determine major value clusters. For example, the person seeking help can be encouraged to become more aware of the nature of his or her value system by exploring the following key question: What are my basic values? (Values are defined as, what you really know is of importance and worth in the course of your life.) Also basic are the questions To what extent is value structure related to the lifestyle and life goals? and How can values and behavior or functioning be brought into closer consonance? Again, it is recognized that the pressure of the large number of persons seeking therapeutic help prevents many therapists from paying explicit attention to this area. If the aim of treatment is to bring greater wholeness to the person, work in the area of value cannot be avoided.

Finally, *facing death and dying* includes an exploration of fears and concerns related to this area. It has been the writer's observation while working with nonpatient populations that a considerable amount of fear, concern, and anxiety accumulates in relation to this area in the course of a lifetime. Much psychic energy is often expended in keeping this area "walled off" or contained. The writer has been using the Death in Life Experience for over a decade to help people get in touch with and begin to work through some of these feelings.[19] This method is particularly effective when used in groups. There have been consistent reports of a lessening of fear and an increase in self-understanding and serenity, often accompanied by a reassessment of values and lifestyles. At some time subsequently, many participants also reported an increased enjoyment of life which lasts for some time.

It should be clear that the process of assessment of a particular component of the belief system is often inseparable from working with the component. The overriding aim throughout this process is to bring greater wholeness to the person and to determine how the belief system, and components of the belief system viewed as a resource, can be brought to bear on the aims and goals of treatment.

6. The Self-Concept, the Self-Image, and Human Sexuality as Major Factors in Treatment

Members of the helping professions are generally agreed that, regardless of the nature of the treatment process, the self-image and self-concept will be affected and hopefully enhanced. However, in many schools of therapy and treatment programs, the focus on the self-concept and self-image is implicit—i.e., changes in this area are seen as an outcome or by-product of the total treatment process. In contrast, the wholistic treatment program differs fundamentally in a number of respects: (1) *the focus on the self-image and self-concept is explicit*—i.e., throughout treatment, a clear focus is maintained on the enhancement of the self-concept and self-image. At the same time, the person seeking help is also encouraged to explore the parameters of his or her self-image and self-concept, using such modalities as the Self-Image Projection Experience.[20] In addition, he or she becomes

involved in Action Programs designed to strengthen the self-concept.
(2) As a part of the explicit focus on the self-concept and self-image, *the
person seeking help is acquainted with the human potentialities
hypothesis*, namely, that people function at considerably less than ten
percent of their capacity. With its emphasis on the fact that every
person has unrealized powers, abilities, and capacities that can be
developed, the human potentialities hypothesis extends a message of
hope and is generally experienced as ego-supportive. Specific ego-
supportive treatment methods are used throughout the wholistic
treatment program, but especially after the midpoint in treatment.
Such ego-supportive (group) treatment modalities may include the
Strength Acknowledgement,[21] the Shapiro Mirror Experience,[22] and
others.

The perspective of many members of the helping professions in
relation to the area of human sexuality is similar to the one held toward
the role of the self-image and self-concept in treatment. As one
therapist put it, "Hopefully, as a result of treatment, some working
through in the area of sexuality will take place." It is clear, however,
that the great majority of treatment programs, whether conducted by
psychotherapists, counselors or social workers, do not explicitly focus
on the area of sexuality and do not appear to have a marked affect on
the sexual attitudes, sexual functioning, and sexual self-image of the
person seeking help. In contemporary society, with its sex-role stereotypes, the impact of the woman's movement, sex-role change, and the
constant use of sexual stimuli (including subliminal stimuli) by the
advertising media, the need for work in the area of human sexuality
has never been more pressing. Sexologists estimate that approximately
fifty percent of American women are preorgasmic and that three out of
five marriages need help with some type of sexual problem. In the
writer's work as sexologist, particularly with nonpatient populations, it
has become very clear that the average well-functioning person
functions at a small fraction of his or her sexual potential. For example, both the quality and quantity of the sexual experience and the
orgasm can be vastly increased.

Wholistic treatment, therefore, includes explicit attention to the
area of human sexuality and sexual functioning, regardless of the type
of presenting problem. In short, *the wholistic treatment program always includes work in the area of human sexuality*, particularly relating
to sexual attitudes, sexual functioning, and the sexual self-image. In

this connection particular attention is paid to attitudes about elimina-tion and body secretions,[23] attitudes about nudity and masturbation,[24] the area of sex traumas,[25] and sexual communication.[26]

7. The New Eclecticism and the Expanded Therapeutic Team

Over the past three decades, a number of new schools of psy-chotherapy have emerged to enrich and make their contribution to the field. There are some indications that adherents to these new schools appear somewhat less insistent in the proclamation of their conversion and the new orthodoxy. A diminishing of the internecine warfare of the past among followers of different therapeutic schools also appears to be evident. A marked trend toward a *new eclecticism* can be ob-served, with a growing number of therapists using theoretical frameworks and treatment modalities drawn from varied sources.

The hallmark of the new eclecticism is the helping person's acquain-tance with a considerable range of theory and treatment modalities drawn from various schools, coupled with a refreshing willingness to try out and use diverse treatment methods based on the individual needs of the person seeking help. In short, more therapists appear to recognize the principle that different persons may need different treatment modalities to make maximum progress in therapy. Today there is also increasing recognition that, as in the field of medicine, the skills and healing potential of the helping person can be enhanced through new discoveries in the field. To insure optimum progress, all licensing programs for the helping professions need to take this fact into consideration and provide for periodic in-service training as a part of an on-going recertification program.

In the course of the past three decades, some remarkable changes have also taken place in the composition of the therapeutic team. At first, the profession of psychiatry (including the long-dominant con-tingent of analysts and analytically trained psychiatrists) considered itself the entire team. Next, and after much in-fighting, psychologists and social workers were admitted to the therapeutic team. With their admission appeared a pecking and status order. Members of these professions were seen to be in need of supervision by the psychiatrist, who remained the unquestioned and unquestionable authoritative head of the therapeutic team.

With the passage of years, psychologists and social workers became coequal team members and, in some instances, team directors. Some time later, paraprofessionals were at first cautiously and then increasingly being used in mental health clinics, while ward attendants and nurses began to conduct groups in state institutions. Slowly there emerged an awareness that *some people are natural therapists or healers* who, with some additional training, could become valued members of the therapeutic team.

Today we are at a point where the concept of the natural therapist or healer needs to be expanded to include the psychic healer. Although such healers are in short supply, they do exist and can make a marked contribution to the therapeutic program. Psychic healers have been used by members of the helping professions both for purposes of diagnosis and to facilitate healing, i.e., as an integral part of therapy. At this point, a pilot research program to assess the nature and parameters of the contribution that could be made by the psychic healer to the therapeutic team would be of considerable value. Finally, unless a member of the helping professions on the team has body-work training, a body-work practitioner needs to be added to, and considered a member of, the therapeutic team that is committed to the goals of wholistic treatment.

Conclusion

The broad parameters of a wholistic treatment program applicable to the helping professions have been outlined. Based on an extrapolation of existing trends in people-helping programs, it is evident that the wholistic treatment model will be the program of choice in the foreseeable future. It is hoped that this presentation will lead to further implementation and more extensive exploration of the wholistic treatment program concept.

Notes

1. Harold Greenwald, ed., *Active Psychotherapy*, 2nd ed. Jason Aaronson (New York: Atherton, 1974).
2. Herbert A. Otto, *Group Methods to Actualize Human Potential: A Handbook* (Beverly Hills, Calif.: The Holistic Press, 1975).
3. Ibid., pp. 55–64.
4. Ibid., pp. 264–67.

5. Ibid., pp. 345–48.

6. Franz Alexander, *Psychosomatic Medicine: Its Principles and Applications* (New York: W. W. Norton, 1950).

7. Flanders Dunbar, *Mind and Body: Psychosomatic Medicine* (New York: Random House, 1955).

8. Two week training programs in Body Work Systems are offered annually as a part of the Summer Training Institute of the National Center for the Exploration of Human Potential, San Diego, Calif.

9. Alexander Lowen, *The Betrayal of the Body* (New York: Macmillan, Collier Books, 1967).

10. A technique of working with the muscle sheath of the body developed by Dr. Ida Rolf. Dr. Rolf trained several hundred practitioners in her methods.

11. Moshe Feldenkrais, *Awareness Through Movement* (New York: Harper and Row, 1972).

12. Gertrude Beard and Elizabeth C. Wood, *Massage* (Philadelphia: W. B. Saunders, 1968).

13. Albert Pesso, *Movement in Psychotherapy* (New York: New York University Press, 1969).

14. Tokujiro Namikoshi, *Shiatsu* (San Francisco: Japan Publications, 1974).

15. J. H. Schultz, *Das Autogene Training* (Stuttgart: Geo. Thieme Verlag, 1964).

16. Herbert A. Otto and Roberta Otto, *Total Sex* (New York: New American Library, Signet, 1973): 82–113.

17. ——, "The Personal and Family Resource Development Programs—A Preliminary Report," *International Journal of Social Psychiatry*, 8, No. 3 (Summer 1962): 185–95.

18. Obtainable from the Holistic Press, 8909 Olympic Blvd., Beverly Hills, CA 90211.

19. Herbert A. Otto, op. cit., pp. 108–16.

20. Ibid., pp. 127–31.

21. Ibid., pp. 55–64.

22. Ibid., pp. 90–93.

23. Herbert A. Otto and Roberta Otto, op. cit., pp. 197–225.

24. Ibid., pp. 126–52, 179–94.

25. Ibid., pp. 40–50.

26. Ibid., pp. 162–75.

9

Herbert A. Otto and James W. Knight

Wholistic Healing and Aging

SINCE THE TURN of the century, better health and increasing numbers have brought about shifts in the age distribution of the U.S. population. Whereas in 1900 only 3.1 million of the total population was over sixty-five years of age, today 21.8 million people, or approximately ten percent of the population, falls into this age classification. Furthermore, while the population has doubled during this century, the number of people over the age of sixty-five has multiplied five times. It is anticipated that in the year 2000 over fifteen percent of the population will be sixty-five or older.

Although the aging constitute a minority and suffer the consequent discrimination and neglect, the larger society must understand that everyone is destined to join this particular minority. Any improvement in the life of the aging should be seen as a valuable investment in the future. We believe that wholistic healing has particular applications to aging because it is directed at improving the overall quality of life, not just the quality of personal health.

The wholistic principles and concepts presented in Chapter I can be adapted to apply to the individuals in that one tenth of our society that is getting old. They are here so restated. Perhaps with practice and in time, the majority of these people will be, and will be seen as, "growing" old.

The Principles and Concepts of Wholistic Healing

Wholistic healing is not simply a form of health-care delivery. In fact, more than attempting to deliver externals, the wholistic approach seeks to preserve or restore health by drawing on the resources inherent in every human being. The applications of wholistic healing to the condition defined as "aging" rest on eight basic concepts.

1. Every human being has untapped potentials, resources, and powers. Recognition and development of these capabilities should continue throughout life.
2. Self-awareness and self-understanding play an important role in the healing process and in maintaining health and vitality.
3. Reliance on the capacities and resources of the individual is a key factor in mobilizing the healing processes and in maintaining health.
4. Interpersonal relationships and physical environment should have a life-supportive and life-enhancing function.
5. Self-regulatory processes and therapies need to be implemented before any illness reaches the point at which chemotherapy or surgical intervention is required.
6. The dynamic therapeutic forces inherent in group interaction and work are effective in developing and sustaining the life-affirmative attitudes and perspectives that are associated with health and longevity.
7. A lifestyle that permits the harmonious integration of goals, aspirations, and values with day-to-day living is essential both to healing and to maintaining good health.
8. Spiritual resources and belief structures continue to play a supportive role in the life of the aging person.

From these concepts, a wide variety of wholistic programs for the aging can be created. Preretirement plans, programs for residents of nursing homes and of retirement homes and communities can be established on the basis of these principles. Before we go into the need for such programs and possible ways of implementing them, it may be helpful to consider the principles of wholistic healing in light of the attitudes of aging individuals and the society in which they have lived to grow old.

Personality Growth and Self-Actualization

The human potentialities hypothesis, which states that every human being is functioning at less than ten percent of potential, becomes increasingly important with advancing age. Modern behavioral science research has revealed that personality growth and the actualizing of individual potential can be a life-long adventure. Many persons in their sixties, seventies, or eighties have discovered and developed interests, talents and capacities; some have enrolled in schools and completed degree programs. Clearly, *the advancing years offer an unprecedented opportunity for self-realization and personal growth*. It is important to recognize that awareness of the human potentialities hypothesis and *the process of being involved in actualizing personal potential is deeply vitalizing, energizing and life-affirmative*. The process of self-actualization adds interest, satisfaction, and joy to life and is essentially life-prolonging.

Recognition of the human potentialities hypothesis by the aging person is also of value because the hypothesis furnishes *hope*, builds self-esteem, and enhances the self-image. In this connection it must be recognized that "agism," just as sexism, is a widespread and pervasive form of discrimination in Western cultures. The aging person is subjected to many subtle slights and "put-downs" in the youth-oriented societies. This causes sustained damage to the sense of self-worth and the ego-structure of many people. Such damage often goes unnoticed.

Preretirement Preparation

Wholistic healing recognizes that the abrupt transition from vocational productivity to retirement often results in stress, mobilizes fears and anxieties and, in all too many instances, is experienced as traumatic and as a major life crisis. In a society where gainful employment and productivity are valued highly, identification of the person with his or her work is all too prevalent. For example, most people, when asked, "Who are you?" at a social gathering, respond with their vocational identification—"I'm an engineer." Withdrawal from work and relative inactivity often have a negative effect on self-esteem and the sense of self-worth, which may lead to damage of the ego structure.

The onset of illness is sometimes directly traceable to this sequence of events.

One effective way to forestall the traumatic effects of retirement is through comprehensive preparation for retirement.

1. It provides for a gradual withdrawal from work over an extended period, beginning approximately one year prior to the date of retirement.
2. It helps the prospective retiree and his or her immediate family cope with the emotional and other factors involved in the process, and focuses on the enhancement of self-esteem and self-worth.
3. It assists the prospective retiree to select the appropriate retirement lifestyle. [1]

An important and integral part of this program is *retirement practice*. While still vocationally active, the prospective retiree uses long weekends and more extended periods to live in the lifestyle chosen for retirement. These periods can be used, not only to try out different lifestyles in order to select the one best suited to the needs and circumstances of the retiree, but also to evaluate different locales or environments and their social and human resources.

Recently AIM—Action for Independent Maturity—has created a comprehensive program on retirement planning. A division of the American Association of Retired Persons, AIM's seminar is available to employers and organizations to help those approaching retirement more effectively help themselves. [2]

A Program of Wholistic Health for the Advancing Years

Basic to the philosophy of a framework for wholistic health in advancing years is the following from a bicentennial editorial in the *Western Journal of Medicine* by Malcolm S. M. Watts:

> There is growing talk of something called quality of life, and of making this something available to every person. . . . there are unmistakable signs that a new humanism has appeared on the American scene, a new and apparently genuine concern with one's fellowman, particularly with those who have been deprived or repressed for one reason or another. . . . There is a new awareness and deep concern

with the long-range bioecological viability of the environment—local, national and worldwide. In another dimension a new social, economic and political interdependence among people is becoming clearly evident everywhere modern technology has been applied to any significant degree. . . . This interdependence will need to become a framework within which cooperation will gradually gain ascendancy over competition as the dominant mode of human interaction. . . .

One wonders what might be the role of medicine. Obviously quality of life is something physicians seek for their patients. But beyond this, what other profession is any closer to the concept and meaning of quality of life—which is so intimately linked to the physical, mental and . . . social well-being of every person? It would seem that medicine could and perhaps should prepare itself for a role of leadership, a role of physician to a society groping for a new purpose in what is already becoming a new era for mankind in world history.[3]

An evolving and ever-expanding program of wholistic health for people of advancing age will necessarily reflect a synthesis of society's continually changing attitudes toward one of its greatest natural resources—its older citizens. The root concepts of the wholistic philosophy should be considered, not only as they relate to the individual members of society, but also as they represent integral facets of the society at large, in all its dimensions and complex interactions.

Areas of a program for wholistic health that will be discussed in this section include: (1) identification and activation of existing and latent talents and potentials; (2) psychological attitudes and self-help; (3) spiritual and interpersonal relationships; (4) lifestyle and household management; (5) economic and legal counseling; (6) education, recreation, and new experiences; (7) creativity and art mobilization; (8) physical awareness and activity; (9) nutritional counseling and education; (10) preventive medicine and home safety; (11) terminal illness and death preparation; and (12) research on aging. We acknowledge, of course, that, in the limitations of this chapter, an overview and brief description are all that is possible; resources listed at the end of the chapter provide specific and in-depth information for continuing action.

Identification and Activation of Talents

Activation of latent interests and talents is an important aspect of a program for wholistic health in the advancing years. A program to help individuals find areas of interest, identify desires, and recognize talents is greatly needed and certainly could be developed. Older persons whose life work and expertise is in these areas can continue to be involved by teaching others to develop their latent talents and interests. This use of manpower is an extremely important function of such a program. Also, challenging aging individuals to serve in areas of community need, even without pay, will both fulfill the need and give the workers a sense of self-respect and self-worth. Existing programs include volunteer service in hospitals, recreational areas, blood banks, churches, and community projects.

Psychological Attitudes and Self-Help

In the development of programs for the aging, counseling toward self-help is important in evaluating factors that may inhibit the individual's life process. Such factors are (1) loss of goal or sense of purpose for living; (2) loss, or fear of loss, of a loved one; (3) feelings of unworthiness; (4) fear of death; and (5) guilt associated with "the rewards of heaven or the punishments of hell." These kinds of feelings often produce negative attitudes toward life in general and toward family, friends, community, and world.

The major pitfall to be avoided in the aging process is depression, which is often associated with feelings of self-pity, a loss of self-worth, and the absence of a life goal. Many elderly persons suffer mental health crises each year. The crisis usually is a culmination of the long-term experiencing of negative attitudes. To aid in such situations, crisis intervention teams can operate on a community-wide basis to aid individuals referred by police, apartment managers, or neighbors and relatives. One such program operating in King County, Washington, is based on the outreach concept. The intervention team is composed of a physician trained in internal medicine and psychiatry, a registered nurse, and a social worker. Those involved in the establishment and maintenance of the program believe that its success rests on its wholistic approach and its professional orientation. Older people trust the medical and health professions, and when a doctor, nurse, and social worker come directly to the individual's home when there is need, the problem is being met head-on. More passive programs, such as health clinics for the mentally or emotionally disturbed, are not utilized widely by people in a potential crisis situation.[4]

Another helpful approach to the problems of aging is based on the concept of reality orientation. A program introduced by a team headed by Dr. James C. Folsom at the Veterans Administration Hospital in Topeka, Kansas, demonstrates the effectiveness of reality-oriented care in a geriatric setting. The implementation of reality orientation has been credited with reversing psychologically induced senility in individuals without documented physiologically caused dementia.[5]

Spiritual and Interpersonal Relationships

Spiritual help and counseling must be readily available to the aging members of society; pastoral counseling programs need to be publicized widely throughout the community. The support provided through the ministry and the availability of opportunities for community worship are of great importance to people in the advanced years. Such support is often found in group workshops in which willingness to share and openness are emphasized. In such group situations, all participants are offered opportunities for spiritual fulfillment. Sharing such an experience also provides a strong foundation for individual interpersonal relationships.

Companionship is very important to the aging, who often find themselves alone, either through the loss of a life partner or through the fear of such loss. Many others are emotionally and socially trapped in marriages that no longer live. Often, one or another of the partners in such a marriage has given in to self-pity, and the relationship itself is slowly dying. In such instances, counseling is often helpful in restoring a sense of growth in companionship or in encouraging changes in direction for individuals who are no longer fulfilled in their partnership.

Lifestyle and Household Management

Counseling in lifestyle management is particularly useful to retirees who seek to maintain an independent way of life. In cooperation with programs to educate the aging to the possibilities of growing old with dignity, social services need to be developed and expanded to allow the elderly to maintain the lifestyle they have chosen. Such community services are of great significance to people who can no longer carry out all the responsibilities of running a household. Among the most valuable of these programs are such homemaker services as Meals on Wheels, Friendly Visitors, and Foster Homes for Grandparents. All these systems are designed to provide assistance to the elderly in preserving their identity and independent lifestyle.

Without assistance, many people are forced to abandon the lifestyle they prefer to the institutionalized environment of the nursing or retirement home. It is important to recognize that people who *choose* an institutional way of life are generally well adjusted within a matter of months. On the other hand, those who are forced to enter such institutions are very unlikely to adjust well, and they go rapidly into withdrawal from the "unchosen" society in which they find themselves. Before such a move becomes a necessity, the person involved should learn about the institutional alternatives in the region in which he or she wishes to live. Both the physician and family members can offer information and guidance preparatory to such a move. A current report provides a "shoppers' guide" to the selection of an appropriate nursing home environment.[6,7] It is most important to include the individual in the planning of the move and the selection of an establishment with the appropriate environment and policies for that person's specific needs.

Maas and Kuypers, on completion of an extensive longitudinal study, insist that basic policy must provide different alternatives for different types of aging people.[8] It is an essential responsibility of the larger society to provide social resources that leave alternatives open to the aging.

A wholistic technique useful for the aging is the Intensive Journal, developed by Dr. Ira Progoff. Especially valuable for persons who are moving through a time of transition where readjustments or difficult decisions must be made, the journal is a process that enables one to restructure life goals in one's own tempo and in one's own terms.[9]

Economic and Legal Counseling

The economy is a factor that plays a tremendous role in the later years of an individual's life. Many people of retirement age have not saved and provided for the remaining years of their lives. Many others have planned carefully, only to find that inflation has reduced their buying power so much that they cannot afford even the barest necessities.

For those in our society who have not been able to provide economic security for themselves, government offers inadequate Social

Security programs. The false hope offered by these federal plans serves only to dehumanize the aging process. Privately operated homes are very expensive and are therefore beyond the reach of those who must rely solely on Social Security benefits. Those unfortunate people with limited financial resources who have been unable to maintain their health must therefore turn to state and county programs, which also are inadequate and incapable of humanely meeting the needs of the disabled and impoverished aging population.

A positive solution to the financial ills that beset many individuals in later years is a program of economic cooperation. The success of such programs should be examined, and those systems that have proven effective could then serve as models for governmental policies in economic cooperation, not only for the provision of goods, but also for such essential services as health care, counseling, transportation, and recreation.

Education and counseling in legal matters, often a confusing subject, could be provided through community resources. Too often services and economic benefits provided by local and federal programs are unused by the aging because they lack information or because no one takes the time to follow through. In Washington, D.C., a pilot project of the American Association of Retired Persons utilizes qualified volunteers as paralegals to assist with questions and counseling in areas of government benefits, estate matters, and simple contractual agreements.[10] On-going courses, providing ample opportunity for individual questions and answers, could also be presented by local community colleges or organizations.

Education, Recreation and New Experiences

U.S. Secretary of Commerce Juanita Kreps stated, "Older people find that the opportunities open to them for experiences . . . are very limited. These options are reduced by reason of the older person's limited income, his health problems, his own lack of interest, his habitual patterns of living. . . ."[11] In addition to challenges to intellectual growth through education, the aging must be offered recreational and cultural alternatives and opportunities for new experiences. Such opportunity does not simply mean that diversions and entertainment be available within the community, but that special efforts be made that implicitly encourage the elderly to participate.

Decreased mobility is a problem for many aging people. Special buses can provide transportation for the elderly to scheduled events throughout the community or region. In addition, social service agencies, public and private, can provide group plans and rates for day trips or brief vacations to points of general interest in the surrounding area. The British government has subsidized such programs for pensioners for many years. Special rates for railroad and coach tours are available to aging persons who wish to expand their horizons, and the very existence of the opportunity is incentive to less mobile individuals to take trips and enjoy recreational events that otherwise they might miss.

Creativity and Art Mobilization

The aging population is a singular group that could derive much benefit from creativity and art mobilization. These persons have a wealth of experience and knowledge. At this time in life, many of the aging persons are freed from their mundane commitments and are able to tap into their creative and artistic abilities. Some have expanded creative hobbies into businesses and second careers, providing an economic base for themselves and jobs for other aging persons.

When the individual is provided the opportunity to be relaxed and unattached, this can stimulate the flow of creativity expressing itself, not only in such art forms as music, poetry, painting, crafts, and ceramics, but at every level of being. Such creativity results in a sense of self-worth and acceptance, as well as a more positive and expanding sense of reality.[12] These personal programs of creativity can be expanded into programs for the collective, and designed in such a way to enrich the lives of those who otherwise would remain unproductive and unfulfilled.

Physical Awareness and Activity

Physical activity should be encouraged with advancing age. In most communities there is great need to organize programs designed to meet the capacities of the aging. Such programs can be personalized to bring individuals to their full capacity for fitness, but competition should be avoided. The point to be stressed is that without optimal health and strength, mental and emotional functioning may be impaired. The word "optimal" is the key in this regard because it denotes the recognition that physical ability decreases with advancing age.

Programs in physical fitness therefore need to be adapted for the development of the greatest possible degree of fitness, within the limitations imposed by the process of aging.

In like manner, specialized programs should be offered to those among the aging population who are physically handicapped, including victims of progressive diseases of the respiratory and vascular systems as well as those afflicted with arthritis, paralysis, or loss of limbs, sight, or hearing. Many such programs can be directed toward rehabilitation of the disabled.

All programs of physical training and rehabilitation should concern themselves with the psychology of sexuality in the aging. With decreasing or impaired physical strength, sexual activity may be reduced or eliminated. What must be emphasized is that sexual expression is not limited to genital expression. Mental, emotional, and physical contact are closely interrelated. An understanding of the need for physical expression without sexual climax is important to the aging. Programs of body awareness and sensitivity as well as sex education workshops can be helpful in this connection.

In addition to a lack of physical activity, our consistent finding has been that older persons suffer from acute touch starvation. They do not have enough stroking, touching, affective, and sensual-sexual satisfaction in their lives. For these reasons, wholistic programs for the aging need to incorporate not only ego-supportive individual, dyad or group experiences, but also exercise or physical fitness regimes as well as massage or stroking programs. One organization, SAGE (Senior Actualization and Growth Exploration), uses the small-group approach and a variety of bioenergetic and other types of body awareness and human potential experiences to help older people regain and maintain vitality, energy, and enjoyment of life. Biofeedback was initially selected as the modality by which people could observe, in relative privacy and in their own timing, that "their minds had something to do with their bodies . . . they saw that they could initiate better health, and that they were potentially in control of that process . . ."[13] Gay Luce, Ph.D., author of *Body Time* and Director of SAGE, adds:

> We did a number of exercises and used a very eclectic approach [in groups] . . . We used Alexander-method techniques for mindfulness of the spinal column. We did body sensing, listening to sounds through the body, getting used to physical contact. We started doing a lot of

massage. . . . This is very important, because touch is an [essential] source of emotional nourishment. . . . if you live in isolation and nobody touches you anymore, there is a message that is lacking in your life. . . . we used Tai-chi exercises which are especially good for developing confidence and grace . . . a kind of smorgasbord so that each person could choose the appropriate methods for himself . . . *to create a program to decondition ourselves from lifeless activity and to get back to a more natural state of beingness* . . . Health and inward growth is an ongoing process . . . As long as people continue to grow, they will continue to explore their reawakened potentials. [14] [Emphasis added.]

Nutritional Counseling and Education

Realistic programs in nutrition education need to be presented to the aging, with particular emphasis on the quality and quantity of food necessary for their activity levels and health. Nutritional guidelines should be simplified and published in multiple languages, with specific reference to the implications of various disease processes in aging. For example, specialized dietary information is essential to those persons affected by diabetes, hypoglycemia, hypercholesterolemia, or cardiovascular diseases. Interesting and informative publications describing various disease states and the dietary adjustments that can reduce their impact could supplement physician instruction and alleviate anxiety and confusion about the nature of these diseases.

Preventive Medicine and Home Safety

Nutritional balance is but one means of avoiding disability with increasing age. Preventive measures must be instituted early in life if health care in the advancing years is to be most effective. Informed but relaxed attitudes toward diet, exercise, lifestyle, sexuality and mental health can be affirmed early in life and reaffirmed throughout the aging process. A longitudinal study initiated in the 1930s among a group of young parents was concluded in the late 1960s, when these people were in their early seventies. The following conclusions emphasize the need for preventive habits: "Being in good health was crucial to allowing old people to lead the type of life they wanted. . . . early adult health care may pay multiple dividends for old age—not only for health status, but also for aging personality dispositions and aging lifestyles." [15]

Another area that has great implications for people of advanced age is accident prevention. As we know, most accidents occur at home, and for people of advancing age, an injury can have catastrophic effects. Media presentations initiated by the National Safety Council or other information agencies can improve levels of awareness of what constitute hazards in every household. For the aging themselves, increased awareness can lead to improved mental acuity, and this may well encourage improvement in physical fitness and reaction time.

Underlying all these concepts and proposed aids is the fact that ill health and disability are not the unavoidable companions of advancing age. Many health problems might be alleviated or even eliminated if the public were better informed of the advantages of early diagnosis and medical treatment. Health care education should focus on precautionary approaches. including recognition of risk factors for certain disease states and broad-range diagnostic screening programs to identify incipient disease. Wholistic health care emphasizes such programs, but further, encourages utilization of the benefits to be gained from such techniques as biofeedback, acupuncture, Autogenic Training, body awareness and psychic healing.

Terminal Illness and Death Preparation

In recent years, extensive efforts have been made toward developing positive attitudes toward death in a society that has, through fear, come to deny the fact of death as part of life. In the mid 1960s, Dr. Elisabeth Kubler-Ross discovered that medical professionals, including physicians, were reluctant to admit that any of their patients were near death. Recognition of this taboo led Kubler-Ross, a psychiatrist, to give a seminar on dying.[16] In the intervening decade, a great deal of attention has been focused on attitudes toward death and dying, and this very attention has effected radical changes in attitudes and approaches toward the terminally ill.

Increased emphasis on helping the dying in their preparation for death has resulted in various types of programs designed to accommodate the terminally ill patient and his family on the road to death. The changes in the concept of death have precipitated the development of new approaches to care of the dying. In the past, the terminally ill have had to rely on the resources of a hospital. By its very nature, a hospital is designed and oriented toward the preservation of life and the restoration of health. Care of the dying patient has quite different goals and perspectives. Recognition of these differences has led to the development of a therapeutic program designed to meet the needs of the terminal patient. Termed *hospice*, this new type of care emphasizes the patient's point of view and is family oriented. The model hospice, St. Christopher's of London, was opened in 1967 by Dr. Cicely Saunders. The hospice is a way station for the dying where humane care and good medical practice combine to ease the suffering, both physical and emotional, of the patient and his family. But hospice is not merely a facility—it is a concept that is applied equally to the patient who wishes to remain at home and to those who are no longer able to do so. In the United States, the concept has been put into practice in New Haven, Connecticut, and construction of a facility for this use is now in the planning stages.[17]

A second type of program for the dying is one that is designed to meet and deal with the emotional-psychological problems associated with impending death. In San Francisco, an all-volunteer agency, Shanti, is directed by Charles Garfield, Ph.D., and staffed by a core of committed counselors trained to meet the terminally ill patient and to help him or her to accept and understand feelings and life attitudes in the face of death. The services offered by Shanti are also helpful to the relatives of such patients.[18]

Yet another aspect of care for the terminally ill is the question defined as "the right to die." The recent publicity attendant upon the controversial Quinlan case in New Jersey has focused public attention on the use of "heroic" or "extraordinary" measures to maintain life processes in terminal cases. Recently, two Boston hospitals, Massachusetts General Hospital and Harvard's Beth Israel Hospital, confronted the question and publicly issued statements of policy on the question of withholding or removing life-support measures when death is imminent.[19] Then, in September, 1976, the State of California legislature became the first to pass a bill defining the right to die.[20]

These changing attitudes and approaches to care of the terminally ill have great impact on the aging population in our society. *Growing acceptance of death as a part of life is significant in the context of wholistic care.* By its very definition, wholistic health care is devoted to the individual in the life process, not simply as an isolated organism afflicted by disease. The mature understanding of life sees death as a part of living, not as its counterpart. In her book *Men in White*

Apparel, Ann Ree Colton voices it well: "Death, seemingly far from life, is ever-present within our life. Men with greater dimensions of the soul look upon death as an inevitable act in the drama of life; they play their parts in the drama of living and of the dead with equal acumen, integrity, peace, and joy. Such men reassure the doubtful, the fearful."[21] It is this attitude of peace and tranquility in the acceptance of death as yet another aspect of life that brings individuals to a point at which they are capable of greater fulfillment.

Research on Aging

Current programs to aid the aging and to improve social understanding of the process of growing old have their roots in on-going medical, psychiatric, and sociological research. Changes in approach to, and improved methods of care for, the aging and terminally ill rely on investigations into the conditions, problems, and successful lifestyles and environments experienced by the elderly in our time. Research in geriatric medicine and social gerontology is extensive, and more programs are being developed and initiated annually to deal with the problems of aging described in this chapter.

A national organization supportive of on-going research and pilot projects in the field of aging is the National Council on Aging. Headquartered in Washington, D.C., the NCOA maintains regional offices to support state and local agencies involved in developing programs for the aging. The emphasis of NCOA research programs is on the findings concerning aging itself and the services, policies and programs best suited to meet the needs of the aging in society.[22]

Nursing Homes, Retirement Homes, and Senior Citizen Communities from the Perspective of Wholistic Health

Again, the application of wholistic principles and concepts can make a major contribution both to maintaining health and vital living and to fostering healing, regardless of whether the setting is the nursing home, the retirement home, the senior citizen community, or the community at large.

Nursing Homes

Numerous investigations and studies of nursing homes in all parts of the United States have revealed the deplorable conditions that prevail in many such facilities. Operators of nursing homes seem to be motivated largely by the income they can derive from their enterprises. Although many facilities have programs scheduled and equipment available for them, there is often a lack of trained personnel or staff time to devote to those programs. For the most part, schedules and services are arranged for the convenience of the staff with the objective of providing only the minimum services needed by the residents. Most nursing homes appear to be locked into a rigid framework of schedules and routines supported by numerous rules and regulations. The physical environment is characterized by overcrowding, starkness, and monotony. The interpersonal relationship environment suffers from a similar bleakness. Often the residents lack opportunities to establish any but superficial relationships with one another. Also, the staff pays little or no attention to the patients' psychological needs. There are, however, many well-meaning, loving, concerned, and dedicated individual staff members who are frustrated by the limitations imposed by the system and the attitudes of their fellow workers.

The application of wholistic principles and concepts to nursing homes focuses on four essential areas.

1. Staff help is given whenever possible to establish supportive and nourishing relationships and relationship clusters among the residents. This involves the use of sociometric methods or surveys to determine which residents like to be in social contact and then making the physical arrangements that permit these people to share a room, have adjoining quarters, or otherwise have access to each other.
2. Maximum focus is on self-help and self-regulation and helping patients help each other, not with the motive of saving on services and maximizing profits, but *to establish a climate of caring and love among residents that is basically life-affirmative*. The necessary first step in this connection is the formation of an advisory committee of residents who will encourage their fellow residents' involvement in a program of wholistic health.[23]
3. The physical environment is transformed so that it will be life-supportive and a source of positive reinforcement. With optimum

resident involvement, the aesthetic environment of a nursing home often can be transformed at minimal cost through the addition of colorful posters, prints, and reproductions *that can be rotated from room to room*. Sometimes the residents themselves want to create drawings or collages or otherwise participate in personalizing their life environment. At a time of redecorating or repainting, the findings from color psychology can be utilized, and the residents should be involved in the selection of paint colors or wallcoverings. Posters gaily illustrated with cutouts from magazines often can be created by residents who wish to offer positive reinforcement with such messages as, Doing Your Exercises in Bed or Out of Bed Helps You To Build Health and Vitality, or, By Helping and Caring for Others, You Help and Care for Yourself. Again, this material needs to be rotated periodically for maximum effect.

4. The greatest possible involvement of community resources in the nursing home program should be a primary goal. This can be achieved through a program of *outreach*. Such a program can be started with letters to local service clubs, churches, and other organizations and by making concrete suggestions as to how clubs and individuals can be of help. Often local senior citizen communities or retirement homes have active members of organizations that will furnish helpful services. Such simple programs as afternoon tea served twice a week, *on-going* visiting and conversation hours, and the showing of slides or films on a room-by-room basis can do much to help residents regain a renewed interest in life and maintain or regain good health. In some communities, psychology or social work students or interns can be interested in conducting motivational sessions either individually or on a room-by-room basis.

Retirement Homes

All too many retirement homes have become human parking or storage places where people spend, or, more accurately, "expend," their remaining time on earth. Most residents of retirement homes have little to look forward to other than the next meal, the next bowel movement, and the next TV show or bingo game. Superficial relationships among residents are the norm, and they are usually caught in a network of schedules and regulations promulgated to serve the best interests of the service and administrative ends of the operation.

Most retirement homes can make direct application of the suggestions presented in the above discussion of nursing homes. Since most residents of retirement homes are ambulatory, however, there is a much greater possibility of creating a supportive community within these institutions. *The process of transforming a retirement home into a supportive community usually begins with the sincere interest of the administrators in such a project.* The inception of the program should be followed by a meeting for all residents at which several key questions need to be considered: (1) What can we do together to make this place an even better place to stay, with the idea of helping us to become more of a community? (2) What can we do to give more help, caring, loving, and understanding to one another?[24] (3) What can we do to stimulate and enlarge our interests, our *creativity*, and our curiosity, and how can we bring more creativity and enjoyment to this place?

With the support of the administration and personnel, as many residents as wish can then be involved, through participation in committee activities, to implement positive change. In many communities, skilled discussion leaders can be found to volunteer their services for such an exciting and pioneering project. *Emphasis, however, always needs to be to draw on and to develop the resources and strengths present in the resident population.* A large part of the skill and effectiveness of good leadership lies in identifying and bringing these strengths and resources to bear on the process of building a community.

Finally, retirement homes offer an opportunity for the organization of life-affirmative groups, such as the Developing Personal Potential program. These groups, which can be conducted by trained, non-professional facilitators, focus on the enhancement of the self-image and self-concept.[25] They help participants become aware of their personality strengths and resources and to decide what potentials to develop further. The Developing Personal Potential groups also create a caring and supportive interpersonal environment and help members to develop positive attitudes toward themselves, toward others, and toward the years ahead. In this connection, research conducted by Dr. Robert Samp of the University of Wisconsin is of interest. His study of 2,000 long-lived people revealed that good health is associated with the personality components of moderation, optimism, serenity, interest in others, and interest in the future. It is clear that these psychological components or attributes also can be acquired in the course of a group experience such as the Developing Personal Potential program.

Retirement Communities

Many contemporary retirement communities are communities in name only, and most lack organizational structures that permit open lines of communication, which are so necessary. Most important, however, they lack the sense of belonging, cohesion, and togetherness that makes a community. A large number of these "communities" also practice a form of segregation by barring younger people and children. They have minimal ties to nearby larger communities and foster a ghetto mentality of isolation.

Yet most retirement communities today offer a singular opportunity for the implementation of wholistic healing principles and concepts. A strong basic motivation to achieve and maintain health and healing is usually present, and the physical and truncated social structures that already exist can *form an excellent base for a retirement community dedicated to wholistic health.* This process usually has its beginnings in a community meeting, perhaps preceded by a lecture presentation by an expert on wholistic health.[26] Following this event, open community dialogue is invited and, if interest warrants, goals are defined, and committees are set up to achieve these goals.

Minimal goals might be: (1) the establishment of support groups to which community members can turn for help at a time of crisis; (2) the organization of on-going classes, lectures, or workshops on wholistic health, wholistic healing, nutrition, diet, and health, and similar topics; (3) the organization of outreach teams to help less fortunate older people in the larger community; (4) the organization of *life-affirmative groups* (such as the Developing Personal Potential program described in the previous section) that focus on the development of life-supportive attitudes, health practices, and perspectives; (5) organization of local chapters of such national organizations as AARP or the Gray Panthers (see Appendix B, Directory of Organizations).

It is necessary to recognize that most retirement communities represent a vast reservoir of skills, talents, knowledge, and resources that, for the most part, remain fallow until their owners take them to the grave. Utilization of even a small portion of these resources by the members of the retirement community and bringing these to bear on the surrounding larger community could result in vast benefits to all concerned. Bringing such resources to the larger community in an outreach program, for example, could do much to establish positive attitudes about aging. The best way to combat stigma and stereotypes is through positive action and through projects that both contribute to the commonweal and have wide community visibility.

In his visits to a number of retirement communities, one of the authors (H.A.O.) has found that aesthetic elements are generally neglected in retirement communities. Yet with minimal expense and maximal utilization of the talents and resources available within the community, most such communities could be transformed into places of outstanding beauty and appeal. In turn, a beautiful community environment enhances self-esteem and community pride and spirit and creates an excellent image of the retirement community vis-à-vis the larger community of which it is a part. *The possibilities that exist in the many retirement communities remain to be explored and constitute one of the neglected challenges of our time.*

Conclusion

In its applications to aging, wholistic health is directed, not simply toward longevity, but toward enhancing the quality of life with progressive age. This calls for emphasis on positive values and the development of self-worth among individuals involved in an on-going life process. Educational programs are key factors in developing talents that vitalize individuals who might otherwise see age as a burden. In a broader sense, education of society may also contribute to positive attitudes toward old age and the aging segment of our society.

What needs to be realized is that the later years of life can be a time for synthesis and new focus. The quality of life that permits the aging the freedom both to synthesize past experience and to find further goals relies on the continued activation or reactivation of interests, talents, and dreams, avoidance of the pitfalls of depression, continuance of physical activity, and maintenance of physical, emotional, mental, and sexual fitness. The wholistic health program is consistent with education toward prevention and rehabilitation and with a strong emphasis on minimizing major disabling disease processes.

The attitudes of society are significant if the aging are to find the supportive environment in which to achieve fulfillment. The experience and knowledge of people of advancing age, if properly channeled, can bring about great advances in every aspect of our society. Even when individuals are ill or disabled and must live in nursing homes or retirement facilities, emphasis on their capabilities, not their disabilities, will help them toward a life of dignity and fulfillment. Realization of human possibilities and recognition of the unique individuality of every person lie at the very heart of the wholistic program for the advancing years.

Notes

1. Dr. Otto for some years has been involved in the development of a wholistic preretirement program and functions as a consultant in this area.
2. For more detailed information on the AIM Seminar Program, contact Action for Independent Maturity, Division of AARP, 1909 K Street NW, Washington, DC 20049.
3. M. S. M. Watts, "A Bicentennial Editorial: Quality of Life—A New National Purpose?" *Western Journal of Medicine* 124 (1976): 55–56.
4. Murray A. Raskind, et al., "Helping the Elderly Psychiatric Patient in Crisis," *Geriatrics* 31 (June, 1976): 51–56.
5. "Government and Geriatrics," *Geriatrics* 31 (August, 1976): 9–12.
6. E. Virginia Beverley, "Helping Your Patient Choose and Adjust to a Nursing Home," *Geriatrics* 31 (May, 1976): 115–20, 125–26.
7. A nursing home rating guide is also available from the Institute of Gerontology, University of Michigan, Ann Arbor, MI 48104.
8. Henry S. Maas and Joseph A. Kuypers, *From Thirty to Seventy* (San Francisco: Jossey-Bass, 1974): 208.
9. Jack Fincher, "Dialogue in a Journal," *Human Behavior* 4 (November, 1975): 17–23.
10. "AIM News: Volunteers Man a Center for Free Legal Advice," *Dynamic Maturity* 11 (May, 1976): 13.
11. Juanita M. Kreps, quoted in "On Growing Old in America," *AAUW Journal* (April, 1972): 19–25.

12. Wolfgang Luthe, *Creativity Mobilization Technique* (New York: Grune and Stratton, 1976): 236.

13. C. C. Elwell II, "The SAGE Spirit," *Human Behavior* 5 (March, 1976): 40–43.

14. Gay Gaer Luce, "Reawakening Age-Old Energies," *Gesar*, 3 (Winter, 1975): 17–20.

15. Henry S. Maas and Joseph A. Kuypers, op. cit.

16. "Elisabeth Kubler-Ross on Death and Dying," *Practical Psychology for Physicians* 3 (February, 1976): 13–22.

17. Constance Holden, "Hospices: For the Dying, Relief from Pain and Fear," *Science* 193 (1976): 389–91.

18. Charles A. Garfield, "Consciousness Alteration and Fear of Death," *Journal of Transpersonal Psychology* 2 (1975): 147–75.

19. "Helping the Dying Die: Two Harvard Hospitals Go Public with Policies," *Science* 193 (1976): 1105–06.

20. California State Legislature, A.B. 3060. Bill effective January 1, 1977. It is entitled the "Natural Death Act."

21. Ann Ree Colton, *Men in White Apparel* (Glendale, Calif.: ARC, 1961). Currently used as a textbook at the University of California, Berkeley.

22. National Council on Aging, 1828 L Street, N.W., Washington, DC 20036.

23. Elliott Carlson, "Nursing Homes: Look How Good They Can Be," *Dynamic Maturity* 11 (May, 1976): 18–22.

24. The Developing Personal Potential program and many of the two-person experiences of this program are suitable for building a caring climate. The experiences are contained in the book *Group Methods to Actualize Human Potential* by H. A. Otto, available from Holistic Press, 6363 Wilshire Blvd., Los Angeles, CA 90048. ($13.50 postpaid).

25. Leadership training seminars are designed both to develop group facilitators and to equip them with professional skills. Summer training programs are offered under the auspices of the National Center for the Exploration of Human Potential, 222 West Bourene St., La Jolla, CA 92037.

26. The authors, Drs. Otto and Knight, are available as a resource for recommending qualified lecturers in the fields of wholistic health and healing.

Bibliography

Davis, Richard, ed. *Aging: Prospects and Issues.* Los Angeles: Ethel Percy Andrus Gerontology Center, University of Southern California, 1973.

Eisdorfer, Carol, and Lawton, M. Powell, eds. *The Psychology of Adult De-*

velopment and Aging. Washington, D.C.: The American Psychological Association, 1973.

Kalish, Richard A. *Late Adulthood: Perspectives on Human Development*. Monterey, Calif.: Brooks/Cole, 1975.

Le Shan, Eda. *The Wonderful Crisis of Middle Age: Some Personal Reflections*. New York: David McKay, 1973.

Nesselroade, J. R. and Reese, H. W., eds. *Life Span Developmental Psychology: Methodology*, New York: Academic Press, 1972.

Palmore, Erdman, ed. *Normal Aging: Reports from the Duke Longitudinal Study 1955–1969*. Durham, N.C.: Duke University Press, 1970.

Riley, M. W., Foner A., and associates. *An Inventory of Research Findings*. Aging and Society, vol 1. New York: Russell Sage Foundation, 1968.

Strauss, Anselm L. *Chronic Illness and the Quality of Life*. St. Louis: C. V.Mosby, 1975.

Taylor, Renee. *Hunza Health Secrets for Long Life and Happiness*. Englewood Cliffs, N.J.: Prentice-Hall, 1966.

10

William A. Tiller

Rationale
for an Energy Medicine

MAN'S VIEW OF reality, or "world picture," locks him into a perceptual mode that is an effective jailor. This has its beneficial and stabilizing aspects, but it also has its strongly limiting aspects. At this time, our growth is being severly limited by our prevailing world picture, but we stand poised on the threshold of transition to a new world view that will be much more effective for mankind's next stage of evolution. This paper outlines some experimental data that violate our present world picture and suggests directions of change needed for generating a more appropriate world picture. One of the consequences of the new world picture will be the development of medical therapeutics based upon controlled energy fields. Here, we lay the foundation of the rationale for such therapeutics.

Basic Hypotheses for a New World View

People have come to look toward science as the vehicle for changing their world picture, and, to this author, the potential scientific knowledge of the universe available to man is like a huge iceberg with only a small exposed tip. From the past several hundred years of study, we have come to know the exposed tip fairly well; however, most of Nature still lies hidden from us. Psychoenergetic experiments presently being conducted around the world suggest some fascinating aspects of the hidden portion of this iceberg. From these studies, one can construct six profound hypotheses that have a dramatic bearing on the structure of our new world picture.

1. There are energies functioning in Nature completely different from those known to us via conventional science and upon which our present technological society is built.
2. The universe organizes and radiates information in other dimensions than just the physical frame that we sense with our five senses. We appear to have latent sensory systems for cognition in these other dimensions.
3. At some of these dimensional levels, we are all connected to each other and to all things on this planet. It is as if we are all part of one vast organism and are just beginning to come awake to ourselves.
4. Time, space, and matter are all mutable; i.e., they can all be deformed. We can perceive events out of our fixed location in space; we can perceive events out of our fixed location in time; we can dematerialize and materialize objects.
5. We do not actually perceive reality at the level of perception of the five physical senses; rather, we perceive the "world of appearances." All we can ask of our science is to provide a set of consistent relationships concerning Nature at this level.
6. At this time, mankind seems to be making the final stages of integration of another sensory system; from observation of his behavioral capacities, it appears as if a biological mutation is taking place.

To briefly illustrate the rationale for the new "world picture," let us consider how medicine, biology, and agriculture have looked at the function aspect of living organisms.

Some of the Cracks Appearing in Our World Picture

Up to the present, medicine, biology, and agriculture have largely viewed living organisms as operating via the following sequence of reactions:

$$\text{function} \rightleftarrows \text{structure} \rightleftarrows \text{chemistry} \rightleftarrows. \qquad (1)$$

As a modification of eq. 1, there is some growing awareness of the interaction between chemical states and electromagnetic fields; this interaction would be added to the right of eq. 1.

Generally, flaws in the function area have been traced to structural defects in the system, arising from certain chemical imbalances. The rectification procedure has usually been via an adjustment of the chemical environment, with more and more sophisticated chemical complexes being utilized to trigger the organism's defense and repair mechanisms. The dilemma that arises is that both the organism and the threatening invaders adapt to the new chemical complex, becoming progressively less sensitive to it, and so the escalation of potency must continue. One very deleterious aspect of this procedure is that the unnatural chemical content of the organism increases and begins to influence other levels of functioning of the organism than the one being corrected. The effect is particularly serious in the agricultural area, where the method of application of the chemicals is via the soil, so that a chemical equilibration develops between the plants and the soil, percolation of water through the system spreads the chemicals over a large area, and the whole ecosystem begins to suffer from chemical pollution. Clearly, mankind must find a better way of understanding and dealing with flaws of function in living organisms. However, so long as he continues to view living organisms via eq. 1, he is stuck with his present methods.

In searching out alternative procedures for influencing the well-being of living organisms, one must first question the validity or completeness of eq. 1. Are there effective physical, as distinct from chemical, techniques for modifying organismic functioning? Can potential techniques for doing likewise be found in the domain of what would presently be called nonphysical energies? Let us look at a number of observations that reveal the total inadequacy of eq. 1.

The most obvious discrepancy is the neglect of applied electromagnetic fields as a way to influence muscles and organs in the human body. Everyone is familiar with the use of X rays for tumor treatment and of diathermy for muscle relaxation, and we know that osteopathic physical manipulation techniques have had great success with improving human functioning for the past hundred years. In addition, researchers in neuropsychiatry have learned that small electric currents between certain specific points in the brain give rise to the same behavioral changes that are observed with certain specific brain-stimulating chemical intakes.[1] More recently, Becker has shown that small direct electric currents ($1 \ \mu\mu A/mm^2$ to $1000 \ \mu\mu A/mm^2$) cause cell regeneration, tissue repair, and fracture rehealing, whereas direct currents greater than 10,000 $\mu\mu$A/mm^2 cause cell degeneration.[2] Thus, the first step in modifying eq. 1 is:

$$\text{function} \rightleftarrows \text{structure} \rightleftarrows \text{chemistry} \rightleftarrows \frac{\text{electromagnetic}}{\text{energy fields}} \rightleftarrows. \quad (2)$$

In addition, the human body under hypnosis has been found to exhibit truly remarkable feats of strength and endurance attesting to a mind/structure link. In Aikido, Zen, or Yoga disciplines, we see a conscious rather than a subconscious link between mind, structure, and function. On another front, modern psychotherapy shows us that certain chemical treatments influence mental states and certain mental treatments influence chemical states.[3] Recent studies have indicated that human acupuncture points, of ancient Oriental description, have different electrical characteristics than the surrounding skin.[4] It is very easy to show that significant changes occur in the skin electrical potential and impedance when a person shifts among waking, drowsy, and sleep states as well as other hypnogogic states.[5] In fact, some Soviet investigators utilize concentration techniques to enhance the voltage difference between two acupuncture points from ~50 mV to ~500 mV as a training technique for developing psychokinetic abilities.[6] Finally, the recent development of biofeedback techniques shows us that the directed use of mind can allow us not only to exercise control over a variety of autonomic body functions like skin temperature, and pain but also to effect considerable repair of the vehicle.[7,8] Certainly the experiments in which Jack Schwarz thrust needles through his body and mentally controlled the bleeding attest to this. From the foregoing, there is little doubt that "mind" must be included on the right of our reaction equation; i.e.,

$$\text{function} \rightleftarrows \text{structure} \rightleftarrows \text{chemical} \rightleftarrows \frac{\text{electromagnetic}}{\text{energy fields}} \leftrightharpoons \text{mind} \leftrightharpoons. \quad (3)$$

Now the going gets a little tougher; for the human body, we have shown a link between what we have called mind forces and the other elements of our reaction equation. We have not demonstrated that these mind forces influence inanimate matter, nor have we demonstrated whether there is an intermediate reaction component between mind and physical energy fields, nor have we shown any unique and distinguishable characteristics of mind. What follows gives an indication of these missing pieces to the puzzle. However, we must begin to go farther afield to find published supporting data.

Careful studies of the enzyme trypsin have shown that its activity can be altered by placing solutions of it between the poles of a strong magnetic field or between the palms of a "healer."[9] The effect of the healer's hands was comparable to that found with fields in the range of 10^4 gauss. A more recent study has shown the healer's ability, not only to influence the growth of plants, but also to influence cloud formation with the hands held (a) adjacent to a small cloud chamber or (b) adjacent to a visualization of the same chamber from 600 miles away.[10] Reference to other healers, from Jesus to Arigo, continue to appear in our publications,[11] and one study has even noted a change in the electrical impedance of specific acupuncture points on both the patient and the healer as a result of a laying-on-of-hands type of treatment.[12]

Motoyama placed a person who showed psi-ability and a second, ordinary person, in separate rooms shielded by concrete walls lined with lead. Then he had the subject possessing psi-ability concentrate his mind on the other individual while Motoyama made measurements to determine if any changes in bodily functions of the second (ordinary) person had occurred during the period of concentration by the psychic subject. Motoyama found that remarkable changes in the pulse and respiratory rate of the ordinary person were evident during the period of mental concentration by the psychic person (see Fig. 10.1.). Since the two rooms were shielded against physical energy, he deduced that the psi-ability responsible for bringing about these modifications was essentially nonphysical in nature.[13]

From experiments directed towards man-plant communication, we gain more support for the interaction between nonphysical energies and physical energies. One of the most remarkable experiments is taking place in Findhorn, Scotland, where, in barren sandy soil and with a hostile climate, the small community has succeeded in producing dozens of vegetables, flowers, and trees unexcelled in size and beauty. Everything is based on the philosophy that views plants, soil, the natural forces of sun, rain, and wind, plus people, as collective parts of the community of life. Via community meditation, talking to and expressing love and thanks to the plants themselves, and invocation of the aid of elemental nature spirits, the people have created agricultural products that defy conventional explanation.[14] Backster's

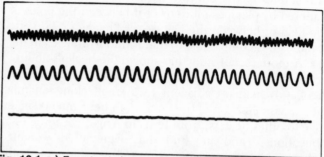

Fig. 10.1 a.) From top to bottom, Plethysmogram and respiratory and galvanic skin resistance recordings in ordinary person occupying shielded room before period of mental concentration by psychic person. (see text)

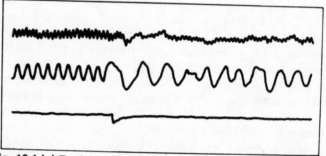

Fig. 10.1 b.) Tracings comparable to those in Figure **a** after the psychic person's period of mental concentration has begun.

initial work and that of Vogel indicate that an electrical response can be obtained from a plant consistent with the experimenter focusing his mind to project (a) the acts of damaging another plant, (b) the destruction of another life form, or (c) a positive thought form, such as love or healing. [15,16] Backster postulated the existence of primary perception as a signal linkage between cellular plant life. However, Vogel postulated that the plants must be charged or sensitized by the experimenter's mind energies before being receptive to thoughts and emotions. Since a recent study showed an inability to reproduce the Backster Effect without a plant sensitization step in the protocol, the Vogel approach may be the more relevant one.[17] Finally, to show our connection to the earth, we note that the Schumann resonance of the global capacitor between the earth and the ionosphere is in the 3 to 14 hertz (H) range, which encompasses the α, β, and θ ranges of the dominant human brain wave patterns.[18] Recent studies have revealed that 10 H electric fields control the human circadian rhythms and that human reaction times are strongly dependent on the specific ELF (extreme low frequency) field being propagated in the local earth environment.[19] In this series of experiments, we see a connectedness developing between living things at more subtle levels of energy than those associated with our physical chemistry.

Turning to the area of psychokinesis (movement of objects with the mind), we find an even greater confrontation with our present world picture. This author observed, firsthand, psychokinetic demonstrations in the Soviet Union by two different people.[20] Swann performed two significant experiments in this area: (1) he mentally altered the temperature of a thermister, located a fixed distance from his body, in a pattern consistent with a prescribed coding of hot, cool, neutral, etc.; and (2) he seemingly influenced the decay rate of a very sensitive magnetic field detector at Stanford University, which was located behind vast metallic and concrete shielding.[21] For fifteen to twenty years, Forwald conducted psychokinetic experiments on small wooden cubes coated with different materials of different thicknesses. He showed an exponential dependence between psychokinetic force and coating thickness plus a proportionality to the neutron number of the coating material.[22] Most recently, the demonstrations of Uri Geller led to the identification of groups of children in England, Germany, Switzerland, Japan, and elsewhere who possess similar and perhaps even greater abilities. Taylor has recently described the experiments he has conducted with the young children in England. Perhaps most striking is their ability to mentally bend aluminum bars placed inside sealed transparent perspec tubes. The 1-foot-long, straight bars are seen to change into an S shape that fills the cross section of the 1-inch-diameter perspec tubes; the end cap seals remain unbroken.[23] Clearly, the mind forces can be used to influence not only living systems but inanimate ones as well.

Recent experiments on "remote viewing" have shown that an individual can (a) perceive and accurately describe objects placed at a removed location from the perceiver and his line of sight, (b) be given the longitude and latitude coordinates of a location on the earth and accurately describe the terrain of that location even though it is thousands of miles away, and (c) tune in on a specific individual and view a remote locality through that individual's eyes. Interestingly enough, the sensitive individual sometimes perceives the scene before the target individual actually arrives there. The reverse of this process —wherein one chooses a particular target, like a potential oil well, and seeks to know the specific earth coordinates—has also been accomplished.[24,25] When one uses instrumental assistance, the technique falls in the category of "radionics" and the specific sub-category is called "map dowsing."[26,27] Radionics is an instrumental form of radiesthesia (defined as sensitivity to radiations covering the whole field of radiations, physical and nonphysical, from any source either living or inert) and, as such, deals with the interaction of mind and matter and with the complete interrelationship of all things.[28]

Conventional dowsing studies, wherein a type of wand is used and one walks over the ground being scanned, have shown that the dowsing response is a muscular action connected via a sequence of biological processes to the cause which, in many cases, is a magnetic field gradient. One individual has shown himself to be sufficiently sensitive to respond to a 1-microamp current flowing in a wire imbedded several feet in the ground, as he walks across the wire's location with the magnetic field at the wand level being about 10^{-10} gauss (earth field strength is 0.5 gauss). The seat of the sensing ability in the body appears to be the adrenal glands.[29] More recently, a number of U.S. osteopathic practitioners, investigating a subject called kineseology, have shown that specific body muscle tonus changes occur when specific minerals or chemicals are merely held in the left hand or placed on the stomach (the ingredients may be in a glass container). This result is very similar to that which this author has found using a type of dowsing wand called a biomechanical transducer.[30]

Many studies have been carried out in the areas of telepathy and clairvoyance, and the results attest to their state of function in the human being and in animals.[31,32] Karagulla has utilized subjects with clairvoyant abilities to observe the "auric" fields around patients and thence describe their state of physical and mental health. These auric fields are perceived as patterns of light of different colors extending outwards from the body. With some subjects, the patterns can be viewed with the eyes closed or in total darkness.[33]

Studies of precognitive awareness are also widespread, and a precognition teaching machine has been developed that allows one to train this ability into subjects, or rather, to enhance the present operating level of this human capacity.[34] Experiments being conducted with pyramids of specific shape suggest that such structures are useful for preserving cellular tissue and enhancing the healthy growth of plants, even in total darkness.[35,36] Combinations of specific shapes and specific materials have been shown to form devices called "psychotronic" generators, which can be charged with biological energy and perform an array of functions that confound conventional understanding.[37] This author has directly observed such devices in operation and accepts that they most probably respond to a "new physics."

The foregoing list could be made much longer; however, I hope that the point has been made that eqs. 1 and 2 are inadequate to account for a variety of new (and old) experiences that have occurred in the family of man. Acceptance of this work is difficult for those who have not had experiential awareness of these "other" energies of Nature, and it is somewhat understandable that the results are vehemently rejected in many quarters as violating our collective picture of the universe. Some of the natural criticism about sloppy experimental procedures is justified in specific cases, because it is extremely difficult to develop a completely "clean" protocol for these experiments (we do not yet understand all the key elements of that protocol). In addition, one may be justified in quibbling about the quality of a particular experiment or about the veracity of a given experimenter. However, the body of experimental data of this type is so vast and is growing so rapidly that it cannot be denied much longer. The weight of mounting evidence is so strong as to readily merit a wise man's reflection.

Incorporating the foregoing experimental results, eq. 1 takes the form

$$\text{function} \rightleftarrows \text{structure} \rightleftarrows \text{chemistry} \rightleftarrows \begin{array}{c}\text{positive}\\\text{space-time}\\\text{energies}\end{array} \rightleftarrows \begin{array}{c}\text{negative}\\\text{space-time}\\\text{energies}\end{array} \rightleftarrows$$

$$\rightleftarrows \text{mind} \rightleftarrows \text{spirit} \rightleftarrows \text{Divine}. \qquad (4)$$

Electromagnetic, gravitational, and other physical energies function in the positive space-time frame. Other nonphysical energies function in the negative space-time frame, which is conjugate to the positive space-time frame but in a higher frequency band.[38] The mind frame is distinguished from both of these in that energies and pattern formation at this level are not limited by space and time. Thus, we live in a multidimensional universe and are, ourselves, multidimensional beings functioning on many different levels of Nature simultaneously. Man is mostly unaware of these levels of self and cannot grasp the visualization that he has an extended energy structure that interconnects and integrates his beingness with seemingly separate localizations of beingness. We are so chained to our view of reality as perceived by the five physical senses that we are unable to give credence to our true nature. We must come to realize the potential of man as expressed by eq. 4 and to recognize that, if man's energy structure is perturbed at any one of the indicated levels, ripples of effect flow out in all directions to produce corresponding perturbations at all other levels. However, the magnitude of the effect and the time of manifestation of the effect will depend upon things like the intensity of the original signal, the conductivity of the medium of the original signal, and the degree of coherence of wave structures at the boundaries between different levels.

A Perspective on Healing

The foregoing leads quite naturally into a perspective on healing: that pathology can develop at a number of levels and that healing is needed at all of them to restore the system to a state of harmony. The initial pathology begins at the level of mind and propagates effects to both the negative space-time and positive space-time levels. We then perceive what we call disease or malfunction at these levels and try to remove the effects by a variety of healing techniques. The best healing mode is to help the individual remove the pathology at the *cause* level and bring about the correction by a return to "right thinking." The next best healing mode is to effect repair of the structure at the negative space-time level. The third-best level of healing is that which medicine practices today: repair of the structure at the positive space-time level. Since the energy structures at these different levels are coupled, repair at a lower level will still produce some feedback modification of energy structure at a higher level. However, if harmony is not restored at the higher level, then a force will continue to exist for pathological development in the energy structure at a lower level. Of course, this force is basically like a thermodynamic potential to produce change so that the effects may be manifested or materialized in very different forms depending upon what alterations have already been made to the energy structures of the positive and negative space-time frames. The closest analogy to this can be found in the field of 'phase equilibria' of materials. If a complex alloy containing a number of chemical constituents is heated until it melts and then cooled again, there results a thermodynamic driving force for a phase change, to one of several possible solid forms. By making very slight but specific modifications to the chemistry or cooling rate or other variables in the process, it is possible to change the type of solid phase that initially develops and the crystalline form that results.

When one is healing another, use is made of this extended energy structure of self to channel the needed frequency components of the needed energy at the particular dimensional level into the one to be healed. Since the particular pathology is represented by a particular energy pattern and all patterns are formed by the superposition of waves, a pattern can be altered or completely eradicated by the input of the appropriate wave components at the appropriate intensity level. To do this effectively, a number of conditions need to be satisfied: (1) one must be able to generate or tap the needed wave components of the requisite type, (2) one must be able to tap these wave components from his extended energy structure at the specifically needed ratios of relative intensities, (3) one needs to tap the requisite correction energy pattern at a high overall intensity so that the healing needed is of short duration, (4) one needs to be sharply attuned to the one to be healed so that these energy components can be brought into his extended energy structure without scattering losses and (5) one needs to have the confidence of the one to be healed so that he doesn't mentally distort or undo the healer's efforts because of fears or doubts.

To understand how this is possible and to gain an appreciation for the implications of such healing events, let us consider the necessary structure of an electrical system designed to deliver electrical energy to a load over a broad frequency range with a specific intensity distribution of frequencies. The individual components in the system will be resonators having a restricted band width of frequencies and restricted

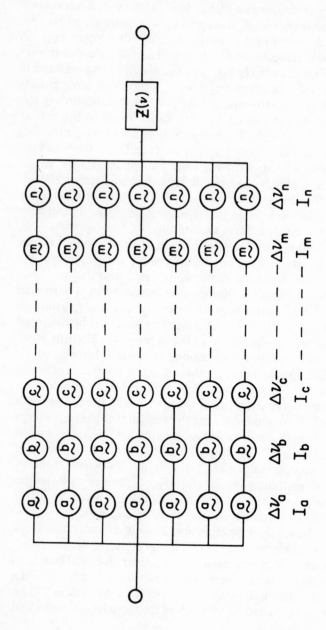

DISTRIBUTED POWER SOURCE

Fig. 10.2 Illustration of a composite healing power supply providing broad band and high intensity characteristics

176

output intensity. Thus, to obtain the required frequency range, a number of different kinds of resonators would need to be coupled in series. To obtain the required output intensity distribution, many resonators of the same kind need to be coupled in parallel. Finally, for this energy to reach the load, the supply must be properly coupled or impedance matched to the load. Such a situation is illustrated in Fig. 10.2. The same type of situation must obtain when we are using biological resonators in the healing mode. The implication is that the extended energy structure of the healer must include a number of different biological resonators functioning on basically different but overlapping frequency bands integrated into a functioning energy system. Further, as the healer expands his consciousness to resonate over a larger frequency range and builds himself to transmit energy at higher intensities, he will become more effective as a healing channel.

In concluding this paper, we note that energy patterns at different dimensions of the universe sustain the chemical patterns we observe at the physical level. In the future, to alter the chemical pattern that we perceive as disease, we may input a hierarchy of energies to the body. We shall see that the energy pattern, rather than simply the energy amplitude, becomes the important consideration. As we develop monitors and eventually generators of these "other" energies, we will be in a position to develop medical therapeutic devices for benefiting mankind at more subtle levels than those associated with present conventional medicine.

Notes

1. D. E. Woolridge, *The Machinery of the Brain* (New York: McGraw-Hill, 1963).
2. R. D. Becker and D. G. Murray, "The Electrical Control System Regulating Fracture Healing in Amphibians," *Clinical Orthopedic and Related Research* 75 (1970): 169.
3. D. Hawkins and L. Pauling, *Orthomolecular Psychiatry* (San Francisco: W. H. Freeman, 1973).
4. M. A. Reichmanis, A. Marino, and R. O. Becker, "Electrical Correlates of Acupuncture Points" *IEEE, Transactions on Biomedical Engineering* BME 22 (November 1975): 533.
5. W. A. Tiller, "Some Physical Network Characteristics of Acupuncture Points and Meridians" (Paper delivered at the Symposium on

Acupuncture, Academy of Parapsychology and Medicine, Stanford University, Palo Alto, Calif., June, 1972).

6. V. Adamenko, private communication, Soviet Union, September, 1971.

7. E. Green, "Biofeedback for Mind-Body Self Regulation: Healing and Creativity" (Paper delivered at the Symposium on Varieties of Healing Experience, Academy of Parapsychology and Medicine, De Anza College, Cupertino, Calif., October, 1971).

8. B. B. Brown, *New Mind, New Body—Biofeedback: New Directions for the Mind* (New York: Harper and Row, 1975).

9. Sister M. Justa Smith, "The Influence of Enzyme Growth by the 'Laying-on-of-Hands' " (Paper delivered at the Symposium on Dimensions of Healing, Academy of Parapsychology and Medicine, Los Altos, Calif., 1972).

10. R. N. Miller, P. B. Reinhart, and A. Kern, *Thought As Energy*, ed. W. Kinnear (Los Angeles: Science of Mind Publications, 1975).

11. A. Puharich, "The Search for a Common Denominator in Medicine and Healing" (Paper presented at the Symposium on Dimensions of Healing, Academy of Parapsychology and Medicine, Los Altos, Calif., 1972).

12. W. A. Tiller, "Some Psychoenergetic Devices" (Paper delivered at the Seventh Annual Medical Symposium on New Horizons in Healing, A.R.E. Clinic and the Edgar Cayce Foundation, Phoenix, Ariz., January 1974).

13. H. Motoyama, "The Mechanism by which PSI-Ability Manifests Itself," *Impact of Science on Society* 24 (1974): 321.

14. P. Tompkins and C. Bird, *The Secret Life of Plants* (New York: Harper and Row, 1972).

15. C. Backster, "Evidence of Primary Perception in Plant Life," *International Journal of Parapsychology* 10 (Winter 1968): 329.

16. M. Vogel, "Man-Plant Communication," in *Psychic Exploration*, ed. E. D. Mitchell and J. White (New York: G. P. Putnam's Sons, 1974).

17. K. A. Horowitz, D. C. Lewis, and E. L. Gasteiger, "Plant 'Primary Perception': Electrophysiological Unresponsiveness to Brine Shrimp Killing," *Science* 189 (1975): 478.

18. W. O. Schumann, "Über die Strahlungslosen Eigenschwing ungen einer leitenden Kugel die von einer Luftschicht und einer Ionosphärenhülle umgeben 1st," *Z. Naturforsch* 7a (1952): 149.

19. H. König, "Biological Effects of Extremely Low Frequency (ELF) Electrical Phenomena in the Atmosphere," *Journal of Interdisciplinary Cycle Research* 2 (1971): 317.

20. W. A. Tiller, "A.R.E. Fact Finding Trip to the Soviet Union," *A.R.E. Journal* 7 (1972): 68.
21. I. Swann, *To Kiss Earth Good-Bye* (New York: Hawthorn, 1975).
22. H. Forwald, *Mind, Matter and Gravitation* (New York: Parapsychology Foundation, 1969).
23. J. Taylor, *Superminds* (London: Macmillan, 1975).
24. I. Swann, op. cit.
25. R. Targ and H. Puthoff, "Information Transmission under Conditions of Sensory Shielding," *Nature* 252 (1974): 602.
26. L. Day and G. de la Warr, *Matter in the Making* (London: Vincent Stuart, 1966).
27. L. Day and G. de la Warr, *New Worlds beyond the Atom* (London: Vincent Stuart, 1956).
28. W. A. Tiller, "Radionics, Radiesthesia and Physics" (Paper delivered at Symposium on the Varieties of Healing Experience, Academy of Parapsychology and Medicine, Los Altos, Calif., 1972).
29. Z. V. Harvalik, "Sensitivity Tests on a Dowser Exposed to Artificial D. C. Magnetic Fields," *American Dowser* 13, no. 3 (1973): 85. Ibid. 14, no. 1 (1974): 4.
30. W. A. Tiller and W. Cook, "Psychoenergetic Field Studies Using a Biomechanical Transducer" (Paper delivered at the A.R.E. Medical Symposium on New Horizons in Healing, Phoenix, Ariz., January, 1974).
31. R. Targ and H. Puthoff, op. cit.
32. S. Ostrander and L. Schroeder, *Psychic Discoveries behind the Iron Curtain* (New York: Prentice-Hall, 1970).
33. S. Karagulla, *Breakthrough to Creativity* (Los Angeles: De Vorss, 1967).
34. H. Puthoff and R. Targ, "Psychic Research and Modern Physics," in *Psychic Explorations*, ed. E. D. Mitchell and J. White (New York: G. P. Putnam's Sons, 1974).
35. S. Ostrander and L. Schroeder, op. cit.
36. G. Milne, *The Pyramid Guide* 18 (1975): 5.
37. D. Hawkins and L. Pauling, op. cit.
38. W. A. Tiller, "The Positive and Negative Space-Time Frames as Conjugate Systems" (Paper delivered at the A.R.E. Medical Symposium, Phoenix, Ariz., January, 1975).

11

E. Stanton Maxey

Some Biophysical Aspects of Wholism

Doubt is not a very agreeable state,
but certainty is a ridiculous one.
—François Marie Arouet (Voltaire)

CLAIRVOYANCE, clairaudience, precognition, psychokinesis, telepathy, and poltergeist phenomena seem mysteriously akin to a newly discovered passive volitional control of such involuntary internal processes as limb temperature, blood pressure, heart rate, brain rhythms, and the growth of malignancies.[1,2] Since these various phenomena are elicited within a framework of psychobiophysical processes, doubts have assuredly been evoked pertaining to the laws of physics and chemistry. We perforce must accept ours as presently "not a very agreeable state."

Some Problems of Science

Let us briefly examine the *certain* sciences—the other side of Voltaire's coin. The Greeks of Aristotle's time philosophized in terms of atoms, and since the days of Newton, science has tended to become ever more rapidly structured. Scientific concepts demanded the consistent replication of phenomena by all researchers. An electrical charge of one volt across a resistance of one ohm must inevitably result in an electrical current of one ampere. No exceptions. Science infers that an adequate comprehension of basic particles will permit an explanation of all existence—including life—since multiple and increasingly complex configurations of such basic building blocks can be envisioned.

Within her own self-proclaimed domain, science has developed her problems. She has been unable to even conceptualize an end to the infinity of increasingly diminutive particles, while at the same time, the cost of defining each newly discovered subatomic particle goes up as the particle size decreases. The Brookhaven National Laboratory supported Dr. Raymond Davis in sequestering 100,000 gallons of cleaning fluid a mile deep in an abandoned gold mine—thus was the elusive particle the neutrino discerned. K-mesons, psi particles, muons, and dileptons are among dozens of particles in the presently conquered subatomic family.

Physics has had other problems. Light failed to behave as self-respecting particles (photons) should, and some other theory was needed. Physicist Louis de Broglie filled that gap by approaching atomic structure from a wave-form viewpoint, and science subsequently settled on two convenient ways of viewing matter; particle structure and wave form composition. Subsequently it was demonstrated that electrons (negatively charged particles forming atomic shells) when transiting through crystalline structures also behaved as if moving in waves.[3]

Other physical phenomena continued to evade explanation by either particle or wave and field theory; the problem led to the brilliant field theory of James Clerk Maxwell. Albert Einstein, in commenting on it, noted that—

> after Maxwell they conceived physical reality as represented by continuous fields, not mechanically explicable. . . . This change in the conception of reality is the most profound and fruitful one that has come to physics since the days of Newton.

Presently the modern physicist rides these three conceptualizations with great dexterity, even though they often appear mutually antagonistic. Like circus stunt riders, physicists jump from one concept-horse to another when called upon to explain phenomena for which a single theory is inadequate. This theory-jumping activity has even achieved consensual formalization into the law of complementarity—but physics obligingly admonishes that the purview of this law should be utilized only as a sort of court of last appeal.

Curiously, the religion of physics on the one hand admits that its laws afford no insight into life's origin and on the other affirms that all life's energies must derive from some conglomerated intermix of the particle, wave and field theories. Biology is now menacing physics even as Galileo's pronouncement of the heliocentric solar system disquieted Pope Urban VIII's Roman church. Life particles, life waves and life fields have not been defined by the material sciences, and it is beginning to look as if life will explain physics instead of the other way around; a sort of cart-before-the-horse complementarity. Let us explore this life-particle dialogue a bit further.

Transmutation: An overview

Physics allows that elemental atoms can be transmuted one into another and that the energies exchanged in such reactions are, for the most part, precisely known. Since the discoveries of the Curies the spontaneous decay of radioactive substances has been widely researched, and radioactive decay rates are considered to be not variable—i.e., they are constant like the speed of light. Contrariwise, scientific observations have revealed inconsistencies in radioactive decay (variations in half-life) with modifications of pressure, temperature, chemical state, electric potential, and stress of monomolecular layers.[4] Presumably there is a complementarity here of some sort.

A more difficult enigma appears when the activity of nonradioactive atoms, especially those in which the nucleus of the hydrogen or oxygen atom may form a constituent, are examined in living processes. Living systems, from bacteria through the largest mammals, are now known to have been ubiquitously alchemizing such elemental transformations throughout untold eons and at energy levels that contemporary physics considers impossibly low. Physicists fear for the edifice of their conceptual castles should living systems perform as they do. The story of this yet unrecognized discovery is a fascinating one.

Albrecht von Herzeele wrote "The Origin of Inorganic Substances" over one hundred years ago (1873) after observing that living plants grown in distilled water mysteriously produced potash, phosphorus, magnesium, calcium, and sulfur. His plants seemed able to transmute phosphorus into sulfur, calcium into phosphorus, magnesium into calcium, and nitrogen into potassium.

Professor Pierre Baranger, Director of the Laboratory of Organic Chemistry of the École Polytechnique in Paris, confirmed such alchemical life processes and noted their relationship to light and moon phasing. His language reveals the man:

> I have been teaching chemistry at the École Polytechnique for twenty years, and believe me, the laboratory which I direct is no den of false science. But I have never confused respect for science with the taboos imposed by intellectual conformism. For me, any meticulously performed experiment is a homage to science even if it shocks our ingrained habits. Von Herzeele's experiments were too few to be absolutely convincing. But their results inspired me to control them with all the precaution possible in a modern lab and to repeat them enough times so that they would be irrefutable. That's what I've done. [5]

More recently, Louis Kervran has studied biological transmutations very extensively in France, and Hisatoki Komaki in Japan observed that twenty-four strains of microorganisms alchemize phosphorus. The former suggested the atomic reaction:

$$Na_{23} + O_{16} \text{------} K_{39}. [6]$$

Professor Olivier Costa de Beauregard, Professor of Theoretical Physics, Poincaré Institute, Paris, has shown theoretically how such biological atomic transformations can be accommodated within physics's presently recognized laws, and he further postulates the rate of transformations as being dependent on the neutrino flux. [7]

It is difficult to comprehend how science has for so long avoided worldwide recognition of these biological atomic transmutations, for no discovery is of greater potential relevance to man's well-being. Millions of acres of land might become suitable for various crops were specific alchemical bacteria (capable of creating missing minerals from those found locally in excess) seeded into the humus of the soil. Saline soil might be desalted biologically with needed potash as a by-product. Since some bacteria thrive in radioactive climates (up to 120,000 times beyond human limits), it seems also possible that atomic wastes might be biologically degraded into innocuous elements and, possibly, even into commercially useful chemicals.

The Nature of Man

What about man? Man originates biologically as a unicelled organism within the mother's womb. Darwinian theory postulates a similar phylogenic beginning. Adult man is an extraordinarily complex organism of some 350 trillion cells so affixed to an internal skeleton that great geographic mobility is allowed. Contact with the environment is provided by the specific senses: touch, taste, hearing, sight, and smell. Consciousness—man's awareness of his own biological structure, his environment, and of the fact that he is aware—might be viewed as man's sixth sense. This sixth sense of awareness uniquely distinguishes man from all other life forms on earth. A seventh sense—man's awareness of his own psyche—seems now to have evolved somewhat beyond the budding stage. Psyche means soul. The sciences of psychology, psychiatry, parapsychology, metapsychiatry, and psychotronics were birthed out of man's compelling need to explain his own soul awareness.

Lest we become obsessed with our abundant knowledge, let us immediately confess that we've very distinct limits. Man's biological structure is by weight about 80 percent water in one form or another. What do we know of water? Some water freezes only at $-196°$ F.[8] Chemically pure water after exposure to a 1,000 oersted (formerly gauss) magnetic field effectively dissolves scale from within industrial boilers but only at specific lunar phases.[9] Such magnetically treated water fed to guinea pigs causes them to diurese and then become ill, and their progeny remain undersized through three subsequent generations.[10] When the water is broken up into small particles, the droplets exhibit either positive or negative charges, depending on droplet size. Nobel laureate Linus Pauling proposed a clathrate hydrate structuring which explains many of water's properties, but not all. How may we comprehend man while failing to fully understand the nature of his most abundant constituent chemical?

Let us extend our humility. If science be true, man's function can be explained through a sufficiently complex intermix of the functions of his various specialized cells. Let us consider one of them, say a leuko-cyte. This cell has a negative electrical charge at the nucleus with respect to the cellular protoplasm and cell membrane (cancer cells have deficient charges). It is as if the cell mimics in a micro-microcosmic way the terrestrial electrical surface charge as compared to the ionosphere. Cellular metabolism consumes oxygen in the process of pumping sodium ions; thus we have a high sodium concentration in extracellular spaces and the maintenance of a high potassium level in intracellular fluids (cancer cells have excess intracellular sodium). The result is an ionic electric charge differential at the cell membrane. Indeed, as long ago as 1943, Dr. George Crile, founder of the Cleveland Clinic, stated, ". . . each living cell [is] a tiny electric battery generating its own current by chemical action."[11]

Precisely so. Yet this concept, though now confirmed and expanded by numerous researchers, was largely ignored in his time. Dr. Albert Schweitzer labeled Dr. Max Gerson "a medical genius who walked among us," for the latter observed aberrations of sodium (Na^+) versus potassium (K^+) in cancer versus normal cells and developed a demonstrably effective dietary cancer therapy.[12] Subsequently, laboratory applications of electron spin detectors were used by the Nobelist, Albrecht Szent-Györgyi, to reveal the biological work function of the cellular electron transfer. He concluded, "The fuel of life is the electron or, more exactly, the energy it takes over from photons in photosynthesis; this energy the electron gives up gradually while flowing through the cellular machinery."[13]

If man is composed of individual electrical battery components, cells, the total organism ought also to have electrical characteristics. This too has proven to be the case but, regrettably, knowledge of organismic bioelectrical phenomena remains largely without medical application. Indeed, Dr. H. S. Burr measured various skin potentials in the mid 1930s and correlated abnormal electrical values to cancer of the female reproductive tract with a reported accuracy of 90 percent.[14] In physiological sleep the human skin resistance may suddenly increase by an order of magnitude and the polarity of the head versus the feet may reverse itself. (The terrestrial electric field polarity often reverses at night). Dreaming is accompanied by distinctive electrical brain rhythms and by an associated penile erection. Human electrical fields, like those of trees, were observed to be phase related to the cyclical modulations of the terrestrial electrical field, and this leads us to suspect that Nature mysteriously links all living things through electrical phenomena.[15]

Cyclical planetary configurations accompany sunspots and solar flares,[16] and these in turn govern our terrestrial electrical events; Eureka—man *is* governed by his celestial bodies! Life within the universe is a WHOLISTIC process!

Contemporary Concepts About the Nature of Man

But let us return to earth and note the dawning of a conceptual revolution of the very greatest moment in man's knowledge of himself. Work on biofeedback has sprouted from laboratories throughout all the world as if the hand of God had broadcast the seed. Many findings of this research derive from electrical skin phenomena, and these enigmata are strangely arresting. On occasion the human will can control skin resistance, while contrariwise, the monitoring of skin resistance modulations allows researchers to query the subconscious itself.[17] Often in laboratory settings the skin denotes its knowledge of facts that the conscious mind can in no wise call forth. The point to be made before passing on is that the will, the psyche if you like, seems inextricably bound up in the internal and external electrical qualities of the whole human organism and the entire body's response to outside terrestrial electrical events.

Happy is the union when the very new and the very old find themselves complementing each other. Such now is the case with modern skin resistance detectors and acupuncture.

Acupuncture, rooted some five thousand years back in history, has long postulated some twelve hundred points on the body surface organized variously into between twenty-four and twenty-eight meridians systems. These systems correlate to specific internal organs and their respective homeostasis. Modern volt-ohm meters readily detect these points because of their characteristically lessened resistance. Hiroshi Motoyama noted variations in electrical conductivity at seiketsu points (acupuncture points at the tips of fingers and toes where the various meridians terminate) in health versus disease. He then invented a computerized machine that measures the electrical activity from all fingers and toes in twenty-eight seconds, compares the data against electronically stored normals, and within moments prints out comparative values.[18] Abnormal values appear in red. It is indeed striking to witness this device print red values for the left-lung meridian in patients with known left-lung disease. It is equally fascinating to watch the device print more normal values for the same patient shortly after appropriate acupuncture needle therapy.

What are we to make of it? Are acupuncture points in fact the "nadis" of the aetheric body as proposed by the many ancient but occult Eastern schools of wisdom? Is the physical body actually precipitated or laid down on an aetheric substratum? Are the aetheric meridian systems subservient to a system of multiple chakras—bundles of radiating psychic energy—which, within its own realm, conveys psychic power and perceptivity? Does psychic healing involve an aetheric phenomenon? Is there an aether?

The Aether and Related Concepts

Let us define the term before proceeding: *Aether* is a medium of unusual qualities postulated in the undulatory theory of light as permeating all space and as transmitting transverse waves.

The presence of such a medium was a pressing question of physics at the turn of the twentieth century and it was addressed by the famous Michelson-Morley light interferometer experiments. Because no variation in the speed of light was satisfactorily demonstrated as the earth spun through our solar system, physics decided that there was no such medium. Morley contested the decision and, up until his death, felt that he had demonstrated a variability in the speed of light.[19] Einstein throughout his various brilliant calculations simply affirmed that his conclusions did not require an aether.

Presently, Dr. H. C. Dudley, professor of radiation physics at the University of Illinois Medical Center, has authored many papers equating the aether to an ubiquitous neutrino sea that contemporary science fully recognizes. Energy calculations reveal 10^{19} electron volts per cubic centimeter within this medium, and Professor Dudley warns that energy fluxes of the aether may well explain the otherwise unexplained energy yield variations observed in atomic detonations. His work cautions that man could unwittingly ignite our globe.[20] As we have seen, Professor Olivier Costa de Beauregard suspects that the biological alchemical transmutation phenomena might be influenced by the neutrino sea and therefore by proximity to atomic reactors where the neutrino flux is elevated.[21]

Occult philosophy indicates that aerions are aetheric in nature; therefore let us also define this term: *Aerion* is one, or a group, of atmospheric molecules carrying an unbalanced charge.

Positive aerions are shy one or more electrons and negative aerions carry extra electrons. Aerions are further defined as small, medium, and large, depending on their mobility in an electric field.[22] The processes whereby aerions are formed in the environment are extremely complex; suffice it to say that positive aerions are found concentrated overhead and in the innermost Van Allen belt and that negative aerions are formed naturally within the earth's crust. Solar activity plays heavily upon this complicated phenomenon in many complex ways.

One need not be abstruse in denoting some biological properties of aerions, for they have been extensively researched. Dr. A. P. Krueger for many years studied the effects of aerions and discovered that levels of serotonin (5-HT), a neurotransmitter chemical of the brain, rise when persons breath air rich in positive aerions.[23] Dr. F. G. Sulman at the Hebrew University in Jerusalem has done similar work in connection with adrenal exhaustion.[24] Adverse positive aerion-rich winds (Föehn in Germany, Sharov in Israel, Santana in California) produce headaches, irritability, rhinitis, and exhaustion, which often can be ameliorated by breathing air treated by negative aerion generators. Mouth breathing of air enriched in negative aerions is followed by an elevation of the blood's pH and an increased resistance to surgical shock. The literature on this subject is very extensive and the best research is said to be from Leningrad, in the USSR.

Associated with the complex aerion mechanics, one finds a terrestrial electric field averaging 60–150 volts per square meter.[25] Values up to 3,000 volts per square meter have been recorded. By consensus, when the polarity of the field is positive overhead and negative at the surface, a positive field is said to exist. As previously noted, the field may shift to a negative polarity briefly at night. Because the ionosphere versus the terrestrial surface acts as a resonant cavity in conducting radiowaves, there is a natural frequency, called the Schumann resonance.[26] It peaks at approximately 7.1 and 14 cycles per second (hertz). Much longer cyclical electric field modulations accompany moon phasing. Many studies have revealed that the absence of the normal

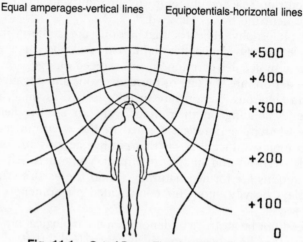

Fig. 11.1   Out-of-Doors Electrical Environment

electric field evokes circadian desynchronization (commonly called jet lag by air travelers) in humans[27] and that in rats the electrolyte changes parallel those experienced by astronauts in space capsules.[28]

Let us see how some of these factors integrate, psychobiophysically speaking. One standing out of doors is subject to his environment, and physics dictates that aerions being propelled within the electrostatic field gradient would flow to the body as lightning to a lightning rod, though not so intensely. Because acupuncture points have a low electrical resistance, the electrical currents derived from traveling aerions must run predominantly through these spots. The currents (amperes), though very low, depend on the intensity of the electric field, the density of aerions, and the dynamic resistance (ohms) of the various acupuncture points. As we have seen, the terrestrial factors evolve from the varying relationship of our earth, sun, and planets—perhaps also some stars—but psychoemotional factors tune the variable resistance of acupoints. The will seemingly influences how man links himself into Nature's forces. The concept is abstruse and we will return to it.

Let us now turn to magnetics, that force that causes a compass to point northward. The average field strength lies between 0.2 and 1.2 oersted, and lines of force, except at the poles and equator, emanate from the surface at about 60°. Smaller units called gammas are em-

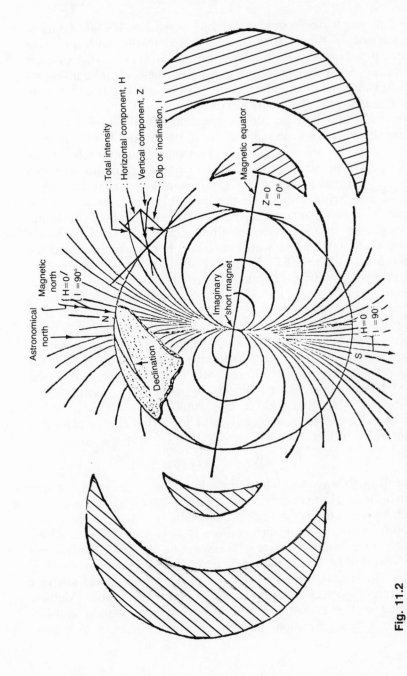

: Total intensity
: Horizontal component, H
: Vertical component, Z
: Dip or inclination, I

Astronomical north

Magnetic north

$H = 0$
$I = 90°$

N

Declination

Imaginary short magnet

Magnetic equator

$Z = 0$
$I = 0°$

$H = 0$
$I = 90°$

S

Fig. 11.2

Schematic diagram illustrating magnetic field produced by an imaginary bar magnet at the Earth's center plus Van Allen zones; inner protons and outer electrons.

191

ployed in much biophysical research; 1 oersted = 100,000 gammas. The strength of the magnetic field varies diurnally, with the lunar month, and seasonally. With solar storms, changes of 500–600 gammas may occur. Such variations in the magnetic field seem strangely related to variations in the precipitation of bismuth chloride,[29] human sedimentation rates,[30] human bleeding tendencies, the incidence of homicides,[31] and biologic atomic transmutations.[32] Low-frequency electromagnetic waves accompany most storm and frontal weather systems, and they are associated with prolonged human reaction times if at 3–5 cycles per second (hertz).[33] The magnetic component of such storm systems may run to 60–100 gammas, but the magnetic component of the Schumann resonance probably never exceeds 0.002 gamma.[34] No living organism is immune to magnetic field effects and the frequency of modulation of these fields. V. N. Mikhailovsky showed that 1,000 gamma waves of 0.01–5 H remarkably altered the human brain rhythm (EEG),[35] and A. P. Dubrov has written an entire book on geomagnetic field effects.[36] Our laboratory found that some subjects' brain rhythms locked into the same frequency as that of applied magnetic waves of 3–13 H at strengths of only 30 gammas.[37] This suggests that the moods of all the earth's peoples may be to some degree controlled by the terrestrial magnetic modulation. G. A. Sergeyev observed that Ninel Kulagina's brain rhythm (EEG) was coupled to the terrestrial resonance (Schumann frequency) at critical moments when she caused objects to move at a distance (psychokinesis).[38] He describes a bioplasmic field (aetheric body?) confirmed by Kirlian photography and feels that the bioplasma is concentrated in the brain. He provides the formula

$$W_1 = W_m/2,$$

where through wave mechanics the will of this gifted person acting through the bioplasma taps a cosmic power source and causes specific objects to move despite any electromagnetic or other shielding. Significantly, Kulagina could not perform if storms were about, which suggests some common factor with respect to the prolonged reaction times observed by König; the magnetic modulation frequency is then adverse. In similar vein, Dr. J. L. Whitton did computer analyses comparing the power spectrum of EEG's of psychic persons (Mathew Manning and others) at rest and during psychic attempts and disconvered a "ramp function" phenomenon in the latter: at that time, most of the energy lay in the lower EEG frequencies.[39] In contrast to Kulagina, Manning produces "exceptional" amounts of phenomena just before thunderstorms.

X-rays are generated when Kulagina moves objects; from the point of view of physics, this indicates that atomic nuclei are to some degree subject to the will. Significantly, Professor Olivier Costa de Beauregard has lectured widely on the Einstein-Podolsky-Rosen paradox of physics and theoretically resolves the enigmata by indicating that atoms of substance avoid the probabilities of chance through responding to the will of the researcher.[40]

Psychic Phenomena and Some Speculations

Having digressed into various related sciences, we may now frame a major question: Are psychic persons—those with telepathic, clairaudient, clairvoyant, and psychokinetic abilities—so gifted because they can at will resonate with a cosmic power? It appears that simultaneous frequency monitoring of brain and terrestrial electromagnetic rhythms is a fertile field for serious psychic research. Science can not for long ignore the Mathew Mannings and Uri Gellers who bend metals by stroking them, the Ninel Kulaginas and the Jan Mertas who move objects by looking at them, the Ted Serios and Ann Gehmans who cause pictures to unexpectedly appear on film and, most importantly, the hundreds of healers who with psychic power relieve their patients' illnesses.

John Pope is a Cherokee shaman.[41] His other, more popular, name fits: the heavens respond with thunder and rain when evoked by Rolling Thunder. Recently he addressed a group of physicians and researchers in Tucson, Arizona, roughly as follows:

> You scientists don't know how those huge stones were put in the big pyramids, but we do. Your doctors practice by a symbolic stick with a couple snakes and wings on it and they don't know what it means. But we know!

Let us accept for now that there is an aether (neutrino sea) and an aetheric body (bioplasmic body) and that mind-over-matter phenomena are transacted via aetheric mechanisms. Is there a corollary

Chakra	Location	Organ affected	Petals	Psycharacteristics
1. Muladhara	Spine base	Adrenals	4	
2. Swadhisthana	Sacral	Gonads	6	
3. Manipura	Solar Plexus	Pancreas	10	Trance { Clairaudience Clairvoyance
4. Anahata	Heart	Thymus	12	
5. Vishudda	Throat	Thyroid	16	
6. Ajna	Forehead	Pituitary	96	
7. Sahasrara	Crown	Pineal	1000	Conscious { Clairvoyance Clairaudience

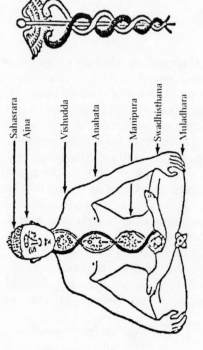

Sahasrara
Ajna
Vishudda
Anahata
Manipura
Swadhisthana
Muladhara

Fig. 11.3

to the physical body's central nervous system, which underlies the aetheric body's function and control?

Serpents in all cultures have symbolized knowledge, and this is equally true within the Judaeo-Christian ethic, wherein a "knowledge of good and evil" was introduced by a serpent. Twin serpents are found entwined in both yogic pictographs and in the hermetic caduceus of the ancient Greeks. According to the tradition of occult wisdom, one of these serpents (the pingala) conveys a positive psychic energy, and its twin (the ida) the negative counterpart. Chakras—bundles of radiating psychic energy—become active as the serpents gradually but progressively uncoil throughout multiple sequential lives; these chakras are pictured as having various numbers of petals (something like lobes of radio energy in modern radar), and they are said to control the various endocrine glands.[42]

When both serpents have fully ascended, their power meets at the crown and circulates back to the base via a central shaft (the sushumna), with the result that all chakras are completely activated: the awakened kundalini.

The petals total 144 + 1000, or, by a Semitic twist, 144,000. St. John the Divine reported of his psychic vision, "And I heard the number of them which were sealed and there were sealed an hundred and forty and four thousand." Coincidence?

World Masters such as the Buddha or the Christ are said to have become omniscient and omnipotent via an evolutionary process of myriad sequential lives.

Lest these arguments be viewed as imaginary flights into improbable Elysian fields, let us remind ourselves that metals are psychically bent and broken; that objects do inexplicably move, appear and disappear; that plants and even atoms respond to gifted individuals' minds; that energy from the various chakras has been electronically registered, and that firm evidence for reincarnation is at hand.[43] In all humility, should we not accept the wisdom of the ancients as at least a working hypothesis? Are not all the pawns of science merely players in life's one game? Is each not potentially a queen? Do not all yield obeisance before one King?

Listen as very ancient echos traverse time's vast reverberating corridors:

> It is true, without falsehood, certain and very real,
> That that which is on high is as that which is below,

And that which is below is as that which is on high,
In order that the miracle of Unity may be perpetual.
—Hermes Trismegistus, *The Emerald Table*

Notes

1. B. Brown, *New Mind, New Body* (New York: Harper and Row, 1974).
2. O. Carl Simonton, "The Role of the Mind in Cancer Therapy" (Paper delivered at the First National Congress on Integrative Health, Tucson, Ariz., October, 1975).
3. Dr. Clinton J. Davidson was awarded the Nobel Prize for ". . . his discovery of the Jekyll-Hyde quality of the electron, which . . . showed that the entire realm of physical nature has a dual personality."
4. H. C. Dudley, "Is There an Ether?" *Industrial Research* 16 (November, 1974) 41–46.
5. P. Tompkins and C. Bird, *The Secret Life of Plants* (New York: Harper and Row, 1973).
6. L. C. Kervran, *Biological Transmutations* (Binghamton, N.Y.: Swan House, 1972).
7. L. C. Kervran, *Transmutations Biologiques à Faible Energie* (Paris: Maloine, 1975).
8. B. D. Allan and R. L. Norman, "The Characterization of Liquids in Contact with High Surface Area Materials" (Paper presented at the New York Academy of Sciences International Conference on Physics—Chemical State of Ions and Water in Living Tissues and Model Systems, 1972).
9. G. Piccardi, "Phénomènes Astrophysiques et Événements Terrestres" (Paper delivered at conference at Pais de la Découverte, 1959).
10. A. S. Pressman, *Electromagnetic Fields and Life* (New York: Plenum, 1970).
11. G. Crile, quoted by Langstone Day and George Delawarr in *New Worlds Beyond the Atom* (London: Vincent Stuart, 1956).
12. M. Gerson, *A Cancer Therapy, Results of Fifty Cases* 1(New York: Dura Books, 1958).
13. A. Szent-György, *Bioelectronics: A Study in Cellular Regulations, Defense and Cancer* (New York: Academy Press, 1968).
14. H. S. Burr, "Biological Organization and the Cancer Problem," *Yale Journal of Biology and Medicine* 12 (1940): 277–282.
15. L. J. Ravitz, "Electrodynamic Field Theory in Psychiatry," *Southern Medical Journal* 46 (1953): 650–60.

16. H. P. Sleeper, *Planetary Resonances, Bi-Stable Oscillation Modes, and Solar Activity Cycles* (NASA Contractor Report CR-2035, 1972).

17. B. Brown, op. cit.

18. H. Motoyama, *Chakra, Nadi of Yoga and Meridians, Points of Acupuncture* (Tokyo: Institute of Religious Psychology, 1972).

19. L. E. Swenson, Jr., *The Ethereal Aether* (Austin: The University of Texas Press, 1972).

20. H. C. Dudley, op. cit.

21. L. C. Kervran, *Transmutations Biologiques*.

22. S. W. Tromp, *Psychical Physics* (New York: Elsevier, 1949): 243.

23. A. P. Krueger, "Air Ion Action on Animals and Man," in *Bioclimatology, Biometeorology and Aerion Therapy*, ed. R. Gaultierotti et al. (Milan: Erba Foundation, 1968).

24. F. G. Sulman, Y. Pfeifer, and E. Superstine, "Adrenal Medullary Exhaustion from Tropical Winds and Its Management," *Israel Journal of Medical Science* 9 (1973): 1022–27.

25. S. W. Tromp, *Physical Physics* (New York: Elsevier, 1949).

26. C. Polk and F. Fitchen, "Schumann Resonance of the Earth-Ionosphere Cavity: Extremely Low Frequency Reception at Kingston, R.I.," *Journal of Research, National Bureau of Standards* 65 (1962): 313–18.

27. R. Wever, "Human Circadian Rhythms under the Influence of Weak Electric Fields and the Different Aspects of These Studies," *International Journal of Biometeorology:* 17 (1973): 227–32.

28. S. Lang, "Influences of an Electric Field of 10 Hz on the Metabolism of Lipids and the Water Electrolyte Balance" (Paper delivered at the Seventh International Biometeorological Congress, University of Maryland, College Parker, August, 1975).

29. G. Piccardi, op. cit.

30. S. W. Tromp, *Medical Biometeorology* (New York: Elsevier, 1973): 318.

31. A. L. Leiber, "Homicides and the Lunar Cycle: Towards a Theory of Lunar Influence on Human Emotional Disturbance," *American Journal of Psychiatry* 129 (1972): 69–73.

32. Rudolf Hauscha, *The Nature of Substance* (London: Vincent Stuart, 1966).

33. H. König, "Biological Effects of Extremely Low Frequency Electrical Phenomena in the Atmosphere," *Journal of Interdisciplinary Cycle Research* 12 (1971): 317–23.

34. C. Polk and F. Fitchen, op. cit.

35. V. N. Mikhailovsky et al., *Toward the Understanding of Weak Magnetic Fields* (Academy of Science USSR, Series B-s-929, 1969).

36. A. P. Dubrov, *The Geomagnetic Field and Life* (Translation No K-5533, Translated April 1975, Headquarters, Department of the Army, Office of Assistant Chief of Staff for Intelligence, Washington, D.C.).

37. E. S. Maxey, "Critical Aspects of Human Versus Terrestrial Electromagnetic Symbiosis" (Paper delivered to the International Union of Radio Science, Boulder, Colo., October, 1975).

38. G. A. Sergeyev, "KNS Phenomenon" (Paper delivered at the Symposium of Psychotronics, Prague, Czechoslovakia, 1970).

39. J. L. Whitton, "Ramp Functions in EEG Power Spectra During Actual or Attempted Paranormal Events," *Journal of New Horizons Research Foundation* 1 (1974): 174–82.

40. O. Costa de Beauregard, *Time Symmetry and Interpretation of Quantum Mechanics Foundation of Physics* (New York: Plenum, in press).

41. D. Boyd, *Rolling Thunder: A Personal Exploration into the Secret Healing Powers of an American Indian Medicine Man* (New York: Random House, 1974).

42. A. A. Bailey, *Esoteric Psychology* (New York: Lucis, 1936).

43. I. Stevenson, *Twenty Cases Suggestive of Reincarnation* (New York: American Society for Psychical Research, 1966).

12

Bernard R. Grad

Some Biological Effects of the Laying on of Hands and Their Implications

Background

The practice of the conventional medicine of modern times has been dominant in the Western world only during the last two centuries, i.e., for less than five percent of the time of recorded history. Conventional medicine is based on observations visible to the ordinary senses. The data so obtained are organized in ways acceptable to the intellect. This type of medicine has the natural sciences of physics, chemistry, and biology as its basis; all are inherently reductionist and mechanistically materialistic. Doctor and patient are clearly separated, with the doctor as the observer and the patient as the object. Conventional medicine claims Hippocrates as its father; however, its real growth began in the sixteenth century with the epoch-making discoveries of Vesalius in anatomy.

For the previous ninety-five percent of recorded history, healing had a magico-religious basis that was wholistic in outlook. Healing leaned more heavily on intuitions, feelings, and perceptions arising from within than it did on the observations of the ordinary senses directed outwards. The healer had to overcome the illness by working on the "inner being" of the patient in this type of medicine, and therefore there was a close rapport between healer and patient. As has the conventional medicine of our own time, traditional medicine has undergone a development, and some aspects of it are operative within the framework of present-day medicine, viz., the dynamic psychiatry of Freud, Jung, Adler, and others.

Early Beginnings

The laying on of hands (LH) was always an important part of traditional medicine and, indeed, there is evidence that it was practiced by Stone Age man about 15,000 B.C. Thus, in a cave called the 'The Three Brothers' in the Pyrenees, there exists a drawing depicting a shaman doing LH. Among the Hebrews, many millenia later, LH was used by the dying Isaac to bless his son Jacob, and by Moses to pass spiritual authority to Joshua. Rabbis still bless by LH.

In the British Museum there is a bas-relief taken from a tomb in Thebes, showing the subject sitting down while, at a short distance from him, a man is standing with hand uplifted, evidently about to make a "pass" over his patient. The goddess Isis, on the Zodiac on her temple at Benderah, is represented as making the same "passes." According to the Ebers Papyrus, medical treatment prior to 1552 B.C. included LH on the head of the patient.

In Greece, the value of LH treatment was known for a long time. Aristophanes saw it being done in Athens about four centuries before the birth of Jesus. It played a part in the cures of the Asklepian temples where a blind man's sight and a barren woman's fertility were restored by the healing hand of the god Asklepios. This experience was attested to in the testimonials left at the temples and by allusions in the literature.

Healing and the Ministry

Many of the healings of Jesus reported in the New Testament were done by LH, which was subsequently carried on by the Christian church, which combined it with the use of water (holy water) and oil (the Office of Unction). This traditional method of healing was continued for many centuries by the Christian churches because, from the beginning, healing was considered as much a part of Christian work as preaching and administering the sacraments. Through the centuries, the healing ministry of the Church declined very considerably. The healing ministry, however, continued to be practiced as the Royal Touch, whereby the kings of several European countries appar-

ently cured scrofula by LH. In England, the practice began with
Edward the Confessor and lasted for seven centuries until it died with
the skeptical William IV. At the same time, inquisitive men such as
Paracelsus, Gul Maxwell, van Helmont, and others continued to test
and inquire about the effects of LH; a peak of interest was eventually
reached with Mesmer in the last quarter of the eighteenth century.

Mesmer Propounds Fluidum

In 1775, Father Johann Joseph Gassner, a modest country priest,
had achieved fame in Wurtemberg as a healer by trial exorcism, which
he conducted by first telling his patient that faith in Jesus was an
essential prerequisite for healing. *However, Mesmer demonstrated at
that time that he could achieve the same results* by means involving,
not faith in Jesus, *but a universal energy that he called Fluidum.*

Mesmer claimed that the Fluidum was a subtle physical fluid that
filled the universe and was the connecting medium between people
and other living things, and between these, the earth and the heavenly
bodies. He also stated that disease resulted from the distortions in the
distribution of this fluid in the body and that health was restored when
the equilibrium was reestablished. With the help of certain techniques
(of which LH was one), this fluid could be channeled to other persons.
According to Mesmer, every human being possesses a certain amount
of this fluid: Gassner possessed it to a very high degree, Mesmer had a
somewhat lesser amount, and the sick have it less than the healthy.
The idea of a universal energy was by no means confined to the West;
the Chinese "chi," the Indian "prana," and the Polynesian "mana"
are impersonal energy of this kind, present in the atmosphere and in
living things.

Fluidum Put to the Test

In 1784, the king of France appointed a commission of inquiry
consisting of members of the Academie des Sciences, the Academie de
Medecine and the Societe Royale. Best known among the commissioners were the chemist Lavoisier, the astronomer Bailly, the physician Guilotin and the American statesman-scientist Benjamin
Franklin. They devised a series of experiments to test the existence of
the magnetic fluid, none of which concerned its medical effects. They
concluded that the Fluidum did not exist and that its medical effects,

which they did not deny, were due to "sensitive excitement, imagination and imitation." One of the commissioners, de Jussieu, disassociated himself from his colleagues and suggested that there probably was an unknown efficient agent at work.[1]

From that time on, Mesmer's personal stock declined, although he had in fact made several important discoveries, many of which were only to be rediscovered later. For example, he discovered the importance of rapport between patient and therapist. Freud later rediscovered it in the form of the transference, but Freud's real contribution here was in utilizing it as a tool of therapy, along with the notion of resistance. Mesmer also discovered the importance of evoking a crisis in the patient in order to effect a cure. Later, Freud strove to uncover in his neurotic patients the specific psychic traumatic event that he believed to be the root cause of their illness and, having achieved this first by hypnosis and later by his free-association technique, attempted to get his patients to relive emotionally the traumatic event. Freud's recognition of the importance of catharsis followed upon Mesmer's experience with the crisis in his patients, though there were marked differences in their techniques for provoking the crisis-catharsis.

Mesmerism Differentiated from Hypnotism

The question of whether mesmerism is the same as hypnotism or different from it needs to be discussed. Certainly, in the minds of most people, including physicians, these two terms are used interchangeably. Yet there are essential differences between the two. Mesmer himself believed that touching the patient played a central role in a cure by his method. This belief can be seen by the motto he gave to his society: *Loge de L'Harmonie*, "Go forth, touch, and cure." His method involved essentially LH.

The identity between mesmerism and hypnotism had long been considered settled by medical organizations, but recently the problem was again raised because of the findings of a series of experiments designed to test the effects of the laying on of hands on animals and plants. The laying on of hands is a biblical expression and is an essential part of what later came to be called mesmerism. As it turned out, these studies were also a critical test of Mesmer's "fluid" or "energy" theory.

Contemporary Experimentation

At the present time, the words *mesmerism* and *hypnotism* are used interchangeably. Thus, the American College Encyclopedic Dictionary (1957) defines mesmerism as "hypnotism" and hypnosis is defined as "a condition or state allied to normal sleep which can be artificially produced and is characterized by marked susceptibility to suggestion."[6] Similarly, the same attitude exists both in the popular mind and amongst professionals at the present time. Thus, Tomlinson and Perret refer to mesmeric sleep as being the same as hypnotism in the article on the history of mesmerism in New Orleans.[3] Even relatively informed biographers of Mesmer, like Frank Podmore[4], and such experienced parapsychologists as E. J. Dingwall[5] rejected the idea that the therapeutic effects of mesmerism were due to a "radiation" coming from the mesmerist (as Mesmer himself claimed), but believed rather "that it was the imagination of the patient himself which was largely responsible for the cures effected," thus in essence equating mesmerism and hypnotism.[4,5] The psychiatrist Ehrenwald who had an interest in the paranormal, carried on the process by praising Braid for denying the existence of a life force in mesmeric phenomena,[6] but Braid's only true claim to fame is for coining the word *hypnotism*. The phenomenon itself was actually discovered decades earlier. Most biographies about Mesmer show an astonishing lack of comprehension of mesmerism. However, recent books about Mesmer by Eden and Wyckoff are more to the point.[7,8]

As early as fifteen years ago, a series of experiments was begun to see whether animals and plants could respond in biologically recognizable ways to the laying on of hands by a man (OE) who claimed considerable success with this ancient method of healing. Mice were selected for the animal studies because of their convenience in handling, ease of maintenance, and relatively low cost: numbers could be sufficient for the accumulation of data for statistical analysis. The plants used in these investigations were barley seeds.

To expose the animals to the treatment by LH, a galvanized iron container resembling an ice-cube tray was devised. The container was divided into compartments, each large enough to contain a mouse comfortably. The size of the treatment tray was adjusted to the size of the healer's hands, and as a result about nine mice could be treated simultaneously. The trays were covered with a fine galvanized wire mesh to prevent the animals from escaping. LH treatment involved placing the cage between the healer's hands, one hand on top of the cage and the other on the bottom; all the mice were covered without the hands touching the mice. Treatment was for fifteen minutes, twice daily, five days a week.

Before beginning the actual experiment, and even before the animals were divided into control and treated groups, the mice were accustomed to the treatment trays by placing them there for an hour a day for one or two weeks. The mice were gently stroked for about a minute before putting them into the treatment trays as a further effort to overcome their nervousness and restlessness and to render them calm. This pretreatment stroking or gentling was stopped when the mice were divided into control and treated groups.

When the LH treatment was begun, both treated and control mice were removed from the cages in which they had been housed and placed in identical trays for the same length of time. The control animals, which received no treatment from the healer, were divided into three groups: (1) some received no treatment at all; (2) some were warmed by insulated electrothermal heating tapes, adjusted to deliver the same amount of heat at the same rate as that produced by the warmth of OE's hands, as determined previously by temperature measurements; and (3) some received LH treatment from people who made no special claim to any gift of healing.

Two types of experiments conducted on the mice will be detailed in this chapter: (1) those involved in studying the effect on goiter and (2) those concerned with the effect on the healing of skin wounds.

The Effect of LH on Goiter in Mice

A series of experiments was conducted to test the effect of LH treatment on goiters produced in mice by feeding them a diet deficient in iodine and dissolving goitrogen and thiouracil in their drinking water. Three groups of mice were placed on this regimen. One group was removed from the cages in which they had been housed and placed in identical trays for the same length of time as the other two groups, without treatment; the second group was heated by tapes as described in the previous experiment; and the third group received LH treatment. This experiment lasted forty days. OE provided the LH treatment during the first twenty days; for the last twenty days, the mice were treated by JB, who was shown to have effects similar to OE's on plants and animals.

The outcome of the experiment was that, while all three groups showed an increase in thyroid size during the forty-day experimental period, *the rate of increase of the LH-treated groups was significantly slower* than that of the two control groups. The heated group showed no significantly different rate of goiter development than did the un-heated controls.

Another experiment involved a treated group that received the LH treatment indirectly—by placing in the cages of the treated mice wool and cotton cuttings that had been held in OE's hands for fifteen minutes, once on the first day of the experiment and twice again during the next few weeks. The duration of the entire experiment was six weeks. Similar cuttings that had not been held in the hands of any person were placed in the cages of the control mice. The cuttings were kept in the cages for an hour in the morning and another hour in the late afternoon, and always the mice, both treated and control, were found sitting on the cuttings at the end of the treatment period. The results were the same as described in the previous experiment: the rate of development of goiter was significantly inhibited by the treated cuttings. Further details of these experiments have been described elsewhere.[9]

The Effect of LH on Wound Healing in Mice

A series of experiments involving LH was also undertaken to see what effect it might have on the healing of skin wounds in mice. To this end, mice were anesthetized and shaven on the back, and equivalent-sized pieces of full skin were removed from each animal. The size of each wound was measured by placing over it a piece of transparent plastic on which the wound outline was traced with a grease pencil. These outlines were copied onto pieces of paper, and the paper "wounds" were cut out and weighed on a sensitive balance. Measurements were made immediately after wounding and on the first, eleventh and fourteenth days after wounding. Statistical analysis of the weights of the paper projections of the wounds revealed that the wounds treated by OE healed at a significantly faster rate than those of the two control groups.[10]

Following two preliminary experiments, a more elaborate double-blind experiment involving a very large number of mice was conducted in collaboration with Drs. E. J. Cadoret and G. I. Paul of the University of Manitoba. The results of this large experiment were essentially the same as the earlier ones: wound healing in mice was significantly accelerated by LH treatment by OE. [11]

The Effect of LH on the Growth of Plants

Barley seeds implanted in soil in peat pots were used for these studies. As in the case of the goiter studies in mice, for LH treatment to be effective the organism did not have to be treated directly. In the case of plants, LH treatment of the solutions used for the first watering was all that was necessary for significant acceleration of growth. Subsequent waterings did not have to be treated by LH.

The plant experiments went through several stages of development. In the first series of experiments, the solution was placed in an open beaker and held between OE's hands for fifteen minutes. [12] In the second series, the solution was treated while in reagent bottles closed with ground glass stoppers, [13] and in the third series, sterile solutions were treated in sealed bottles. [14] In all three types of experiments, plants treated with water that had been "magnetized" by LH grew significantly faster and/or more abundantly.

In the study involving treatment of solutions in sealed bottles, *the emotional state of a person at the time of the treatment* of the solutions *was shown to be of crucial importance* in determining what effect such solutions would have on the growth of barley seeds. The study involved four groups of plants: one group watered by a solution treated by a person who had a "green thumb," two groups treated by solutions held by persons who had been psychiatrically diagnosed as suffering from a depression, and a fourth group watered by a solution that had not been treated by anyone; it served as the control group. The outcome revealed that the plants watered by the solution treated by the person with the "green thumb" grew better than those watered with the three other solutions. Of some interest was the finding that *the plants watered by the solution of one of the depressed persons* grew the slowest of all. (He was diagnosed as suffering from a psychotic depression and was hospitalized full-time; the other depressed patient was diagnosed as suffering from a neurotic depression requiring only visits to the hospital during the day.)

Animal Magnetism vs. Hypnotism

Like LH, hypnotism is an ancient practice that was rediscovered. In 1784, a disciple of Mesmer's, the Marquis Amand Marie Jacques Chastenet de Puységur, attempted to "magnetize" one of his first patients, Victor Race, who readily fell into a trance.[15] Victor did not have any convulsions, so often observed in Mesmer's patients, and in addition, although he was in a trance, he seemed far more alert and more intelligent than in the waking state. Puységur obtained similar effects with other patients.

State of Healer

Mesmer claimed the results obtained by his method were due to the passage of an energy from the healer (magnetiser) to the patient. He makes no mention of need for the healer to exert his will over the patient, as was the case with Puységur, who claimed the necessity to "believe and want."[16] However, as shown by the experiments mentioned above, the therapeutic effectiveness of Mesmer's technique was dependent on some characteristics of the person who carried out the technique. A talent or gift would certainly seem to be involved, and the plant experiment points out the necessity of being in the right frame of mind. Moreover, in these experiments neither OE or JB exerted his will while treating the mice. Nor did they attempt to "concentrate," for it was possible to have a normal conversation with them during the LH treatment of the animals. *Apparently, the passage of the energy from OE or JB to the animal or plant was a natural process that did not involve the will,* as hypnotism does.[17]

In the human situation, the transfer of energy to the patient in mesmerism therefore appears to be a function of the mesmerist's physical and emotional state and not directly of his will or any mental exertion. That is, *success in healing by LH would appear to depend on a certain way of bodily functioning, not yet clearly understood, but involving a certain awareness by the healer of his own bodily energy and the energy around him coupled with a certain way of utilizing that energy.* For example, in those who are able to produce some therapeutic effects by LH, it is likely that the therapeutic situation itself is such as to provoke the streaming of a greater than normal amount of energy down the hands of the healer and thence to the patient, where it can do its work of healing. A critical part of the psychological attitude of the healer is that he be in such a frame of mind that he can receive the energy from a still more powerful energy source—that is, from the atmosphere, according to Mesmer, or from God, according to religion. That is, *the chain of energy flow is from God (atmosphere) to healer to patient, and for the chain to be complete the patient must be open to the healer while the latter must be open to the higher energy source.*

The emotional state of the healer may be decisive in determining whether the outcome for the patient is favorable or unfavorable. Not only are psychological and physical factors involved, but as with any talent, *sociological factors may in fact determine whether or not such an ability will surface to consciousness.*

The *plant experiments* previously reported, involving a person with a "green thumb" and two depressed patients, *revealed that there is a correlation between the qualitative effect produced by the energy transferred by LH and the emotional state of the person "magnetizing" the water.*[18]

LH and Prayer

When LH is not associated with mesmerism, it is associated in the public mind with prayer. This association is due to the fact that much of the healing done by Jesus was by LH. The question as to whether prayer itself is effective in helping sick people recover more rapidly was first tested scientifically by Galton in 1883.[19] Since that time, very few studies in this field have been published, and the findings of those done were not conclusive.[20,21] Of course, the healings at Lourdes have received a great deal of attention.[22]

Although LH is usually associated with prayer, both OE and JB did not pray while practicing LH in the plant and animal studies reported above, nor did they seek to influence the outcome of the results by prayer. However, both were in a positive frame of mind during the LH treatment, and both do have a belief in a Supreme Power.

In one of the plant studies, it was shown that there was a decreased transmission of the LH-treated solution as compared with controls.[23] The implication of this finding is that the internuclear distance between the oxygen and hydrogen atoms had probably been increased by the LH treatment and possibly also the water molecule had been further ionized with a larger charge at one end. This together with the increased internuclear distance should result in an altered dipole moment of the molecule. Thus, either the ionic properties or the dipole moment of a significant number of water molecules in the LH-treated solutions was changed. This process occurred as a result of the transfer of energy to the solution by the subject holding the bottle during the LH treatment.

Robert N. Miller also showed that LH treatment by other subjects lowered the surface tension of water.[24] Miller, Reinhart, and Kern also reported that the healer OW produced anomalous wave forms when she held her hands on either side of a diffusion cloud chamber. Normally, the type of perturbations that appear in the cloud chamber are vapor trails due to cosmic rays, not wave motions. Yet when OW placed her hands on either side of the cloud chamber, a wave motion appeared parallel to the position of her hands. When she positioned her hands at right angles to the first position, the direction of the wave motion also changed so as to continue to be parallel to the position of the hands.[25]

The findings reported here support Mesmer's claim that a fluid (energy) can pass from therapist to patient during the LH treatment, and indeed it is quite possible that this is also true in the case of hypnotism. This possibility is suggested by a number of experiments attempting to influence the outcome of certain biological phenomena by mental concentration, that is, by the influence of the will. These included the inhibition of tumor growth in mice and of fungal growth in petri dish culture[26,27] and the hastening of the resuscitation of anesthetized mice.[28] Also, in this regard, Miller demonstrated that two well-known healers (AW and OW) were able to cause an 830 percent increase in the growth rate of rye grass from a distance of 600 miles by focusing their attention on the plant and willing its accelerated growth.[29]

Thus, it would appear that there is a transfer of energy from the therapist to the patient in both LH and hypnotism. However, from observation of both processes, *it is speculated that the critical difference between the two is that in hypnotism, the energy that is transferred to the patient or subject originates within the hypnotist himself, while during the process of LH, the therapist comes in contact with a source of energy from outside and allows his or her physical body to act as a medium or transformer through which the energy passes to the patient.* Further study of this phenomenon is obviously required.

Notes

1. Later proponents of a vital energy, such as Karl von Reichenbach and Wilhelm Reich, who, more than anyone else, extended our knowledge of life energy, experienced the same rejection as did Mesmer. However, Mesmer was allowed to die at home in his eighties, but Reich died in prison at the age of sixty. Never again in the hundred and seventy-five years between Mesmer and Reich was the idea of a vital energy taken as seriously by so many men of intellect as was the case in Mesmer's time, and never since that time has it come so close to entering the body of science.

2. *The American College Encyclopedic Dictionary*, *s. v.* "Mesmerism."

3. Wallace K. Tomlinson and J. John Perret, "Mesmerism in New Orleans (1845–1861)," *American Journal of Psychiatry*, 13 (1974): 1402–04.

4. Frank Podmore, *From Mesmer to Christian Science: A Short History of Mental Healing* (New Hyde Park, N.Y.: University Books, 1963).

5. Eric J. Dingwall, introduction to *From Mesmer to Christian Science*.

6. Jan Ehrenwald, *From Medicine Man to Freud* (New York: Dell, 1956): 281.

7. Jerome Eden, *Animal Magnetism and the Life Energy* (Hicksville, N.Y.: Exposition Press, 1974).

8. James Wyckoff, *Franz Anton Mesmer: Between God and Devil* (Englewood Cliffs, N.J.: Prentice-Hall, 1975).

9. Bernard R. Grad, "The Biological Effects of the 'Laying on of Hands' on Animals and Plants: Implications for Biology," in *Parapsychology: Its Relation to Physics, Biology, Psychology, and Psychiatry*, ed. Gertrude R. Schreidler (Metuchen, N.J.: Scarecrow, 1967).

10. Bernard R. Grad, "Some Biological Effects of the 'Laying on of Hands': A Review of Experiments with Animals and Plants," *Journal of the American Society for Psychical Research* 59 (April, 1965): 95–127.

11. Bernard R. Grad, Remi J. Cadoret, and G. I. Paul, "An Unorthodox Method of Treatment on Wound Healing in Mice," *International Journal of Parapsychology* 3 (Spring, 1961): 5–24.

12. Bernard R. Grad, "A Telekinetic Effect on Plant Growth," *International Journal of Parapsychology* 5 (Spring, 1963): 117–33.

13. Bernard R. Grad, "A Telekinetic Effect on Plant Growth, II. Experiments Involving Treatment of Saline in Stoppered Bottles," *International Journal of Parapsychology* 6 (Autumn, 1964): 473–98.

14. Bernard R. Grad, "The 'Laying on of Hands': Implications for Psy-

chotherapy, Gentling and the Placebo Effect," *Journal of the American Society for Psychical Research*, 61 (October, 1967): 286–305.

15. Henri F. Ellenberger, "Mesmer and Puységur: From Magnetism to Hypnotism," *The Psychoanalytic Review*, 52 (1965): 137–53.
16. Ibid.
17. Hypnotism was known by a series of names, including the perfect crisis, artificial somnambulism, and finally, hypnotism. At the time of his discovery and later, Puységur thought that Victor's perfect crisis was the same phenomenon that Mesmer obtained in his patients, except that the perfect crisis involved a loss of consciousness and the absence of convulsions. That is, mesmerism and hypnotism were confused from the moment the latter was discovered, even though the discoverer himself saw that there were differences. This confusion was further confounded when the entranced Victor told Puységur that the main agent in hypnotism, now confused with mesmerism, was the influence of the will of one person over another, and not the transfer of a fluid as Mesmer claimed. It would appear that in Puységur's technique, at least, exertion of the human will was indeed important, for instead of proclaiming Mesmer's slogan, "Go forth, touch and heal," he advocated, "Believe and want." In the usual conditions under which the patient encounters the therapist, the relationship between the two readily lends itself to the imposition of the will of the therapist over that of the patient, and this must have been doubly true in the case of Puységur and Victor: the latter's family had served Puységur's for several generations. However, the exertion of the will was far less likely in the case of the nonaristocratic Mesmer treating aristocrats.
18. Bernard R. Grad, "The 'Laying on of Hands' "
19. F. Galton, *Inquiries in the Human Faculty and Its Development* (London: Macmillan, 1883): 277–94.
20. C. R. B. Joyce and R. M. C. Welldon, "The Objective Efficacy of Prayer: A Double Blind Clinical Trial," *Journal of Chronic Disease* 18 (1966): 367–77.
21. P. J. Collipp, "The Efficacy of Prayer: A Triple Blind Study," *Medical Times* 97 (1969) 201–4.
22. François Lauret and Henri Boni, *Modern Miraculous Cures: A Documented Account of Miracles and Medicine in the 20th Century*, trans. A. T. MacQueen and John C. Barry (New York: Farrar, Straus and Cudahy, 1957).
23. Bernard R. Grad, "Telekenetic Effect on Plant Growth, II."
24. Robert N. Miller, personal communication.
25. Robert N. Miller, P. B. Reinhart, and A. Kern, "Scientists Register Thought Energy," *Science of Mind* (July, 1974): 12–16.

26. G. H. Elguin, "Psychokinesis in Experimental Tumorigenesis," *Journal of Parapsychology*, 30 (1966): 220 (abstract).
27. J. Barry, "General and Comparative Study of the Psychokinetic Effect on a Fungus Culture," *Journal of Parapsychology* 32 (1968): 237–43.
28. G. Watkins and A. M. Watkins, "Possible PK Influence on the Resuscitation of Anaesthetized Mice," *Journal of Parapsychology* 35 (1971): 257–72.
29. R. Miller, "The Effect of Thought Upon the Growth Rate of Remotely Located Plants," *Journal of Pastoral Counseling* 6 (1971–72): 61–63.

13

Morton T. Kelsey

Faith: Its Function in the Wholistic Healing Process

FROM EARLIEST TIMES, healing and faith have been interrelated. Whenever an individual was sick, he or she sought out either the temple with its priesthood and sacrifices or the religious person, the shaman, who used his many rites and ceremonies to facilitate health. Indeed, to Western observers the shaman was seen so fully as physician that he was often called the medicine man or witch doctor. One of the reasons for the ancient Hebrew rejection of medicine was simply that most healers or physicians were associated in some way with the pagan temple and its cults and were thus "contaminated."

This ancient connection between religion, faith, and healing would be little more than an interesting piece of historical data were it not for the recent recognition on the part of many physicians that faith is still a crucially important factor in the healing process. When treating the whole person, one becomes more and more aware that the basic attitudes of the individual toward the doctor, the treatment, and the world in general will influence the course of the sickness. However, *the basic place of faith is seldom treated directly in medical education or in professional discussions within the medical community.*

In order to understand this somewhat elusive subject, let us first of all look at some recent written statements by physicians concerning the place of faith in the healing process. Then let us analyze the word *faith* so that we can understand the nature of the quality of life under discussion. Let us then take a quick look at the history of faith and healing so we can understand the strange separation that has taken

213

place between them in Western culture from the twelfth century until recently.

We will conclude by looking at the emotions that seem most antagonistic to faith and make some suggestions for dealing with these obstacles to facilitating the healing creativity of faith.

Faith, Doctors, and Science

It was, of course, the monumental work of Flanders Dunbar that broke open the materialistic medical point of view that reigned supreme in the nineteenth and early twentieth centuries. In 1935, Dr. Dunbar collected a large number of the papers written up to her time in her book *Emotions and Bodily Changes*. Citing reference after reference from scholarly journals, she gives a great deal of evidence to support the satire of current medicine by the British physician F. G. Crookshank. She quotes this telling passage from his article in the *British Journal of Medical Psychology*:

> I often wonder that some hardboiled and orthodox clinician does not describe emotional weeping as a "new disease," calling it paroxysmal lachrymation, and suggesting treatment by belladonna, astringent local applications, avoidance of sexual excess, tea, tobacco and alcohol, and a salt-free diet with the restriction of fluid intake, proceeding in the event of failure to early removal of the tear glands.[1]

The impact of Dr. Dunbar's work was enormous. She expressed the changing spirit of the times and did so with impeccable scholarship and sensitive understanding. Within four years, the journal *Psychosomatic Medicine* was founded. Edward Weiss and O. Spurgeon English produced their textbook, *Psychosomatic Medicine: The Clinical Application of Psychopathology to General Medical Problems*, which has since gone through many editions.[2] More and more, physicians have noted and recorded the importance of patients' attitudes. In my book *Healing and Christianity*, I have discussed at some length the changing attitude toward medicine initiated by Dr. Dunbar.[3]

Once it was understood that emotions could affect the body, it was not long before one's faith was seen as important in maintaining health. Only the most dogmatic behaviorist would maintain that the patient's basic attitude of trust and confidence had no effect upon his emotions. One of the finest statements of the connection between healing and faith was written by Johns Hopkins psychiatrist Jerome Frank in his provocative book, *Persuasion and Healing*. He concluded his study with these words:

> The question of how far a physician should go to meet a patient's expectations is a thorny one. Obviously he cannot use methods in which he himself does not believe. Moreover, reliance on the healing power of faith, if it led to neglect of proper diagnostic or treatment procedures, would clearly be irresponsible. On the other hand, faith may be a specific antidote for certain emotions such as fear or discouragement, which may constitute the essence of a patient's illness. For such patients, the mobilization of expectant trust by whatever means may be as much an etiological remedy as penicillin for pneumonia.[4]

The most recent and one of the most delightfully written discussions of faith and healing is Wimpole Street British psychiatrist R. Alan McGlashan's *Gravity and Levity*, published in 1976. In a chapter entitled Concerning Humbug, he writes,

> It is in fact very difficult to cure anybody of anything by means of a remedy in which you yourself have no faith. The successful doctor, no less than the successful "quack" is the man who is really convinced he has got something. Every medical man has had experiences of achieving impressive results with a certain drug, so long as he believes in it himself. As soon as he has some failures and begins to doubt its remedial powers, the results on patients tail off, and in a few months the "wonder drug" is, as far as that practitioner is concerned, discarded and forgotten.

He goes on to say that the efficacy of the treatment applies not only to drugs,

> but also more alarmingly, to surgical operations. It is within the memory of many of us that a child who had several attacks of sore throat would almost automatically have its tonsils and adenoids removed. Statistics and authorative textbooks of the period "proved" how correct and beneficial this procedure was. Now when belief in this particular measure has dwindled, statistics and authoritative textbooks of today "prove" precisely the opposite. This is not due to deliberate manipulation of the statistics. The procedure is no longer believed in;

so it no longer works. The thing which was officially approved of by one medical generation is then scornfully condemned by the next.

McGlashan then speaks about some of the remedies which have had enthusiastic support in past generations—remedies such as usnea, shoe leather, and urine.[5] One of the most dramatic uses of faith has been developed by Dr. Carl Simonton of Oncology Associates in Fort Worth. His description of the use of meditational practices in the treatment of cancer is a spectacular specific usage of "faith" technique in a specific problem. Dr. Simonton's talk before the Assembly of Episcopal Hospitals and Chaplains is available.[6] The data on healing in which faith is evidently a constitutive element are increasing. One of the best surveys of the material is found in a 1972 symposium transcript, *The Dimensions of Healing*.[7] The research in the area of faith and healing has been well summarized by students of parapsychology who see healing by faith as another example of human openness to a dimension of experience beyond that of ordinary sensory experience. Excellent books have been written from this point of view by Charles Panati, Lawrence LeShan, Lyall Watson, Stanley Krippner, and Claudio Naranjo.[8] One could go on and on giving specific instances of healing by faith. A careful reading of the available materials leaves little doubt that health and healing are related to "faith." What is this quality of life that has so creative and powerful an effect upon human well-being?

The Anatomy of Faith

It is easier to tell what is not meant by faith than to describe it clearly and directly. For many people the word *faith* stands for "the faith," the accumulated propositions of a belief system. It is also understood by some as belief in that for which there is no evidence—for example, a persistent belief in unicorns. Here faith depends simply upon authority. Still others use the word *faith* when it is not appropriate. Some would say that they use faith in believing in the existence of a nonphysical or spiritual world. However, this other dimension of reality is not a matter of faith so much as a matter of experience. It is useless to hold to things by faith when experience is available. Faith is none of these, but rather it is the basic conviction that the world around one is kindly intentioned towards one. This probably springs most often from the kind of childhood in which the child is valued, cared for, and loved. The child is ministered to in hurt and difficulty. Faith is the attitude that one's total environment is supportive and caring, that not only those close to one, but even one's own body, the community and the physical world around one can be counted on. What a difference it makes whether the child learns to suspect and doubt the concern and caring of those around him or her because of parental blunders and lack of consistency, or whether the child learns to expect concern and care. One's attitude acts as a filter selecting and interpreting the data of life. When a child has learned that life is uncaring in the home and family, it takes either the careful attention of a significant other or some breakthrough such as a drematic religious experience to turn around one's basic attitude toward life. Sometimes it takes both experiences.

As the child's horizon expands, the attitudes acquired in childhood are widened to take in the whole world encompassing the individual. The one with faith sees the universe as essentially friendly and caring, accepting the evidence to the contrary as one of the necessary problems of life. The one who finds it difficult to find reason for trust and confidence in the universe sees the difficulties and pains as normative and moments of caring as chance or coincidental occurrences. To such persons the universe is either essentially meaningless or hostile.

Many who have been solidly indoctrinated in the materialism of the nineteenth century see human beings as totally irrevelant, purely epiphenomenal chance products. There is nothing to have faith in. Reality is an inexorable, blind mechanical process. If it goes wrong and one cannot right it mechanically, there is no changing it. For such a person to have faith, he must be shown that the best of modern scientists no longer think they know enough to believe in such certain mathematical materialism. If the physician is to facilitate the faith process in a patient, he must certainly have some alternative to that materialistic and mechanistic conviction. This can be learned and taught.[9]

There is also an attitude that is found among most primitive peoples—that the universe is not just meaningless, but more accurately hostile with demonic and destructive tendencies. Either the universe is essentially capricious, or else it is like a punitive and demanding parent, punishing us when we do not live up to its impossible standards! Since this is the way most parents do, in fact, treat their children, it is easy to see how they are readied for such an attitude. This point of view is even more difficult to turn around than the former one.

Faith, then, is an attitude that is a part of one's central frame of reference. It views the world and its inhabitants as essentially friendly and concerned. If there is a belief in a world beyond this, it is seen to be as well intentioned toward the individual as the physical world is. In the last analysis, the realities and powers of the universe are supportive of the one who has faith; they can be reached out to and depended upon.

This does not mean that there will be no fear or anger or striving for success. To have faith does not mean that one is carried about in an eternal womb. However, the fear and anger will be appropriate to the individual situation in which the person finds himself or herself. The person with faith is convinced that life and reality are plastic and difficulties can be overcome because the core of reality is kindly disposed toward human beings. Psychosomatic medicine emphasizes the dangers of anger, fear, depression, and stressful ego striving on the health of mind and body. These are the emotions that tend to predominate in the individual who has little faith. When one has no confidence in his close family world or in the less personal total environment, one tends to become either fearful or angry, depressed or pressured with stress. This is the natural psychological reaction to being an alien in a family, a community, or a universe.

Religion, Faith, and Healing

From the time of prehistoric shamanism and the historical religious cults all over the world right up to Edgar Cayce, healing, medicine, and religion have been closely related. Mircea Eliade has provided the definitive study of the shaman in his carefully researched study, *Shamanism.* [10] The basic task of the shaman was to find his own healing and then share his secret. Most often he was one who had been afflicted by some sickness seen as a visitation of evil spirits. As he struggled to free himself from the domination of evil forces, he came in contact with positive spiritual powers and became instrumental in leading others to these healing forces and so to health. On this level, it is impossible to separate religion, faith, and healing. This kind of practice is far from dead, as seen by the renewed interest in the American Indian shaman. We have descriptions of modern practice from Hosteen Klah, Black Elk, Lame Deer, and David Villasenor, as well as from Carlos Castaneda's books.[11] The U.S. Department of Health, Education and Welfare appropriated funds to support the training of Navajo shamans because it was evident that they were able to touch some diseases that ordinary medicine did not affect.[12]

The basic point of view of shamanism is found all over the world. There are evil and destructive forces, forces of disharmony and division; and there are spirits (complexes) and forces of wholeness, restoration, and healing. (In many languages the words for these two ideas are related.) *The religious task and the healing task are essentially the same: to release the individual from the destructive realities and bring him or her into relationship with the protecting, positive, healing realities.* This is true in nearly all primitive religions all over the world and in the more sophisticated cultures of China, India, and Persia.[13]

The same understanding was common in the Mediterranean world from which Western culture arose. This point of view about healing was stated philosophically by Plato, who erected a world view that integrated the fundamental elements of shamanism. For Plato, it was almost unthinkable to treat the body without treating the soul. He wrote in the *Charmides* a line that could have been written by Flanders Dunbar: "For this is the great error of our day in the treatment of the human body, that physicians separate the soul from the body."[14]

With this pervasive history of connection between faith, religion, and healing, one wonders how the separation between them took place in Western culture. The development of rational materialism came too late to account for the division that took place in Western culture. As one reads the documents of the New Testament, one is even more puzzled upon discovering that Jesus acted more in the role of shaman than of moral teacher or even traditional Hebrew prophet. He is frequently misunderstood because it so seldom occurs to modern interpreters to see him in the role of shaman. Jesus healed because he saw sickness as destructive in itself and caused on the whole by a destructive, demonic force from which he came to rescue humankind. The same tradition was continued in early Christian history as recorded in the book of Acts and records of the first five centuries of Christian life.[15]

What has happeened? As Western society disintegrated with the incursions of the Barbarians and the collapse of the social structures in the fifth century A.D., men and women lost hope and turned back to the religious ideas of the Old Testament, in which God is sometimes seen as the giver of illness and destruction as well as healing. He punished disobedience with all manner of illness and destruction as described in Deuteronomy 28:22 ff. The Old Testament is one of the few religious books having few positive references to the physician. Indeed, the Old Testament states that what God gave in sickness should seldom be taken away. Healing then became connected with the pagan temples and was thus all the more taboo. It is true that in order to be declared clean of certain diseases, one still went to the priests, but healing could only come through a gift from God *after* moral change. It must be emphasized that this was not the later Jewish point of view nor is it the current one. The Jews have found it necessary to interpret the Old Testament through the Talmud, the Mishna, and other sacred books. The Christian Fundamentalist is about the only person today who takes the Old Testament literally.

In the Middle Ages and later, the attitude that one is really not holy unless he is sick became quite common. The healing sacrament was turned into extreme unction to help one die in a holy way. In the English *Book of Common Prayer* the authors went so far as to state that unless one was sick, one was a bastard (the exact word used), since one did not know the loving correction of the Father.[16] In lecturing all over the Western world, I have been amazed to discover how deeply this idea of sickness is imbedded in the unconscious attitudes of Western Christians, both Catholic and Protestant.

In the thirteenth century, the Church developed a logical and invariant theological system, especially through Aquinas, based upon the thinking of Aristotle (who had a materialistic view of healing) and the Christian Scriptures. When the thinking of Copernicus, Kepler, and Galileo questioned the geocentric cosmology of the Church, she withdrew into her fortified walls of dogma. Thus science and religion came to a tragic split, and Christianty developed with almost no critical or scientific point of view, and science with little or no moral or religious orientation.

Science (from which modern medicine grew) became almost entirely materialistic and rational. The body was treated as another material object, and so the point of view parodied by Dr. Crookshank developed. Such a split never occurred in Greek Orthodox or Oriental religions. As we read the latest developments of modern science, it becomes quite clear that such a materialistic point of view is no longer tenable. On the whole, medical persons are far more open to the relationship of faith and healing than the clergy, who are still largely caught in the nineteenth century religion/science split. Thus it is often difficult for the physician to find dialogue with Christian clergy on the relationship between faith and healing, and there are few other religious experts available.

Facilitating Faith

Several destructive emotions arise when an individual is faced with a meaningless or hostile world. In such cases there is usually a sense of helplessness, powerlessness, and threat, to which human beings react in four basically different ways. One can react to this threat with agitated fear, the flight response, and then the whole of life is covered with a pall of anxiety. The physiological and psychic damages of this attitude are legion. On the other hand, one can stand essentially by the fight response and turn against the world and those around one with anger, hostility, rage, and violence. Any human being under this kind of constant stress will also sustain damage. Similar to the fight response is the egocentric approach, in which the individual becomes "God" and sees it as his or her responsibility to take care of the problems of the whole world. This is a heavy burden and results in often unbearable stress, with all the psychological and physiological concomitants that go with it. The fourth response is simple collapse before the threat. There is neither fight nor flight, just hopelessness, depression, loss of meaning. There is no point in doing anything, one feels. Simple depression of this kind is the common cold of modern psychiatry, and the physiological results of this kind of "giving up" are found in every doctor's office.

Obviously, when this kind of meaninglessness and hopelessness is an element in disease, the symptoms can be ameliorated, but confidence in some helping, redeeming factor is necessary before health is restored. This is the function of faith. How can the physician facilitate this kind of attitude toward life?

In the first place, the physician's own basic attitude will most certainly be picked up by the patient. If he or she finds himself or herself in a position of helplessness and stress, this will be communicated to the patient. If, however, he or she truly sees the world as meaningful, valuable, sustaining and promoting human fulfillment (in spite of the realistic evidence to the contrary), then this attitude is likely to be conveyed to the patient. This is most obviously true in psychiatry, but it is true of all long-range relationships with others, and with patients in particular. Jung once wrote that a psychiatrist is a physician whose only scalpel is his own personality. This influence extends beyond psychiatry to all the helping professions.

One of the most effective methods of demonstrating to another that this is a meaningful universe is to treat the other person with care and concern. It is difficult to believe that the universe is basically disposed in a kindly way toward one until one at least discovers a human being who treats one in this way.

And how does one show that one truly does care? How can one communicate that his caring is an instrument of a more universal caring? Seldom can we show care unless we can listen to another person. Few human beings feel truly cared for unless they are listened to. Then one can respond with positive and caring words. How deeply such words strike into the human psyche! The physician is then in a unique place to provide actions of caring in healing treatment. Human touch is also healing, as it demonstrates caring concern far below the verbal level. Perhaps this is why Dolores Kreiger's experiments with healing touch have been successful. [17]

There are some people who are so locked into a meaningless world view that they also need cognitive understanding that there is a way out of their intellectual, emotional, and physical problem. The more intelligent the individual, the more likely it is that the intellectual viewpoint of hopelessness will affect the mind and body. Jung discovered that he had to attack this problem with patients himself because so few of the clergy were competent to do so. *It may be necessary to provide the "faithless" one with a world view that offers some hope for meaning.* If one has worked at developing his own faith attitude, he will be better able to help another through meaninglessness to faith and health. I have written some suggestions on how this can be accomplished in *Finding Meaning: Guidelines for Counselors.* [18]

Surveying the history of religion and medicine, we see that there is a close relationship between an attitude of confident faith and a belief in the meaningfulness of the universe, and healing. The physician interested in permanent healing will consider the world view and the emotional state of the patient and will try to provide the kind of atmosphere in which faith is facilitated in the patient.[19] This will involve a total physician, a whole physician, dealing with the total patient—mind, emotions and body. It is an approach that offers greater wholeness to both the patient and the physician.

Notes

1. Flanders Dunbar, *Emotions and Bodily Changes*, 4th ed. (New York: Columbia University Press, 1954): 83.
2. Edward Weiss and O. Spurgeon English, *Psychosomatic Medicine: The Clinical Application of Psychopathology to General Medical Problems*, 3rd ed. (Philadelphia: Saunders, 1957).
3. Morton T. Kelsey, *Healing and Christianity* (New York: Harper and Row, 1973), particularly chapters 1, 2, 9, 10, 11, 13. Complete references are provided in these chapters.
4. Jerome Frank, *Persuasion and Healing* (New York: Schochen Books, 1969). In addition, another excellent study of the interrelationship of healing and emotions and faith is found in William Sargant's *Battle for the Mind* (Baltimore, Penguin Books, 1961).
5. R. Alan McGlashan, *Gravity and Levity* (Boston: Houghton Mifflin, 1976): 37–38 ff. Dr. McGlashan also mentions healing which seems to flow from the individual with no desire on the part of the healer, a kind of natural healer. In 1960 a British physician wrote a book entitled *The Nature of Healing*, anonymously, on this subject. Another such book was called to my attention by C. G. Jung: *The Reluctant Healer: A Remarkable Autobiography* by William J. MacMillan (New York: Thomas Crowell, 1952).
6. The Institute of Religion and Medicine, Bishop Anderson House, 1743 W. Harrison Street, Chicago, IL 60612, 1975.
7. *The Dimensions of Healing, A Symposium* (The Academy of Parapsychology and Medicine, 314 Second Street, Los Altos, CA 94022, 1973).
8. Charles Panati, *Supersenses: Our Potential for Parasensory Experience* (New York: Quadrangle/The New York Times Book Company, 1974).
   Lyall Watson, *Supernature: A Natural History of the Supernatural* (New York: Bantam Books, 1974).
   Lawrence LeShan, *The Medium, the Mystic and the Physicist: Toward a*

General Theory of the Paranormal (New York: Viking, 1974).

———, *Alternate Realities* (New York: Evans, 1976).

Stanley Krippner, *Song of the Siren: A Parapsychological Odyssey* (New York: Harper and Row, 1975).

Claudio Naranjo, *The Healing Journey: New Approaches to Consciousness* (New York: Pantheon, 1973).

9. One of the best recent discussions of alternative world views is found in Alan McGlashan's *Gravity and Levity.* Several other books have been helpful in freeing my students at Notre Dame from the grip of this faith-denying world view:

Thomas S. Kuhn, *The Structure of Scientific Revolutions,* 2nd ed. (Chicago: The University of Chicago Press, 1970).

Bob Toben, *Space-Time and Beyond* (New York: Dutton, 1975).

Werner Heisenberg, *Physics and Philosophy: The Revolution in Modern Science* (New York: Harper and Brothers, 1958).

All of the above books break through many common scientific prejudices and open many doors. Jung's *Memories, Dreams, Reflections* gives an alternative world view which I have summarized and diagrammed in my own *Encounter With God* (Minneapolis: Bethany Fellowship, 1973).

C. G. Jung, *Memories, Dreams, Reflections,* Recorded and edited by Aniela Jaffé (New York: Pantheon, 1963).

10. Mircea Eliade, *Shamanism: Archaic Technique of Ecstasy* (Princeton, Princeton University Press, 1970).

11. Franc Johnson Newcomb, *Hosteen Klah: Navaho Medicine Man and Sand Painter* (Norman: University of Oklahoma Press, 1964).

John G. Neihardt, *Black Elk Speaks: Being the Life Story of a Holy Man of the Oglala Sioux* (Lincoln: University of Nebraska Press, 1961).

Lame Deer and Richard Erdoes, *Lame Deer: Seekers of Visions* (New York: Simon & Schuster, 1972).

David Villasenor, *Tapestries in Sand: The Spirit of Indian Sandpainting* (Healdsburg, Calif.: Naturegraph Company, 1966).

Carlos Castaneda, *The Teachings of Don Juan: A Yaqui Way of Knowledge* (Berkeley: University of California Press, 1968).

———, *A Separate Reality: Further Conversations with Don Juan* (New York: Simon & Schuster, 1971).

———, *Journey to Ixtlan: The Lessons of Don Juan* (New York: Pocket Books, 1974).

———, *Tales of Power* (New York: Simon & Schuster, 1974).

12. The *New York Times*, July 7, 1972, p. 33 has a full-page article on this subject.
13. For a survey of Persian thought, see *Healing and Christianity*, p. 38 ff., and my *Myth, History and Faith* (New York: Paulist Press, 1974), pp. 52 ff. For China, Japan and India, see *Half the World; The History and Culture of China and Japan* (New York: Holt, Rinehart and Winston, 1973), particularly Chapter 4, "The Path to Wisdom," pp. 95 ff.
14. Plato, *Dialogues*, trans. B. Jowett (New York: Random House, 1937). Further references to Platonic theory, which became the basis of Graeco-Roman thought and Christian theology, are to be found in *Healing and Christianity*, p. 45 ff. There was little difference between this point of view and that of the healing shrines of Asklepios in which Greek medicine was born and grew.
15. A full account of this development is found in chapters 3 to 9 of *Healing and Christianity*. There is no other account of these data available.
16. See *Healing and Christianity*, p. 15 ff., for a full exposition of this point of view.
17. Dolores Kreiger, *American Journal of Nursing* (May, 1975). See also my pamphlet, *The Art of Christian Love* (Pecos, N.M.: Dove Publications, 1974), for a more extensive discussion of how to express concern to another human being.
18. Morton T. Kelsey, *Finding Meaning: Guidelines for Counselors* (Pecos, N.M.: Dove Publications, 1974).
19. Dr. J. Andrew Canale has written a paper expressing a similar point of view in an article published in the first issue in 1977 of the *Unitarian Universalist Review*. It is entitled "Dealing with Pain from the Perspective of Wholeness."

Part III

Western Approaches
to
Wholistic Healing

14
Norman S. Don

Four Self-Regulatory Therapies in Wholistic Health

Self-Regulation

INHERENT IN THE philosophy of wholistic health is the possibility that people can sense and regulate their own bodies, thoughts, feelings, and behaviors, and their relationships with people and with their environments. This notion only a few years ago would have been greeted with extreme skepticism if not outright rejection in the Western world. The present volume attests to the dramatic change in the Western world view and to a convergence between Western science and Eastern and other esoteric traditions.

The acceptance of the possibility of self-regulation has come about largely through laboratory tests. They have shown that people can influence physiological functions that ordinarily are autonomic, or not consciously controllable—for example, heartbeat, blood pressure, brain waves, and many other "involuntary" bodily processes.

It is most interesting that, although the possibility of self-regulation has been known to Western science for at least forty years, only recently has there emerged a significant self-regulatory philosophy and world view to encompass this human potential. It was in 1929 that the first edition of Jacobson's classic book, *Progressive Relaxation*, appeared.[1] This work elaborated a voluntary method of self-regulation of muscle tension and reported the effects of this relaxation on stress-related pathology. In 1954 Jacobson reported that patients in training with his system of Progressive Relaxation could learn to control their muscle tension when this was displayed to them on an oscilloscope.[2] In 1934 the distinguished neurophysiologist Lord Adrian fed back his own alpha waves to himself, thus performing the first biofeedback experiment in the contemporary sense.[3] Despite these clear harbingers by recognized scientists, the possibilities of self-regulation did not start to capture the imagination of Western science until the late 1960s. There is clearly such a thing as a valid idea waiting until its time has come.

The concept of self-regulation often invokes the image of the stern Victorian will. In that tradition, the will was thought of as a force that could and should be employed on both one's self and the world. Will in this sense was cold, coercive, and a force to be used in a repressive and domineering manner. Apropos of this attitude, Dr. Roberto Assagioli has stated that

> such a misconception might be called a caricature of the will. The true function of the will is not to act against the personality drives to *force* the accomplishment of one's purposes. The will has a *directive* and *regulatory* function; it balances and constructively utilizes all the other activities and energies of the human being without repressing any of them.[4]

It is clear that any real degree of self-regulation must entail some procedures or methods of exercising voluntary control over one's physical, mental, and emotional states or behaviors. Dr. Johann Stoyva, in his introduction to the first issue of the journal *Biofeedback and Self-Regulation*, has suggested that there exists a common feature in a host of seemingly unrelated practices, including biofeedback, Autogenic Training, Progressive Relaxation, behavioral techniques, meditation, hypnosis, chanting, and various esoteric religious practices. This common feature he has identified as self-regulation: "the endeavor to modify voluntarily one's own physiological activity, behavior, or processes of consciousness."[5]

Defined in this way, Stoyva has explicitly included among the self-regulatory methods the operant conditioning techniques first laid down by B. F. Skinner.[6] Behaviorism and the techniques of operant conditioning would seem to be antithetical to the theme of wholistic healing; however, Stoyva has pointed out that some contemporary methods of behavioral self-regulation are the counterpart to biofeedback of physiological functions. For example, a person may learn how to change his attitudes about himself by rewarding himself for certain kinds of statements.[7] Within the content of wholistic healing, however, the concept of self-regulation generally takes on a broader connotation than it does when applied to self-reinforcement procedures in behaviorism.

In a feedback model elaborated by William T. Powers, the groundwork has been laid for an understanding of self-regulation that is both applicable to scientific research and consonant with the philosophy of wholistic health.[8] It is this model of self-regulation that I wish to use in dealing with the self-regulatory therapies because it has shifted the ground for understanding behavior—especially self-regulatory behavior.

In the older scientific models of behavior there was a stimulus, an organism, a response to the stimulus, and perhaps a reward or punishment for the behavior. Behaviorism and operant conditioning in particular are based upon this model. Powers has pointed out that in most natural settings a person's responses are experienced by the person himself, and so there is a feedback *to* the person *from* his own responses. The effect of this feedback is to maintain the person's own internal states in some stable mode of functioning. What a person perceives is not a stimulus or input from the outside, but a weighted function of the input and feedback. The responses operate to produce feedback that modifies external information so that the stability of the person's internal states is maintained. This is called negative feedback and it functions so as to reduce the effects of change.

Powers has proposed that the central nervous system functions like a set of feedback-controlled loops, hierarchically ordered. In such an arrangement, a feedback-controlled loop sends a signal to the next lower level of the hierarchy, thus controlling it, and this effect is passed on down to still lower levels. This signal is called a "reference signal." A "reference signal" or "reference level" is an internal perception or standard of how things should be working. The higher up in the hierarchy the reference signal issues from, the more global the control over the entire system. Powers proposes that there are at least nine levels in the hierarchy representing the functioning of the human central nervous system. The seventh level deals with the system's "programs," which constitute our ordinary cognitive functioning. The levels above this—which deal with the system's principles and concepts and perhaps even higher levels—exert an even more global effect than the cognitive level of functioning.

It is characteristic of the four self-regulatory therapies I have chosen to discuss—biofeedback, Autogenic Training, the Alexander Technique, and the Feldenkrais Method—that one masters them by letting go of one's usual way of learning and functioning. In biofeedback training and Autogenic Training, one shifts to an attitude of "passive volition," and "the body will comply, so long as the accompanying emotional stance is detached, non-anxious, merely expectant."[9] In biofeedback and Autogenic Training, cortical control supervenes normally involuntary subcortical and autonomic processes. In these methods one *intends* and then *allows* the desired effect.

In terms of the hierarchical model, one shifts up to hierarchical levels above ordinary cognitive functioning or processing (seventh level) and intends or selects the desired action. Then one suspends ordinary seventh level modes of functioning so as to allow the desired result to occur. However, this process of "passive volition" is "passive" only in the sense that we must not pursue goals in our *usual* "active" way. Powers points out that there must exist hierarchical levels that allow us to form *concepts and images* of what is or what we intend to happen, and from these are passed down ways of selecting *principles* consistent with these concepts and images. At the seventh level, programs are selected that will gain the results consistent with our original concept of the goal. The process of this reorganization is not, however, passive. It involves an ongoing reorganization guided by the concepts, images, and principles we have selected as our desired goal: "once we have learned to perceive in terms of some particular principle, we become able to see the state of that principle in all our lower-order perceptions having to do with it, and we can learn to behave in such a way as to control that state."[10] In other words, the reorganization initiated by our concept or image proceeds and is maintained by feeding back the results of the reorganization—a completely active process of self-regulation. However, this comes about first by forming the intention and then by allowing the effect to occur. One seems to *wait* for the result since control by higher order levels is slower than control from more familiar lower order levels. Furthermore, this process involves the simultaneous, interrelated functioning of all levels of the system. The more one learns to function from these higher levels, the greater the scope of self-regulation and thus the more global and wholistic the effects on our functioning.

Biofeedback Training

The uses of biofeedback training in healing are presented in Chapter 15 of this book. I would, however, like to discuss some aspects of biofeedback training that relate to self-regulation and conscious experience. In terms of the feedback model, what biofeedback allows us to do is to shift the reference levels of our internal states. Reference levels are the internal criteria that control what these states should be like. For example, a person attempting to lower the muscle tension level of the frontalis muscle of the forehead may observe a meter and intend the meter reading to go down. As just discussed, this intention occurs at a high level of the person's being. The information "fed back" to the person by the meter on the EMG feedback machine gives an indication of the system's "error": the difference between the intended tension level and the actual level. The system reorganizes so as to minimize this error. That is, there is a shift in the internal reference levels for muscle tension of the person using the biofeedback machine.

Biofeedback training to a large extent involves the training of attention. Feelings, subtle shifts of internal states, and other covert processes often become more experienceable by the biofeedback trainee. Also, it is not uncommon for biofeedback training in one modality, e.g., brainwaves, to generalize to and enhance self-regulatory ability over other physiological functions. In an experiment in our laboratory concerned with shifts of affect and cognition, it was found that all these events coincided with brief stabilizations of brainwaves (EEG). When this happened, the person's dominant alpha wave frequency (most commonly around ten cycles per second) and the theta waves (four or five per second) and/or delta waves (two or three per second) would simultaneously stabilize and increase to high levels of amplitude.[11] Changes in conscious experience coincided with these specific brain wave events; this replicates the result found by Banquet in a study of the EEG of transcendental meditators. These studies and associated evidence suggest that these EEG stabilities are associated with specific levels of the feedback-controlled hierarchy and thus with different types of conscious experience.[12] Our laboratory is presently using a biofeedback EEG trainer designed to train people for these multiple, coincident-frequency events. It is expected that this training may lead to new types of conscious experience and to enhanced self-regulatory abilities stemming from higher and therefore more global levels of the person's system.

Autogenic Training

While biofeedback training uses electronics in teaching self-regulation of physiological functions, Autogenic Training relies on the person's natural abilities to focus attention on various body parts, paired with phrases that are repeated silently; most of the phrases suggest heaviness, warmth, or other aspects of a relaxed state.

Autogenic Training was first introduced in 1910 by Johannes Schultz, a German physician, and grew out of his interest in hypnosis and yoga. The term *autogenic*, meaning self-generating, reflects Schultz's conclusion that failures in hypnotherapy were in large measure due to the patient's resistance to the hypnotherapist or too-passive role in the process. Schultz noticed that successful hypnotic patients experienced a feeling of heaviness in the body and warmth in the limbs. He decided that quieting the body and mind were keys to successful therapy, and so he taught his patients first to induce a state of physiological quietness and then to tell their bodies what to do, using what he termed "organ specific" formulas. Dr. Elmer Green has analogized this process to taking a tape recorder out of the "active" playback mode and putting it into the "receptive" record mode, so it can take in instructions. [13]

The Autogenic system has been used extensively in Europe, where several thousand research articles on it have been published. In 1969 the first of a set of six comprehensive volumes appeared in English translation edited by Dr. Wolfgang Luthe. [14] The Autogenic system has attracted wide interest in the United States since then, especially among biofeedback practitioners, who often use relaxation methods along with biofeedback training.

The Autogenic trainee is first taught the Autogenic Standard Exercises, consisting of six parts. In my clinic these exercises are usually introduced and practiced at the rate of one a week. At the same time, biofeedback training is in progress. In the first of the Standard Exercises, the person assumes a relaxed posture, turns his attention first to the right arm, and silently repeats, "My right arm is heavy," several times. Each limb is treated in similar fashion until it is possible for the person to experience heaviness in the limbs merely by being aware of the arms and legs and repeating to himself, "My arms and legs are heavy." Next, warmth is induced in the arms and legs in exactly the same manner, so that with mastery of the first two of the Standard Exercises, the trainee can induce heaviness and warmth—which means that the muscles are relaxed and the peripheral blood vessels are dilated—by attending to the arms and legs and repeating the phrase, "My arms and legs are heavy and warm." Next attention is turned to the heartbeat, the phrase here being "Heartbeat calm and regular." The remaining three exercises involve passively observing the breath, warming the solar plexus, and cooling the forehead. As one practices this system, both during the training period and afterward, he or she may experience muscle twitches, jerking of the limbs, sensations of floating, or a person may burst into tears. All these effects are regarded as therapeutic discharges and are part of a process of the body's seeking and maintaining a new balance of nervous system functioning. Luthe reports that an astonishing variety of somatic problems are alleviated by this practice.[15] For example, the systematic practice of the Autogenic Standard Exercises tends to reduce the insulin dosages necessary to maintain diabetics. We have replicated this finding in our clinic.[16] In a pilot study on hypertension, we found that all five hypertense patients in a group practicing the Standard Exercises substantially lowered their blood pressures. At the end of eight weeks, three of the five people had blood pressures well within normal limits. In the case of chronic back pain, the neurosurgery department of Johns Hopkins University is teaching the Autogenic Standard Exercises to patients so that they may learn to self-regulate pain.

As mentioned earlier, there are other parts to the Autogenic system, such as the Organ Specific Formulas. These involve, first, putting the body into a quiet state through use of the Standard Exercises and then focusing attention onto a specific organ or a troublesome area of the body. For example, in the case of colitis, the phrase "My lower abdomen is warm" has been used. In addition to the Standard Exercises and the Organ Specific Formulas there are several other parts to the system which are used either to deepen the Autogenic state of homeostasis or to induce the cathartic discharge of tension.

The attitude of "passive volition," mentioned earlier in connection with self-regulation, is maintained during the Autogenic exercises. Luthe has likened this attitude, and indeed the whole underlying philosophy of Autogenic Training, to that of Taoism—the ancient Chinese philosophy that articulates as an ideal the harmonious relating of man to Nature, in a nonstriving, "flowing" manner.[17] From this angle, healing involves a rebalancing and a harmonization of one's self, both internally and with the world.

The Alexander Technique

While the most common clinical applications of biofeedback and Autogenic Training aim toward the reduction of hyperaroused physiological functioning, the Alexander Technique aims toward a global reeducation in the way we use our bodies. This involves learning to be aware of kinesthetic impressions—sensations of weight, position, and movement of the organism and its parts—and then learning to use the body in an effortless and flowing manner.

About seventy years ago, F. M. Alexander, who was an actor at that time, developed serious vocal trouble that was not helped by the various physicians he consulted. He then started to observe himself in a mirror as he practiced recitations and found that his voice worsened when he assumed certain stances and positions that he considered appropriate for what he was reciting. Over a period of years, he set about to improve what he called the "use" of the voluntary musculature of the body, in all its postures and movements. Eventually Alexander regained control of his voice and decided to teach his "technique" to other people—he did not refer to this training as a therapy.

Central to the Alexander Technique is the head-neck-torso relationship, and during Alexander lessons the teacher imparts their correct relationship and kinesthetic sense to the student by a subtle method of touching and guiding the student's body. The results of this training can only be appreciated by experiencing it. Aldous Huxley, who was an enthusiastic advocate of the technique, refused even to try to describe the kinesthetic experience, saying that it would be like trying to describe color to a person blind from birth.

The results of Alexander training go beyond the kinesthetic sense of lightness and effortless movement. The amelioration of a host of joint and muscle problems has been reported,[18] and in 1974 Dr. Nokolaas Tinbergen devoted half of his Nobel Prize acceptance lecture to the Alexander Technique. Among the results that he and his family experienced from their own lessons were "very striking improvements in such diverse things as high blood pressure, breathing, depth of sleep, overall cheerfulness and mental alertness, resilience against outside pressures, and also in such a refined skill as playing a stringed instrument."[19]

The limbs are also worked on, although the method focuses mainly on the head-neck-torso postural and kinesthetic relationship, since it is considered that this is the key to the correct use of the body. The head-neck reflexes have been studied by a host of investigators, one of the earliest being R. Magnus, who demonstrated that the position of an animal's head in space or relative to its body affects tension pattern in the neck, back, and limbs.[20,21] Magnus summarized this by stating that the head leads and the body follows—exactly the phrase often uttered to Alexander trainees during lessons. Two types of head-neck reflexes were identified by Magnus: (1) the *attitudinal* reflexes used to maintain special postures, during which the head position imposes an attitude upon the rest of the body, and 2) the *righting* reflexes involved in returning to normal upright posture. Besides these effects, there are derivative effects on respiration, circulation, and eye position.[22] These effects come about when a person learns to inhibit his usual head-neck-torso relationship from its habitual attitude, thereby facilitating the righting reflexes that impart a lengthening, uprightness, and lightness to the body. Dr. Franklin P. Jones, an American physiologist who did laboratory experiments and also taught the Alexander Technique, stated that "the changes in breathing, in circulation, and in the use of the eyes, which are sometimes reported, take place automatically by reflex facilitation when the head moves into its new relationship to the trunk."[23] Consistent with this claim, after three months of Alexander lessons, I was able to discontinue the use of eyeglasses in most situations.

In order to maintain proper use, or "direction" as it is often termed, one must first learn to inhibit the usual reflex patterns, since people have typically acquired a sense of their functioning that is actually not proper. Secondly, the student is instructed to be aware of how he performs motor acts—"the means whereby"—rather than focus on just the desired result, such as getting out of a chair—"the end gain."

As Jones states, "the only satisfactory way to achieve such a control is to reorganize the field of attention, so that when a stimulus to move is received, the focus of attention remains within the organism."[24] The goal, such as standing up, is not ignored but is not allowed to dominate the field of attention.

In terms of our model of self-regulation, this method involves becoming aware of higher-order reference levels and learning to shift reference levels of the lower-order kinesthetic loops in accordance with these higher levels. Writing in 1925, Magnus claimed that the righting reflexes were located beneath the cortex and were thus incapable of conscious self-regulation; however, by learning to inhibit postural responses that interfere with the righting reflex, indirect control could be established.[25] However, the recent work on biofeedback has amply documented the ability of people to learn cortical control over subcortical processes, and so it may well be that the Alexander trainee does learn to self-regulate these reflexes. Moreover, it is now known that there are feedback loops between the skeletal muscles and the central nervous system, and so the musculoskeletal system has a regulatory effect on the central nervous system. The righting reflex may be triggered or controlled first by learning to control musculature from a high reference level.

The Feldenkrais Method

In 1949, Dr. Moshe Feldenkrais, an applied physicist who had made an intensive study of the use and mechanics of the human body, published his first book, *Body and Mature Behavior*. The goals of the Feldenkrais Method are completely consistent with those of the Alexander Technique, although the methods of training are very different. More than 1,000 exercises, with several variations possible on each, have been elaborated, reflecting Feldenkrais's scientific background. Writing about his use of the method, Robert Masters has stated that there is an experience of "lengthening and lightening of the body," "easy, flowing movements," and "breathing that is free."[27] Joints and movements become free, the body is experienced as light, effortless, and flowing in its use, and the energy required to execute movement is minimized. Through this process, the psychological conception of one's body image changes, as does one's psychological functioning in general. During the training, the Feldenkrais exercises are practiced in a way that is experienced as pleasurable. Feldenkrais agrees with Alexander that, because of man's great increase of cognitive capacity over that of animals, he has learned methods of self-use that are far less than ideal, and these must be changed in order for his potential to be realized.

A guiding principle in correcting patterns of poor use is to first exaggerate the poor pattern. One could see this as a positive feedback effect that amplifies the derivation from the optimum state so greatly that the stability of the old pattern of poor usage is quickly destroyed. At this point the optimum mode of functioning can be introduced and practiced. This practice may also involve visualizing the desired results of the practice. Feldenkrais states that after fifteen to thirty repetitions of a practice movement, the effort of the movement becomes very small; the thought of the movement and the movement itself becoming practically identical.

Again there is an increase of awareness and of the body's capacity for conscious self-regulation. Moreover, the unity of mind and body is experienced because one learns to perceive at a higher level in the feedback-controlled hierarchy.

Conclusion

We have seen how the principles of self-regulation are articulated in four self-regulatory therapies and how the methods of these therapies can be related to our feedback-controlled, hierarchically organized model. The methods all involve a change of high order: one involving functional concepts and principles.

As powerful and contemporary as this model may be in accounting for the *flow of control*, it does not definitively account for how we attend to these high-order functions in the first place. It does not, ultimately, account for the underlying basis of self-regulation: the focusing of awareness itself. Consonant with the outlook of positivistic science, we can claim that there must be a biophysical basis for this and that in due course scientific research will find it. Scientific studies are increasingly unearthing physiological correlates of conscious experience, without, however, revealing how a person attends to *any* experiential state in the first place.

An alternative to the positivistic approach is a transcendental one, which regards attention as a metaforce, connected with, but distinct from, psychophysical reality.[28,29] There are some very serious theoretical problems with such a view;[30] however, it is the only one that can begin to account for some of the findings of parapsychology and altered-states-of-consciousness research.[31] One can theoretically justify a metaview of attention if it is seen as part of an energy continuum that also includes ordinary psychophysical reality. One then gets a layered continuity of levels of reality that can intercommunicate under certain conditions.[32]

If Powers's model of hierarchical control is correct, then the higher one's awareness, the greater one's self-regulation. What would perception be like at the highest level of complete wholism?

> Perhaps what some see as a universal urge toward Oneness represents the first glimmerings of a mode of perception in which all systems concepts are seen as examples of higher versions of reality, so that system concepts—what we called "realities"—will some day be manipulated as casually as we now manipulate principles in service of systems. Could the human race be in the process *evolving* the capacity to perceive and control tenth-level entities? *Inventing* it?[33]

Notes

1. E. Jacobson, *Progressive Relaxation*, 1st ed. (Chicago: University of Chicago Press, 1929).
2. ——— (Article on electromyographic measurement), *Newsweek* (1 February 1954): 39. Cited by J. Stoyva in "Self-Regulation: A Context for Biofeedback," *Biofeedback and Self-Regulation* 1 (1976): 4.
3. E. D. Adrian and B. H. C. Matthews, "The Berger Rhythm: Potential Changes from the Occipital Lobe in Man," *Brain* 57 (1934): 354–85.
4. R. Assagioli, *The Act of Will* (New York: Viking, 1973); p. 10.
5. J. Stoyva, "Self-Regulation: A Context for Biofeedback," *Biofeedback and Self-Regulation* 1 (1976): 2.
6. B. F. Skinner, *The Behavior of Organisms* (New York: Appleton-Century-Crofts, 1938).
7. D. H. Meichenbaum, "Cognitive Factors in Behavior Modification: Modifying What Clients Say to Themselves," in *Annual Review of Behavior*

   Therapy, ed. C. M. Franks and G. T. Wilson (New York: Brunner/Mazel, 1973).
8. W. T. Powers, *Behavior: The Control of Perception* (Chicago: Aldine, 1973).
9. E. Green and A. Green, "Regulating Our Mind-Body Processes," *Fields Within Fields* 10 (1973–74): 17.
10. W. T. Powers, op. cit., p. 170.
11. N. S. Don, "Cortical Activity Changes During a Psychotherapeutic Procedure: Implications for EEG Biofeedback Training," *Proceedings of the Biofeedback Research Society* (1975): 68.
12. J. P. Banquet, "Spectral Analysis of the EEG in Meditation," *Electroencephalography and Clinical Neurophysiology* 35 (1973): 143–51.
13. E. Green and A. Green, "Biofeedback and Volition" (Paper presented at New Dimensions of Habilitation for the Handicapped, University of Florida, Gainesville, June, 1974).
14. W. Luthe, *Autogenic Therapy*, vol. 1–6 (New York: Grune and Stratton, 1969–1973).
15. Ibid., vol. 2.
16. Ibid., vol. 2, pp. 107–12.
17. W. Luthe (Paper presented at the Conference of the Biofeedback Research Society, Monterey, Calif., March, 1975).
18. W. Barlow, *The Alexander Technique* (New York: Alfred E. Knopf, 1973).
19. N. Tinbergen, "Ethology and Stress Diseases," *Science* 185 (1974): 20–27.
20. R. Magnus, *Korperstellung* (Berlin: Springer, 1924).
21. R. Magnus, and A. de Kleijn, "Abhängigkeit des Tonus der Extremitätenmuskeln von der Kopfstellung," *Pfugers Archiv fur die gesamte Physiologie der Menschen and der-Tiere* 145 (1912): 455–548.
22. F. Jones, "Method of Changing Stereotyped Response Patterns by the Inhibition of Certain Postural Sets," *Psychological Review* 72 (1965): 196–214.
23. Ibid., p. 211.
24. Ibid.
25. R. Magnus, "Animal Posture," *Proceedings of the Royal Society of London*, vol. 98, series B (1925): 339–53.
26. M. Feldenkrais, *Body and Mature Behavior* (New York: International Universities Press, 1973).
27. R. Masters, "The Feldenkrais Method," *Elysium Journal of the Senses*, no. 34 (Winter, 1976): 3, excerpted from *The Psychophysical Experience* by R. Masters, in press.

28. E. Green and A. Green, "Regulating our Mind Body Processes," *Fields Within Fields*, no. 10 (Winter 1973–74): 16–24.
29. R. Assagioli, *The Act of Will* (New York: Viking, 1973).
30. E. Gellhorn, and G. N. Loofbourrow, *Emotions and Emotional Disorders* (New York: Harper and Row, 1963): 139–43.
31. E. D. Mitchell, and J. White, eds. *Psychic Exploration* (New York: Charles Putnam's Sons, 1974).
32. E. Green, "Tibetan Buddhism" (Paper presented at the Council Grove Conference on Voluntary Control of Internal States, Council Grove, Kansas, April, 1969).
33. W. T. Powers, op. cit., p. 174.

Bibliography

Alexander, F. M. *The Resurrection of the Body*. New York: Dell, 1969.

Barlow, W. *The Alexander Technique*. New York: Alfred E. Knopf, 1973.

Barber, Theodore; Dicara, Leo V.; Kamiya, Joe; Miller, Neal E.; Shapiro, David; and Stoyva, Johann. *Biofeedback and Self Control*. Chicago: Aldine-Atherton, 1970.

Brown, Barbara. *New Mind, New Body*. New York: Harper and Row, 1975.

Eliade, M. *Yoga, Immortality and Freedom*. 2nd ed. Princeton: Princeton University Press, 1969.

Feldenkrais, M. *Body and Mature Behavior*. New York: International Universities Press, 1969.

———. *Awareness Through Movement*. New York: Harper and Row, 1972.

Jacobson, Edmund. *Progressive Relaxation*. Chicago: University of Chicago Press, 1938.

Karlins, M., and Andrews, L. *Biofeedback: Turning On the Power of Your Mind*. Philadelphia: Lippincott, 1972.

Luthe, W., ed. *Autogenic Therapy*. Vols. I–IV. New York: Grune and Stratton, 1969–1973.

Penfield, W. *The Mystery of the Mind*. Princeton: Princeton University Press, 1975.

Powers, W. T. *Behavior: The Control of Perception*. Chicago: Aldine, 1973.

Tart, Charles T., ed. *Altered States of Consciousness*. New York: Wiley, 1969.

15

Arthur E. Gladman and Norma Estrada

Biofeedback:
Uses in Healing

Background

IN ATTEMPTING to demonstrate the uses of biofeedback in healing, it is necessary to provide the reader with a brief explanation of biofeedback and how it functions in the practice of medicine. The term biofeedback (body feedback) refers to the use of sensitive instrumentation to monitor internal functions that are below conscious awareness. If a person can be aware of his (unconscious) physiologic functioning, he or she can learn to modify it.

The foundations of the present understanding of the relationship of inappropriate body responses to the development of disease were initiated by the work of Claude Bernard, Ivan Pavlov, Walter B. Cannon, Harold G. Wolff, and Hans Selye.[1] Their observations, as well as those of others, led to the development of "psychosomatic medicine" as a separate branch of the healing arts. Today the category "psychosomatic disease" is no longer a separate entity, since it has been recognized that the patient cannot be separated from his illness and any illness can be influenced by what goes on in the body.[2]

Evolutionary Trends

Biofeedback, an emerging therapeutic modality, provides man with an image of his own physical, emotional, and mental functioning and so

243

with a means by which he can effect change to promote good health. Out of scientific technology comes the opportunity for patients to share with their doctors the process of their own illnesses and to be participatory in formulating their own individual treatment. In this way, the experience of the illness can, in itself, become a lesson to be used by the patient to reevaluate goals and attitudes, to initiate the mobilization of unrealized strengths, and to improve the quality of his or her life.

The brilliant physician and educator Sir William Osler repeatedly observed that the outcome of the disease is dependent upon the person who has it.[3] Research and clinical studies continue to demonstrate the specificity the individual manifests in creating his or her own illness and, conversely, the individuality used in eliminating it. Individuals provided with the proper internal information through visual and audio feedback of their own body processes (biofeedback) learn to make appropriate changes to correct their own dysfunctions and to restore the body to a more homeostatic state. Patients "see" for themselves, and the knowledge gained through individual experience may change their lives. It is important to differentiate here between (1) voluntary control of internal states, as reflected in craniospinal, autonomic, and central nervous system indicators; and (2) conditioned control of such indicators, as in working with animals. Voluntary control moves toward increased inner freedom; conditioned control moves toward loss of freedom.[4]

Healing Potential

In treating psychosomatic illness, using biofeedback, the process of healing has transcendent qualities that are often difficult to define. Clinicians and researchers alike are hard put to formulate the dynamics of what takes place in healing, but the results embody wholistic principles that appear to be complex in nature. Several models have been proposed as a basis for exploring the biofeedback therapies. A. T. W. Simeons's communication model of psychosomatic disease, which proposes a lack of communication between the old (visceral) brain and the new (cerebral cortex) brain, is an excellent model for both professional and lay people.[5] It is based on the concept that the old brain, which includes the autonomic nervous system and the master gland (the pituitary) of the endocrine system, has poor communication with the cerebral cortex. As a result, the day-to-day stress of modern society, which often preoccupies the new brain, is experienced by the visceral brain as threats, which in turn trigger a biological danger alarm. The result is a chronic "fight or flight" reaction, which leads to the inappropriate body responses called psychosomatic illness.

The efficacy of biofeedback as a therapeutic tool in treating both the patient and the illness is gaining considerable attention, not only for the amelioration of the symptom, but for the benefits derived in learning skills that prevent future illness from taking place. Age, intellectual capacity, cultural or ethnic factors present no barriers in learning voluntary control of internal states. Young children are particularly adept at mastery, since they learn how their body works and the ways in which they can modify its functioning. This learned control enhances a child's self-image and makes him aware that he is not at the mercy of external forces.

"The New Medicine": Transitional Process

The use of instrumentation in the process of internal control has relevance at this particular time in history and makes possible the transitional practice of medicine, merging Eastern philosophies with Western technology. The use of biofeedback instruments accomplishes two things: the patient learns to control and quiet internal states, and the physician, as teacher, can use the instrument as a bridge to communicate with the patient in a new and different way.

In the context of the "new medicine," the therapist's role in biofeedback becomes that of teacher and colleague—providing the patient with knowledge and information, encouraging the activation of latent human and biological resources for healing. The healing potential of their relationship depends upon their interaction as human beings and often exceeds the treatment of disease. It is impossible to separate patients from their diseases or for doctors to limit their expertise to medical technology. It is the simple art of medicine teamed with the best of scientific research. In an effort to facilitate this learning in the face of everyday stress, adjunctive techniques are used to help the patient integrate new skills. Constructive introspection fostered by specific techniques is a necessary prerequisite in order for an individual to function with controlled spontaneity.[7] Psychophysiologic processes are subtle, and difficult to detect by the naïve individual, and one task of the therapist is to help the patient develop an awareness of these changes. The therapist can also provide the patient with exercises other than biofeedback that expand individual capacity.

Induction of the mental state of "passive concentration" is relatively easy by means of biofeedback.[8] Once in this state, a person can observe and assess fantasies and thoughts with a measurement of objectivity and detachment. Such a state is clearly the prerequisite to self-understanding and is the basis for constructive alterations in behavior. Once the awareness takes place, the patient proceeds to "get in touch" with those aspects of his or her internal functioning that need correcting and learns how to interpret autonomic reactions more accurately. A competent therapist can help the patient develop an understanding of the particular way in which he or she manifests reaction to stress and, with biofeedback training, develop healthier ways of coping with the stress of everyday life. An individual can then fully participate actively and directly in learning how not to be ill. The body maintains its defenses as long as it is in a state of "ease."

Treatment Setting and Techniques

There are a variety of devices now available to the clinician for monitoring various body functions. In our practice, we use, primarily, a sensitive thermometer for temperature feedback (blood flow), an electromyograph (EMG) for muscle tension feedback, and an electroencephalograph (EEG) for brain wave feedback. Our aim is to elicit the "relaxation response" (integrated hypothalamic response leading to decreased sympathetic nervous system activity)[9] and to acquaint individuals with their internal processes in order that they might gain insight into their psychological and physiological state.

Early observations of the "specificity hypothesis" (the way in which each individual reacts to stress and life events)[10] led us to institute a multiphasic approach to treatment regardless of the symptom for which treatment is sought. Each person seeking treatment must learn to warm his or her hands (control blood flow), reduce and increase tension in the muscles, and control brain wave activity with an adequate degree of spontaneity. Usually a primary instrument for treatment evolves, and the major portion of training will take place on the instrument that monitors the internal state the patient finds most difficult to control.

The use of a team approach, with a male and a female therapist, allows the use of a multiplicity of techniques that are not always possible in a one-to-one therapeutic setting. The use of biofeedback equipment requires that electrodes be placed on the patient, and this touching can be a "laying on of hands" that is very beneficial to many patients. The way that the therapists relate to one another (warm, friendly, noncompetitive) serves as a model for the patient. Conversation between therapists concerning the patient's progress and success with the instruments can have a positive supportive effect. The team's interaction, while offering encouragement and support, can serve to emphasize the fact that patients are expected to make changes in their physiological and psychological functioning.

In order to facilitate a carryover to regular living, the treatment setting is a small, informally comfortable room that is not shielded from ordinary office noise and interruptions. It is made clear that skills learned in the office are to be carried into the patient's everyday living. The many adjunctive techniques used to reinforce learning are tailored to the individual and are dependent upon age, lifestyle, ethnic or cultural influences, economic factors, or personal preferences. These techniques are almost always used in modification and are incorporated in home practice exercises. These might include Autogenic Training, Jacobson's relaxation, meditation, imagery, self-suggestion, operant conditioning, behavior modification, or simple physical exercises to induce muscle tone and body awareness.

Biofeedback, coupled with psychotherapy, helps the individual develop new, more adaptive and satisfying conceptual structures and to find ways of integrating needs with life circumstances. Fundamentally, this involves helping the patient clarify or modify attitudes and values.

Case Histories

The following case studies are presented to serve as an illustration of (1) the potential of biofeedback as a therapeutic agent (2) the diversity of complaints that can be treated effectively, and (3) the variety of other therapies contributing to biofeedback's effectiveness.

Case One

This eighty-three-year-old female was referred for treatment of tension headaches of two years duration. The headaches developed immediately following bilateral cataract surgery. She had had extensive neurological tests with no dysfunctional organic findings and had some relief for a short period with "heat treatments." Three weeks prior to coming for her first visit, she was having headaches day and night.

On her first visit she discussed her problem and explained that her husband, a retired successful engineer, had been ill for some time and required constant care. On observation, she was nicely dressed, looked younger than her stated years, was warm, friendly, and intellectually sharp. Therapy consisted mainly of biofeedback combined with emotional support, instruction, suggestion, and autogenic phrases.

When placed on the electromyograph for the first time, she showed marked tension in the frontalis (forehead) muscle. By the end of the session, she had reduced the tension to three quarters of her beginning level. Her brain wave readings during relaxation indicated a relaxed alpha state. Her statement at the end of the session was, "Calming myself is very helpful." She was given autogenic phrases for home practice and instructed to do them twice a day, morning and night, for ten to fifteen minutes.

As treatment progressed, she was able to reduce her tension in the frontalis muscle and was headache-free by the sixth visit. In the course of treatment, the major portion of training took place on the electroencephalograph (EEG). She was able to maintain mid-range alpha with high amplitude. During the EEG training, we explored the various problems associated with her eyes and worked out a simple solution for inserting the contact lenses, a morning ritual that had contributed to the original tension pattern. Her problems with housekeeping and attending her husband were resolved by simple conversations suggesting possible alternatives. With little assistance, she implemented all suggestions and, by the sixth visit, was having a weekly outing with an old schoolmate and enjoying the weekend ride with her husband that her teen-age grandson had initiated.

The treatment schedule consisted of half-hour, weekly visits. Termination took place by mutual consent after six visits. The patient felt she had absolute control of her tension and was symptom-free. Her parting remark was: "My husband tells me I'm smiling now. This is the first time he's seen me smile in a year."

She returned for treatment one year later, saying that the headaches were under control, she now had help at home eight hours a day, but her husband's condition had worsened, he was now bedridden, and she had strained her back in moving him. Treatment consisted of EMG training on the back muscles while she assumed a reclining position, with the aim of enabling her to maintain a comfortable sleeping position. After the third visit, she felt she had the strain under control, and treatment was terminated with her promise to keep in touch with us.

Case Two

This forty-four-year-old male shipping clerk complained of colitis of four to five years duration and was referred for biofeedback therapy. We treated him on an average of once a week for three months and currently see him once every three to four months for a "checkup" (his term). At first, the patient was significantly apprehensive, so that our first goal was to create a relaxed, friendly, nondemanding relationship.

The experience with this person illustrates several points. It became clear rather quickly that the "colitis" could properly be diagnosed as an irritable colon that was symptomatic of the patient's anxious anticipation of failure on the job and a reflection of his low self-esteem. As he learned to quiet his rather marked muscle tension, he became more confident and was less and less upset with his fellow workers. His wife and son commented on the fact that he no longer had fits of anger at them. The psychotherapy was mainly supportive. He was reassured that he was really quite "normal" (his term) and, in fact, much more creative in his thinking than he was aware of. By the fourth month of the treatment, the patient was able to spend three weeks in Europe without any symptoms.

The therapy consisted mainly of biofeedback, combined with emotional support and reassurance. The fact that this patient learned that he was in control and could reduce his physical tension did much to build his self-esteem.

Case Three

This thirty-three-year-old female was referred for treatment after suffering a stroke with right hemiplegia during delivery of her only child five months prior to her first visit. She had had physical therapy since the date of the vascular accident and had been told that further benefits from therapy were limited. She was wearing a brace on her right arm and on her right leg and was using a cane when she came to see us.

The wife of a minister, she was highly motivated and had a positive attitude about overcoming her present disability. She expressed intuitive feelings about her ability to reactivate the muscles but was having difficulty implementing her feelings. We immediately began work with the extensor muscles on the right arm, using the electromyograph (EMG) to show the presence of electrical activity. During this first visit, while watching the instrument dial, she was able to raise her wrist for the first time since the accident. This positive event was sufficient to convince her that she had found the way to implement her inner feelings of control.

If she consciously concentrated on a training task, she was unsuccessful. (Passive, or inactive, conscious effort is necessary to achieve internal control.) We worked on "letting it happen" while she kept her mind on pleasant thoughts or conversations and maintained a relaxed alpha brain wave state while training on the EMG. EEG training to maintain an alpha state proved helpful for this purpose. Performing the task on the left side of the body was helpful in relearning the skill on the right side. Visual imagery (imaging in her mind's eye) was used to help her develop a conceptualization of what was happening inside her body.

Since she traveled a good distance for visits, we saw her on a monthly basis. Home practice consisted of supportive techniques that she could integrate into her daily housekeeping and child care. These consisted of autogenic phrases during periods of relaxation, the performance of tasks in fantasy, if not in fact, as well as the repeated use of each new skill learned during treatment in practical everyday activities, such as holding a pencil. Due to the infrequency of visits and the severity of the illness, the patient was allowed the use of an instrument for home practice during a two-month period. (Ordinarily, we do not give instruments for home practice. We feel this eliminates any instrument dependency that might occur and encourages the individual to develop body awareness.)

As treatment progressed, she was able to abandon her leg and arm braces. A dramatic occasion was the discovery of her ability to walk perfectly without aid during a shopping tour. When she became consciously aware of the fact, she lost her ability to do so. She gradually regained the ability and is now driving a car, maintaining her home, and caring for her child without outside aid.

With supportive counseling she has prospered, though confronted with periods of crisis in her personal life. With the discovery that it would be necessary for her husband to make a change in his professional life, she returned to graduate school and is currently doing volunteer work with brain-damaged individuals at a local community hospital, using biofeedback and her own experiential learning in helping others.

In all, this patient was seen for a total of twenty-six visits over a period of a year and a half. She is leading an active life with little residue of her disability.

Concluding Perspective

Over the past decade, research in biofeedback has demonstrated that if an individual can become aware of an internal process that is usually outside of awareness, he can modify it. This approach has enabled us to treat a wide variety of illnesses with more than moderate success. The diagnoses include not only the so-called psychosomatic illnesses, but also a wide variety of others.

The research designs attempt to eliminate or minimize personal interaction between subject and researcher. In our use of biofeedback in healing, we have added the ingredients of various psychotherapies: we use the instrument as a bridge between us and the patient, while at the same time adding a close personal interaction which, to us, is the most important element in healing.

Notes

1. R. Dubos and M. Pines, *Health and Disease* (New York: Time-Life Books, Life Science Library, 1975).
2. E. E. Green, A. M. Green, and E. D. Walters, "Voluntary Control of Internal States: Psychological and Physiological," *Journal of Transpersonal Psychology* 2 (1970): 1–26.

3. William Osler, *Selected Writings of Sir William Osler* (Oxford: Oxford University Press, 1951).
4. E. E. Green, A. M. Green, and E. D. Walters, op. cit.
5. A. T. W. Simeons, *Man's Presumptuous Brain* (New York: E. P. Dutton, 1960).
6. A. E. Gladman and N. Estrada, "Clinical Applications of Biofeedback in the Context of the New Medicine" (Paper delivered at the First National Congress on Integrative Health, Tucson, Ariz., October, 1975).
7. Kenneth R. Pelletier, "Diagnostic and Treatment Protocols for Clinical Biofeedback," *The Journal of Biofeedback* 2 (Fall–Winter, 1975): 4.
8. W. Luthe, "Method, Research and Application of Autogenic Training," *The American Journal of Clinical Hypnosis* 5 (July 1962): 17–23.
9. H. Benson, J. D. Beary, and M. P. Carol, "The Relaxation Response," *Psychiatry* (February, 1974): 37.
10. F. Alexander, "The Logic of Emotions and Its Dynamic Background," *International Journal of Psychoanalysis* 16 (1955): 399.

Bibliography

Barber, Theodore; Dicara, Leo V.; Kamiya, Joe; Miller, Neal E.; Shapiro, David; and Stoyva, Johann, eds. *Biofeedback and Self Control*. Chicago: Aldine-Atherton, 1971 (Contains seventy five selected articles on biofeedback prior to 1970). See also later editions of this book.

Basmajian, J. D. "Conscious Control and Training of Motor Units and Motor Neurons. In *Muscles Alive: Their Functions Revealed by Electromyography* by J. V. Basmajian. 2nd ed. Baltimore, Md.: Williams & Wilkins, 1967.

Brown, Barbara. *New Mind, New Body*. New York: Harper and Row, 1975.

Gladman, Arthur E., and Estrada, N. "Biofeedback in Clinical Practice." In *Psychiatry and Mysticism*, edited by Stanley R. Dean. Chicago: Nelson-Hall, 1975.

Jacobson, Edmund. *Progressive Relaxation*. Chicago: University of Chicago Press, 1938.

Karlins, M., and Andrews, L. *Biofeedback: Turning on the Power of Your Mind*. Philadelphia: Lippincott, 1972 (Programmed for the lay reader).

Pelletier, K. R., and Garfield, C. *Consciousness: East and West*. New York: Harper and Row, 1975.

Pelletier, K. R. *Mind as Healer, Mind as Slayer*. New York: Delacorte, 1976.

Tart, Charles T., ed. *Altered States of Consciousness*. New York: Wiley, 1969.

16

Claudio Naranjo

Meditation and Psychosomatic Health

TO SPEAK of the beneficial repercussions of meditation upon soul and body is to speak of the healing virtue of spiritual experience—a fact observed since the earliest times. Indeed, the domains of the sacred and of healing were once, in the story of human consciousness, inter-fused. The shaman, leader of souls, was at the same time a prophet and a medicine man. It is clear that in the spiritual traditions that arose from the shamanistic matrix, too, sainthood and the "miraculous" power of healing have continued to keep company.

The relation between the spiritual and the physical has been particularly stressed in the formulation of esoteric Taoism, in which enlightenment is understood as a condition inseparable from health, and this from a process in which the holy and healing "elixir of immortality" flows unimpeded through the subtle channels of the body. Buddhism, on the other hand, has emphasized the connection between nirvana and psychological health. In Tantric Buddhism it is possible to find the most elaborately perfected body of theory and practice concerning the interdependence between the spiritual (Buddhahood) and the mind-body complex.

In our day, the modern West turns towards the ancient East. And psychology, after a creative season in the field of healing through interpersonal interactions, seems to be rediscovering the healing power of the transpersonal element and the potential of *intra*personal work. Increasingly, I think, psychotherapists are coming to accept the traditional Eastern claim that meditation is, not only the royal road to enlightenment, but also beneficial to physical and mental health.

In Buddhism, which may be regarded as a religion of mind development, two basic types of meditation are usually distinguished: (1) Samatha, leading to the pacification of the mind; and (2) Samapatti or Vipassana, also called insight meditation, involving the cultivation of awareness. In the great meditation traditions of later Buddhism, such as Zen and the Tantric Mahamudra teachings, Samatha and Samapatti become one. Worship and surrender to God's will are, of course, the basic gestures of Western spirituality, and they were emphasized in pre-Buddhist India. There are two ways to union, says Patanjoli: Yoga—in the sense of a stopping of mental agitation (*cittavriti-nirodha*)—and *Isvara-pranidhana*, surrender to the Lord.

When I wrote the chapter Meditation—Its Spirit and Techniques for the book the *Psychology of Meditation*, I proposed a threefold classification of approaches: I contrasted the Apollonian, disciplined style of concentrative meditation (Samatha) with the Dionysian style of surrender, and saw these two in turn as standing in contrast to the path of emptiness, as embodied, for instance, in Zazene. Today I prefer a fourfold classification. In the new model for the dimensions of meditation that I have adopted, there are contrasted, in the first place, (1) nondoing, the basic Yogic maneuver of stopping the mental merry-go-round, and (2) letting go, the equally basic religious nonmaneuver of surrendering. We may place these at opposite ends of a horizontal line, while representing at the ends of a vertical coordinate still another polarity in the domain of meditation: (1) mindfulness, the cultivation of awareness (as in Buddhism or the "fourth way" approach), and (2) God-mindedness, the cultivation of the sense of the holy, which is related to the internal gesture of worship. (See Fig. 16.1.) In mindfulness, awareness is focused on the phenomenal self, but consciousness in God-mindedness is said to rest in the indwelling adamantine Buddha nature, the inner Christ, or the Essence, which is of the nature of the Absolute. This focusing of awareness on the divine, however, culminates in an experience in which the subject-object duality disappears, so that the meditator may be said to be absorbed in the meditation, the I and the Thou, the human in the transhuman—so we may call this practice *absorptive* meditation. It includes those spiritual exercises in which a real or mental object becomes the symbol of divine, cosmic, or

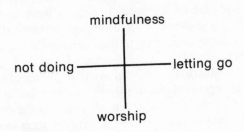

Fig. 16.1

archetypal experience—a blue pearl, the sound of the ocean, a mudra, the scent of jasmine, the taste of honey, and so on.

I am proposing with this scheme that we distinguish, not only four basic types of meditation, but also four dimensions or components of meditation, all of which converge upon and are contained in the experience that constitutes the meditator's ultimate goal. Higher consciousness involves silence of the lower or peripheral mind, a condition of internal freedom and spontaneity, awareness, and sacredness. This implies that the polarities that I have described are not contradictions but *complementarities*, for they are only contradictory on a superficial level of experience. The contrasting gestures of coming to a state of mental stillness and of allowing the free flow of internal processes, for instance, are compatible, and they come together in a mental state that is at the same time one of mental silence and one of inner freedom, as is frequently described in Zen literature.

Without the experience that lies at the hub or heart of meditation, however—the ineffable experience that involves at the same time peace, freedom, consciousness, and numinosity—meditators pursuing the separate paths of not doing and surrender (for instance) are likely to develop contrasting mental attitudes. The path of Wu-Wei (the traditional Chinese term for not doing) can easily lead to a meditation that is "too dry." The path of letting go, on the other hand, can easily become "too wet" in its ecstasies. These two paths, the wet or lunar and the dry or solar, which are the dominant styles of the East and West, respectively, can potentially take the meditator to a common destination, however. This is not to say that the spirituality attained through the pursuit of one path or the other is identical. It would be more exact to say that even though the summit of the mountain can be reached from the east or the west as well as from the north or the south, we must also understand that the experience of the summit will differ in some respects according to the experiential background of the different climbers.

Elaborating on this simile, we can say that the mountaintop will be experienced and expressed differently by one who has come by way of the swamps and by another who has climbed up the rocky cliffs, for each has developed peculiar abilities during the long journey and will now receive the new impressions in a mind that has specialized in a certain way. In the same manner, the experience of enlightenment is differently articulated by those who came to it through mindfulness or through the way of God-mindedness. This polarity, too, expresses contrast of the dry and the wet and the difference between East and West, and is, beyond the apparent contradiction evoked by the terms, a complementarity. To the extent that the way of mindfulness reaches its destination, it is a gateway to spiritual experience, so that even the driest form of Theravada Buddhism rests in a context of religiosity. The pursuit of God-mindedness, on the other hand, can only become a true experience of the Divine (as distinct from intellectual conception) with the assistance of mindfulness. Absentminded prayer is not prayer.

Mindfulness and not doing ordinarily stand out in the Yogic or dry path of the East, while God-mindedness and surrender are stressed in the West; yet both ends of these polarities are important in the most developed manifestations of Eastern and Western spirituality: Tantric Buddhism and Sufism. It could be said that these traditions, which represent the growing tip of the Yogic and prophetic paths, and which have come to rest in adjoining areas at the center of the Eurasian continent, have developed a comparable balance between Yoga and devotion, mindfulness and God-mindedness, self-remembrance and the remembrance of God—as also between internal silence and spontaneity.

It might be confusing to attempt to examine the psychosomatic aspects of meditation without some notion of what its components are, for the forms of meditation are many. Given the dimensions that I have enumerated, however, it is possible to ask about the therapeutic relevance of not doing, letting go, mindfulness, and absorption. I will share my answer at once, in few words: These four internal gestures lead to a single consequence: the dissolution of the ego, or "lower mind," which in turn makes possible the experience of our deeper nature ("higher mind")—Mind-as-such, our True Being. And though the extinction of the ego (*fana*, "emptiness") precedes the realization of Being (*baqa*, "illumination" or "gnosis"), the two may be regarded as aspects of a single event that are simultaneously present in the enlightened mind. We may picture the convergence of not doing, spontaneity or naturalness, awareness, and absorption upon the dissolution of the ego by placing the condition of nonego, or Being, at the center of the fourfold graph—and so could we do in order to represent the convergence of the four mental operations upon the experience of Being, as shown in Fig. 16.2.

More exact, however, is to visualize nonego and Being as the two ends of another dimension that crosses the other two at their intersection (see Fig. 16.3.). In the hexagon that results from this construction, the vertical axis may be regarded as the fruit or consequence of meditation, while the plane of contact between the upper and lower pyramids could be called that of the work of meditation, its process or course. Yet all six concepts that I have enumerated can be regarded as dimensions, aspects, or components of the meditator's mind, whether the plane or the axis is in the foreground, whether the work of meditation or its fruits is more prominent in the field of awareness. (It is interesting to note that, according to tradition, one does not imply more effective or useful meditation than the other.)

When I use the terms *nonego* and *nothingness* interchangeably, I am of course using *ego* in the sense given to the term by the spiritual traditions rather than in that of psychoanalysis or "ego psychology."

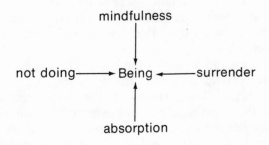

Fig. 16.2

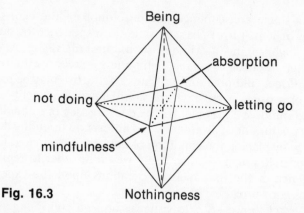

Fig. 16.3

Since a failure to distinguish between these old and new meanings has been the source of some confusion in discussions of the ideal of egolessness, I will be more precise about what I mean by saying that the dissolution of the ego is a common process shared by all meditation. Translating old understandings into psychological language, I would describe ego loss as a melting away of a dysfunctional system within the psyche. The ego, an organization of experience and behavior that was once an emergency operation in the face of pain, has ended in constituting an antiorganismic force, a self-obstructing and deadening factor. The ego may be understood as an insularization of consciousness—in the sense that an island of personality tyranically assumes control over the whole and thus interferes with the more complex and subtle process of wholistic, organismic self-regulation. This is true at both the physical and mental levels, for the psychological ego is rooted in physical processes and may be said to cast a physical shadow. An important aspect of this "body ego" is what has been called, since Reich, the body armor or character armor, a pattern of chronic muscular tensions that bear a relation to the process of instinctual repression.

Conversely, a basic aspect in the psychophysiology of nonego or enlightenment is relaxation; the capacity of relaxing at the physical level may be regarded as a gateway to the subtler relaxation of the mind, first at the emotional level, in the form of nonattachment, and then at the intellectual level, as a suspension of verbal and conceptual activity. According to Tantric Buddhism, the processes of the mind are inseparable from the circulation of *prana* or energy in the body, and the mental condition of *shunyata* (emptiness) is coupled both with relaxation and with certain processes that manifest in deep relaxation, classically described as the perceptions of centers (chakras) and conducts (nadis) in the subtle "enlightenment body." It is a release phenomenon belonging to this domain of experience that Reich described when he spoke of "streamings." By these he referred to a pulsation that he considered the mark of full aliveness. The phenomenon may be regarded as an expression of spontaneity or nonrepression; together with other expressions of "energy," it is a physical concomitant of the mental spontaneity and nonrepression of the oceanic experience.

The intimate connection between relaxation and the activation of the streamings (and other subtle "energy phenomena") is the same that may be seen, in the domain of meditation, between stopping and letting go—which I am claiming are not true opposites, but alternative forms of freedom from conditioned processes. But the traditionally known phenomena of *prana* are precipitated not only by nondoing and by letting go. They are also cultivated through the sharpening of attention and are a concomitant of absorption. The same may be said of the mental side of ego dissolution—dispassion and the cessation of thinking; all four strategies of meditation converge upon them.

If the ego is, at the behavioral level, a fixidity of obsolete conditioned responses that interfere with the spontaneity of instinctual and intuitive self-regulation, at the emotional level it is passionateness. Desire and aversion, narcissism and fear may well be regarded as emotional compulsions that stand in contrast with the enlightened attitude—which is responsive and appreciative yet open, loving yet not craving, abundant yet not deficient. It is because of the passion underlying our behavior that we cannot easily "just sit." As Suzuki Roshi once said, "To work on something is not difficult, but to work on anything is rather difficult." To suspend external activity may be possible—though probably boring—but the suspension of mental activity goes against the ego's craving, compulsion to cope, ambition, and automatisms.

If not doing involves a victory over compulsiveness and habit, the same may be said of letting go. All passion involves clinging, which is opposite to letting go, and to let go, contrary to misconception, involves some courage and ability to escape the grip of passion and be open to the unexpected. Significantly, Shiva, Lord of Yogis, is depicted, not only in meditation, but also in dance, and he is sometimes represented as a *lingam*, or phallus. The condition of nonego is freedom to stop as well as freedom to go, and it is freedom *from* both. Moreover, the experience of egolessness (or, better said, until enlightenment, suspension of the ego) entails, as I have mentioned, an aspect of stability or quiet and one of fluidity and spontaneity, as in a changeless ocean with infinite waves or the reflections of flowing water on a mirror. This, at the experiential level, echoes the physical concomitants of stopping and letting go in the form of relaxation and release phenomena (perceptual, motor, and autonomic). Yet it would not be correct to consider these two aspects of experience a true duality; the state of nothingness entails the cessation of certain mental operations and also a letting go to a spontaneous tendency of the mind, as when we surrender to sleep.

The reciprocal relation between awareness and passion flows from the interdependence, in the function of the ego, between passion and active unconsciousness, repression, and self-deadening. There is repression because there is something at stake in seeing things and ourselves in a certain way, and conversely, repression, by robbing us of our wholeness, feeds dissatisfaction and deficiency motivation.

Awareness, on the other hand, the most evolved form of feedback in the organism, supports proper function. In contrast to passion, which gropes in the dark ("unconscious motivation"), the light of consciousness dispels phantom needs and goes hand in hand with dispassionate abundance. The value of awareness (just as that of letting go) in the cure of neurosis has been rediscovered by contemporary psychotherapy (specifically Gestalt therapy), and awareness may be understood as a goal of therapy as well as a technique. The same is true of awareness in meditation. The *Therevada* practice of insight meditation, for instance, in cultivating watchfulness cultivates also an attitude of nonidentification with the contents of consciousness and dispassionate noninterference; it may eventually lead, in successful cases, to a quantum leap in the transcendence of the ego—the crossing of the "great waters."

The psychology of absorption is that of self-forgetting in the contemplative or theurgic act of creative imagination. (Its physiology is that of relaxation and deep trance.) The affective aspect of self-forgetting is a selfless abandon dispassionate enough to lead to a temporary "death in God." This psychological death involves more than the severance of attachments, however. It entails, in its intellectual aspect, the suspension of conceptualizations, just as is brought about in the practic of *Wu-Wei*, and which may also be brought about by intensive mindfulness, as in Vipassana or Fourth Way schools, or by surrender. For the same four gestures that undermine the ego at the heart, making it dispassionate, undermine its life at the head, making it empty. And they undermine and eventually put poison in the belly of the physical ego, the deepest scar of karma (the impact of the past). The process of the *via purgativa*, throughout which the ego undergoes various stages of dissolution, has not only a mental but a physical aspect, and this not without its agony. "Karmic tensions" well up in meditation in the form of neural processes that may cause sensations such as those of being full or worms, or of burning, among others— just as a psychological cure usually involves temporary worsening, and acupuncture sometimes brings about the symptoms manifesting the body's dysfunction in the form of a therapeutic crisis. As these tensions are meditated through or processed, however, and as faulty conditioning melts away, a regenerative process takes place—the circulation of the "elixir," the awakening of the "serpent power" that is the physical concomitant of spiritual experience.

In some traditions, these physical processes—connected to the "subtle body" as experienced by one who has developed a finer perception or function than the ordinary—are specifically reinforced by concentration on the energy centers and the help of images or words. Such skillful means are, however, something of a luxury, for these release phenomena that supervene when the output (innervation) "noise" of the ego is in abeyance are a natural consequence of "purely mental" meditation: the practice of nonego through a nonconceptual and dispassionate approach to experience.

The most fitting physical support for this practice is that of mere relaxation, so that there is a relaxation of the body and its breathing, a relaxation of grasping (as in *trying* to meditate or seeking to obtain something from meditation) and of thinking (in the form of mental silence). From the removal of obstructions in body, heart, and mind, a new body, heart, and mind come into operation, subtler than those under the control of the ego, in the form of a "body of light," compassion, and openness. It is the process of ego dissolution or ego relaxation that may be spoken of as the psychology of meditation proper, while the emergence of Being from behind the veil—ranging from presence in the here and now to spiritual Presence—lies in the domain of Spirit rather than that of the soul.

To summarize then: *Per aspera ad astra.* Four ways lead to new life and reality through the death of the unreality-creating factor, or ego—a death that is gradual and yet punctuated by quantum leaps. It is this dissolution that makes the experience of Being possible and from this experience virtue flows naturally and the healing potential of the organism is released. The hexagon of meditation is asymmetric: not only does it express a polarity of yin and yang in its horizontal dimensions, but it has a bottom and a top, just as a tree has roots and foliage that are not interchangeable. Self-remembering and self-forgetting, stopping and flowing, lead to Being through the extinction of false being, to awakening and reality through the cessation of the dreamlike state that human culture has come to regard as the fullness of consciousness.

The dissolution or relaxation of ego is the crux of the psychology of meditation and involves, basically, three aspects: (1) cessation of conceptual operations, (2) letting go of attachment-aversion (and defensive unconsciousness), and (3) deep relaxation. The experience of "I am that I am" is its mystical theology: a phenomenon of *gnosis* or revelation that supervenes when psychophysical obstructions have been removed. The work of meditation is a purification and a therapeutic experience that opens the way for spiritual experience and constitutes *our* end of the stick—what is in our hands to pursue.

I have remarked in passing how the value of awareness and of letting go have been rediscovered in contemporary psychotherapy; the same could be said to some extent of the other dimensions of meditation that I have outlined: absorptive identification and a spiritual orientation are prominent in transpersonal approaches, such as psychosynthesis, and not doing is manifest in the purely contemplative attitude of orthodox psychoanalysis and in the injunction against manipulation in Gestalt therapy, for instance.

All this does not mean that meditation and psychotherapy are redundant. In my view, the ideal situation is one in which interpersonal and intrapersonal work are combined and supported by an intellectual context and by some form of attention to the body, so that the individual advances at the same time on all fronts—physical, affective, intellectual, and spiritual. Having in recent years created and directed an integral program in human development comprising these four components (SAT Institute), I have had occasion to appreciate how efforts in the four directions can be mutually supportive and the total effect of the curriculum most substantial. I quote typical response to a questionnaire study on the effects of the program:

> I am calmer, clearer, happier. I know myself better, and I accept myself—and others. I am less manipulative, more open and loving, more relaxed, I regain my balance more quickly when I fall. I play more, allow myself more freedom and fun. I am more childlike and more mature, I have felt more and longer periods of ecstasy in the last year than in all my life before. I feel certain that I am on the Path. I feel a vital connection with the Spirit, and—very often—an at-oneness with the whole of life.

In a situation such as I have described, it is difficult if not impossible to discriminate what results derive from meditation and which from other factors (such as group dynamics or world view), so that the records of personal experience available to me are illsuited to document broad ideas of the kind I have enunciated—such as the effect of meditation in dissolving the ego by undermining conceptual thinking and attachment, or in relation to the relaxation of the body armor and to little-known sensory-motor excitatory phenomena. What I can do, however, is to collate from such material a mosaic of statements that may illustrate psychological and physiological effects of meditation in the words of specific individuals. To this end, I am concluding this otherwise theoretical paper with a clinical colophon consisting of three excerpts from meditation journals:

> I've reread my year's meditation notes. At first the great highs and colors and depressions and body sensations and all kinds of exciting things, energy zipping around my body, etc. Then this spring deep depressions, fear, fighting with ———. But also my experience fasting which seemed to leave me at a higher level. Something changed then, which has remained. After that [May], meditation levelled out. Fewer highs and lows. More silence. The retreat seems to have again moved [my] consciousness to a new level of stillness and love. Openness. You wrote once: "Love is all-there-is and Emptiness," and that seems to say it. Love flowing out of emptiness. Those seem to be my values now, the places I feel right in: Emptiness and a state of open love without wanting. The retreat did something, which came to fruition in the last two days of the retreat. Open love. And ——— and I are more open to each other

Perhaps because it is done in the evening, or maybe because it is just the right antidote for an achievement-oriented person, this meditation bears much fruit for me. The most characteristic experience is a feeling of being entirely balanced and still and at rest. I seem to go to a place that I know or remember. I don't know how to convey the feelings of being *exactly* balanced, at a place that has no dimension, no time like the instant of rest between the excursions of a pendulum. And of course, there is no problem about thoughts or gaze—everything goes and I keep my eyes closed in utter darkness. Another "result" is a feeling of tremendous strength. Sometimes I feel a very delicate and widespread vibration. The sense of poised awareness endures through these other phenomena. The most dramatic symptom I get is a pressure at the back of the head that seems to be made by something hard and flat pressing on my head. It is real. The first time it happened I was terrified. Now I welcome it. There is also pressure on the bridge of the nose. Finally, there [are] localized pressures at the base of the spine, in the area of the mid-back, and a strange, more local and rounded pressure at the very top of my head. I assume that these sensations are related to chakra activities.

One of the things I have been struggling with in my meditation practice, as in all else, is coming to terms with my tendency to be either excessively self-punitive or excessively self-indulgent. In the early months of my meditation practice, I was plagued with the feeling that I was a failure at it, I wasn't doing it "right" or even that I wasn't meditating at all. Dutiful good student that I usually am, I persisted nonetheless, and was considerably relieved by statements from you to the effect that it was the fruit of the effort, not the "success" of the session, that was important. This made sense to me, as I experienced an increasing sense of calm despite the fact that my sittings were so full of thoughts. [1]

Note

1. Phyllis M. Beauvais, "Claudio Naranjo and SAT: A Modern Manifestation of Sufism?" (Thesis, Hartford Seminary Foundation, Litchfield, Conn., 1973).

Bibliography

Longchenpa. *Kindly Bend to Ease Us*. Translated by H. V. Guenther. Emeryville, Calif.: Dharma, 1975. This is a more difficult book than those listed below. It may be consulted for a discussion of the perception of Being.

Naranjo, Claudio, and Ornstein, Robert E. *On the Psychology of Meditation*. New York: Viking, Compass Edition, 1971. This book provides an overview of the various forms of meditation with particular emphasis on the absorptive form and the way of surrender.

Suzuki, Shrunyu. *Zen Mind—Beginner's Mind*. New York: Walker-Weatherhill, 1970. Castaneda, Carlos. *Tales of Power*. New York: Simon & Schuster, 1975. These books may be recommended for discussions of not doing.

Thera, Nyaponika. *The Heart of Buddhist Meditation*. London: Rider, 1969. This is an excellent discussion of the path of mindfulness.

17
Patricia Garfield

Wholistic Health and Dream Work: Using Dreams to Enhance Health*

THE SUN makes dappled patterns on the cool green tile floor as it filters through the lacy curtains and ferns in my plant-filled sunporch. I love this quiet time of day. I recline comfortably with a book in the fan-backed wicker chair, my feet propped up on a reed stool. There's a soft afternoon breeze from the casement window that lifts the deep green spears of the potted palm.

In the still of that sunny-cool afternoon time, I hear a soft rustle. A tiny ruffle. Turning to my right, I see, with a wave of intense pleasure, that a petal of the first gardenia bud has just unfolded. Spellbound, I watch and behold with the same soft flurry the unfolding of the fragrant flower. In one magnificent moment the whole flower is there. One soft whoosh, and the bright white, rich, perfumed presence pervades the room. The petals arch back and push forward the center of the bloom.

Sometimes in the midst of hectic days, rushing to meet someone through heavy downtown traffic, skirting cars, weaving through crowds, thinking of a dozen things to do before dinner, I have an image of that delicious moment when the gardenia unfurled before my eyes. Why does it so fascinate me? Flowers open all the time. Yet to *see* and to *hear* it happen was a kind of marvel, a magic instant. And I carry within me the image of that transformation, which sweetens the most beleaguered days.

---

* "Using Dreams to Enhance Health," Copyright © 1978 by Patricia L. Garfield.

And sometimes that pretty blossom lifts its soft, white head once more in a dream, long after it fell withered and brown. In fact, the condition of my dream flowers and plants often reflects the state of my body. Images like my blooming gardenia, observed while awake and then dreamt about, or images dream-derived and then reflected on while awake can be of vital importance. They have power to heal.

Dream Imagery and the Emotions

We of the Western world have long used dreams to give us messages about our emotional state. We dream of being trapped in a small room with no one to hear our cries and, on waking, know full well that the dream symbolizes our sense of entrapment in a particular relationship. We find ourselves in a dream overwhelmed by great tidal waves and need no interpreter to tell us, after waking reflection, that we do, indeed, feel overwhelmed by a certain situation. We see a dream animal hauling a tremendous load, almost unbearably heavy, and realize as we consider it on waking that, of course, a specific burden of responsibility we carry is too much. We are accustomed to reading the emotional messages dreams contain.

But we have not yet learned to reliably read the messages about our bodies in our dreams. And, more importantly, we have not learned to actively use our dreams to produce the healthful physical conditions we desire.

In fact, our dreams are one of our greatest resources. They can serve our physical as well as emotional needs. Most particularly in the dream state we can express the intricate interconnections between our bodies and our emotions, even better than in the waking state. In dreams, our power to visualize is increased manyfold. Our power to symbolize is superb. When we utilize it, our power to change and to heal ourselves in our dreams may be supremely effective.

Dream Healing in Ancient Times

Using dream images to reinforce health is not new. Ancient peoples sought out special places—rough-hewn caves, sacred temples—where they came to perform rites, worship the local god, sleep, and seek a divine curative dream, or get advice on treatment to obtain a cure.[1]

Ordinary dream images were sometimes used by ancient peoples to diagnose a disease already present or as a warning of an impending disease. Hippocrates, the founder of modern medicine, in the work attributed to him, described a correspondence between the condition of the dreamer's body and the dream images he or she produced.[2] The basic assumption was that the heavenly bodies and all cosmic events were symbolic in dreams of the state of health or sickness of the dreamer. For example, if the stars, moon, or sun shone normally and were in their correct orbits, the dreamer's body was thought to be functioning harmoniously also. If the stars, moon, or sun were clouded or dimmed or fell from their orbit, disease was said to be shaping. Likewise, analogies were set up between the condition of dream trees and the dreamer's body. The movement of dream rivers was likened to the movement of the dreamer's blood.

People of today would not be as likely to symbolize their health by such images, but we can readily understand them when we consider the importance of the starry skies and other natural phenomena for the ancient dreamer.

Disease Prediction in Dreams?

Contemporary Russians feel they have evidence that specific diseases are forecast by specific dream imagery.[3] A consumptive patient, for example, for months before her condition was diagnosed, dreamt she was buried alive. She could feel the weight and cold of damp earth heaped upon her chest, her breathing was labored, and she awoke in panic. In a similar way, patients who were later diagnosed as having cerebral tumors had previously dreamt of being wounded in the head.

Whether such dreams were truly predictive or were magnifications during sleep or already present but minute symptoms that had until then gone unnoticed in a waking state is not yet clear. It may be that, in just such sensitive ways, dreams can be of value in early diagnosis.

However, considering the fact that dreams are often symbolic as well as literal, we cannot totally rely on this approach. The consumptive patient could have been expressing a feeling of being buried in some life situation rather than signaling the development of a diseased condition of the lungs. Nonetheless, such dreams can be significant cues. Either emotional or physical disturbance is a matter of valid interest on behalf of a health state for the whole person.

Finding Health Messages in Dreams

Our best stance in looking to our own dreams, then, may be to consider, at least initially, the general condition expressed, rather than to watch for specific disease symptoms. My own dreams often reflect my general physical health. At times this is symbolic. I may inspect a dream plant to find it is infested with bugs, or find plants that are drooping for lack of water and care. Or, conversely, I may discover some tender new shoots or luxuriant new growth, and my good physical condition often corresponds. At other times, my physical condition is depicted more directly, as in the following recent dream:

> I am in a kitchen preparing dinner. Near me sits a girl on a stool who is very, very tired and cranky. She has dark circles under her eyes. I think how her behavior is not unreasonable considering her state of fatigue. I'll be patient and she'll probably feel better after dinner.

In this case I had in waking life been exhausted from the preparations for a large party and then by the party itself two days before the dream. I still felt physically worn, yet, as the dream suggested, I'd be all right and was. A weary condition is usually expressed directly in my dreams these days; the dreams advise me to be cautious and get additional rest.

On another occasion, however, I neglected a dream warning that might have enabled me to avoid serious inconvenience. I came down with a severe virus that lasted on and off for a month. Some time later, curious to see if my dreams had forewarned it, I looked at the records of the dreams of the two nights preceding my becoming ill. Sure enough, the Sunday night before the Tuesday morning that I woke up feeling sick, there was this obvious warning in my dreams:

> I am with my husband at a party. We are being given hexagrams (symbolic arrangements of six lines given as answers when the *I Ching* is consulted as an oracle) by a psychic who obtained them by an elaborate process. The hexagram given to my husband predicted that

he would not be sick, but he should watch his health. There was nothing else special in it. For some reason I thought there had been a mixup and that his hexagram should have been given to me.

Unfortunately, once awake, I didn't pay much attention to this dream fragment and proceeded to become quite sick. We need to become attuned to our bodies and their feelings enough to learn to recognize such early dream messages.

Could extra precaution based on this dream warning have helped me avoid becoming ill? Perhaps. In fact, if I had known the power of visualization at the time of this dream, I might have been able to use it to alter the course of the disease that followed.

Waking Visualizations Can Heal

Hippocrates not only used dreams in diagnosis; he also anticipated recent findings on the power of images to heal. He believed the following dream images are healthful signs: the sun shining in strength, the stars radiating brightness, the rivers passing majestically, clothing of dazzling whiteness, and in general, the sun, moon, and stars, clear and bright and in their rightful positions. If such dream symbols reflect health, he reasoned, can we not induce them when sickness threatens?[4]

Robert Desoille, a contemporary French therapist, uses this concept as a basis for his "guided waking daydream" therapy. He states that the most efficacious images are Jungian archetypes, including images of natural phenomena that influence our lives. He considers the daily movement of the sun, movement from left to right, from down to up, from darkness into light, to be desirable images to induce. He further believes that the physician should not suggest the images *per se* but should draw them from the dreamer's own personal experience.[5] That is to say, the physician should find the archetypes within the dreamer's own personal dream imagery and then summon these archetypes during the waking state "guided daydream."

Desoille's and Hippocrates's concepts combine readily with the findings of Carl Simonton, a contemporary physician of Fort Worth, Texas, who has demonstrated the power of visualization in affecting the course of terminal cancer.[6] As part of a process that includes traditional treatment, Simonton has his patients visualize a peaceful, natural scene. He has them picture their cancer, and see their immune mechanism working to pick up dead and dying cells, a kind of army of white cells swarming over the malignant ones that have been weakened or killed by radiation therapy. The patients see the white cells break down the malignant ones and flush them out of their bodies. Finally, the patient is to see himself or herself as well. Thus, *the patient is visualizing both the process of attacking the disease and the final goal state of good health.*

Patients are educated about their disease and shown their own X rays and pictures of tumors healing so that they have specific images to visualize. They may wish to visualize these curative events in their own symbolic terms. For instance, one of Simonton's terminal cancer patients (who was given a thirty percent chance to live) pictured his cancer as some despicable animal like a snake or wolverine. He saw his immune mechanism as a pack of white husky dogs who dashed in, attacked, tore apart the vicious animal, and finally licked the area clean. He pictured this scene for ten to fifteen minutes three times a day. After six weeks of meditation, an examination showed his tumor reduced by seventy-five percent and after two months, a cancer scan showed all trace of it had disappeared. Many of Simonton's patients show similar recovery patterns.

We already know that people can learn to regulate their body mechanisms by biofeedback—for example, changing blood flow, heart rate, or amount of acid in the stomach. Yogis have been doing it for centuries without feedback. They control body experience by visualization, for example, producing body heat by visualizing a sun or a fire at certain nerve centers.[7] Such pinpointed visualizations can direct blood flow to a specific spot in the body. Now it seems that we, too, are discovering how imagery can affect bodily change.

The Senoi Confront-and-Conquer Technique

The Simonton visualization technique is, in my opinion, a version of what I have called the confront-and-conquer technique for use in dreams.[8] The usual Westerner's response to a frightening dream image is to try to get away from it. We run from the threatening dream monster, the unknown evil stranger, and so on. As capture becomes imminent, we "escape" further by waking up. The Senoi, a primitive Malaysian tribe, however, teach their children to stay asleep, to face the dream attacker, to fight back, to get help if necessary, to win, and to destroy the negative dream image. Eventually, in their system, the spirit of the conquered enemy becomes a servant to the dreamer and provides him or her with "gifts"—poems, songs, dances, designs, inventions, and so on.

The constant application of this principle during dreams seems to produce a culture that has extraordinarily good psychological adjustment. The pattern of confront and conquer leading to good emotional health is remarkably similar to that of the cancer patient who confronts his disease image, conquers it, and derives the gift of good physical health.

Learning to Read Dream Symbols

Students whom I have taught to confront and conquer negative dream images develop, like the Senoi, greater confidence and ability to cope with problems in waking life. Perhaps we can infer a general rule that a person must always face internal threat head-on in order to overcome it, whether the threat is emotional or physical.

Since a major component of physical illness is emotional (the World Health Organization estimates that, in the United States, eighty-five percent of patients seeking medical help have no organic basis for their symptoms), it seems highly probable that the confront-and-conquer technique may be effective for many types of internal physical breakdown in addition to cancer.

I believe it is quite probable that our dream state offers us unique opportunities for early awareness of our physical as well as our emotional condition and needs. *We must, first of all, learn to read the symbols of our dreams that present messages portraying current physical conditions.* If dream plants droop, if dream characters are weary, or if they receive comments urging them to watch their health, we need to heed such signals. By extra care, we can perhaps reduce the severity of an impending disease, if not avert it.

If our dreams suggest methods of treatment, we, like our ancient predecessors who incubated dreams for the purpose of obtaining advice or cures, may well benefit from advice givers who appear in our dreams. A group of doctors who were consulting in a dream about a sprained muscle I actually had, urged heat, which did indeed help. Of course, such a suggestion is hardly novel. However, *we can at least consider whether treatment suggested in dreams might be helpful.*

The Power of Mental Practice

Most importantly, however, I think, is the potential of dreams to produce new conditions. Waking visualizations are far more effective than most Westerners yet realize. Controlled experiments have demonstrated the value of mental practice. For example, practicing throwing darts by imagination as one sits in front of the target has been shown to improve aim as much as actually throwing the darts.[9] Students who practiced sinking basketballs on free throws in their imagination for twenty minutes every day for twenty days improved their scores on a post test almost as much (twenty-three percent) as those students who spent an equivalent amount of time in actual practice (twenty-four percent improvement). Students who engaged in neither mental nor actual practice showed no improvement.[10] Recent writers in sports fields have urged the value of mental practice and visualization of the desired goal in improving golf scores and tennis performance.[11,12] Oriental weightlifters are said to have long employed similar mental practice. The con man character Professor Harold Hill in the musical comedy *The Music Man* taught his band players to play their instruments by the "think method" to avoid detection of his lack of musical training. As in his case, if the basic skills are not present it is unlikely that any amount of mental practice will help. But *given basic skills it seems we can literally practice them by the "picture method."*

Dream Practice as Optimal Mental Practice

Thus, mental practice of any sort is effective. Dream practice may be even more so. Women pregnant with their first child who had anxious dreams about their upcoming labor experience were likely to deliver their babies more easily and in shorter time than the women who did not have such dreams.[13] Researchers hypothesize that the women who attempted to master the anticipated stress of childbirth by coping with it in their dreams were preparing themselves to perform more efficiently and with less tension. Arnold Schwarzenegger, holder of the Mr. World title for several years, told me that he often dreams the night before a big competition that he is performing well and wins. Shy students who learn to confront and conquer negative dream figures find themselves able to be appropriately assertive in waking life situations.

Dream practice can prepare us to cope with waking stress more effectively. As we confront and conquer in our dreams, we experience the event as though it were happening, even more vividly than if we were imagining it. We *feel* the fear, the action, and the victory as though they were real. Perhaps the physiological changes produced by the dream experiences are more intense, too. At the same time, our bodies are deeply relaxed, even more than in meditation, thus providing a condition of maximum receptivity to the new learning. Furthermore, not everyone can take the time to engage in waking visualizations, but all of us sleep. And we dream about twenty percent of our sleeping time. This is time we can use to develop our visualization skills and our health.

Enhancing Health with Visualization

While awake, we can symbolize our discomfort, whatever it may be, and our immune mechanism attacking it, just as the patient pictured his cancer as a snake and his white cells as husky dogs. Or, we can read our dream language and pick out the symbols of health or illness that emerge from it. In either case, practicing confronting and conquering in vivid picture language in the hypnagogic state prior to sleep, or running through these symbols during a dream, can have powerful repercussions.

Dreamers can even learn to become conscious of the fact that they are dreaming. This so-called lucid dream state can be triggered when a dreamer becomes so frightened that he realizes he is dreaming or when he becomes aware of incongruities during the ongoing dream and deduces that he is in a dream. In the lucid dream state, dreamers can call up desired imagery at will. *We can use lucid dream states to reinforce healthful imagery as well as to cope with specific problems.*

Enhancing Health with Dreams: A Summary

Suppose we have a diseased condition that requires a specific *process of treatment*. We can use our dreams to enhance healing by taking these steps:

1. Become familiar with the healing process required and put this into vivid picture language. For example, one could determine, "I need more white cells to destroy the malignant cancer cells," and picture the cancer as a rat and the white cells as a troop of white angora cats.
2. Practice confronting and conquering the disease symbol (e.g., rat) by the symbol of strength (e.g., cats) in clear pictures. Make every detail of the struggle as clear as possible. Do this in the relaxed drowsy state prior to sleep or during meditation.
3. Become alert to incongruities in ongoing dreams while asleep and try to analyze them during the dream, until you become fully aware that you are dreaming. Summon the desired imagery of successful confrontation.

Supposing, however, we are ignorant of the necessary process to cure ourselves, or indeed, supposing we are not ill but simply wish to reinforce our good health, we can use our dreams to enhance a *desirable final state of health* by undertaking to—

1. Picture ourselves as vigorous and vibrantly healthy. Do this in the drowsy state prior to sleep or during meditation, or conjure up these images in lucid dreams.
2. Symbolize our good health in the manner of the ancients. Use such images as bright sun, moon, stars; clear, majestic, flowing rivers; or clothing of dazzling whiteness. Focus on them while drowsy or meditating or during lucid dreams.
3. Select images that seem to reflect health from our own personal dream language. Deliberately replay them while drowsy or meditating. Summon them during lucid dreams. Examples might be luxuriant foliage, fragrant blossoms, or strong dream characters of our own making.

White Light as a Healing Symbol

The brightness of the stars and dazzling whiteness of clothing mentioned in step 2 above are related to the concept of white light that mystics have associated with healing processes. I find it intriguing that in almost every altered state of consciousness—mystic experiences, drug states, lucid dreams—those people experiencing the altered state mention a change in the quality of the light during the experience.

In fact, the most common perception reported by people who have a mystic experience is a change in the quality of light.[14] People describe the landscape as becoming flooded with a clear, bright light, or they see individual objects and people as radiant, as though glowing from within. Light as a divine symbol in all religions and cultures probably stems from this mystic experience. Halos of the saints, auras of the mystics, the luminous and jeweled landscapes of paradises and fairy tales are thought to reflect this "illuminated" or "enlightened" condition. A contemporary anthropologist suggests that enlightenment is a physical and measurable event in the brain, as well as a psychological experience. He says that "endocranial bioluminescence" may be a literal form of light generated in and by the brain.[15]

When ordinary dreams become lucid, the dreamer often experiences a shift in the quality of light from murky or commonplace to one of brilliant clarity. Objects infuse with color and glow or even pulsate. When we "awaken" to the fact that we are now asleep and dreaming, I believe we are experiencing a kind of "minienlightenment." Theorists are not able to explain why this happens, but the phenomenon occurs so repeatedly it deserves exploration.

It may be that the bright light of lucid dreams has healing properties as well. We may find it beneficial to picture white light in our drowsy states and seek it out in our lucid dreams. We can see ourselves as surrounded by a cloud of brilliant white, like sunshine on fresh-fallen snow. We can direct this light to injured areas. Such visualizations can change the actual flow of the blood.[16]

Personal Healing Symbols

Other symbols of healing and protection are available. Those people for whom religious symbols still hold intense feeling can evoke them.

People who practice transcendental meditation and chanting tell me that they often find themselves repeating their mantra during their dreams whenever frightening images appear. Other people visualize their gurus or saints.

Carl Jung suggested that the most meaningful symbols of all emerge out of our own psychic life experiences.[17] He believed that the major problem for the person in the second half of life (over thirty-five years of age) is to find a religious outlook. He asserted that his patients had lost touch with a sense of value in traditional religions and were not totally healed emotionally until this value was regained or replaced. The outer forms and symbols of religion were no longer satisfying. The archetypal symbols that emerged from their own dreams, however, were possessed of power. "It is from the depths of our own psychic life that new spiritual forms will arise. . . . .[18]

Attending to our dreams and staying alert for the special images, the ones that puzzle and fascinate, will help us get in touch with our inner values. Unusual dream images such as a dancing vegetable or a woman with antler-branches growing from her head are idiosyncratic. These idiosyncratic dream images are ideal for meditation or calling up during lucid dream states because they are tailor-made by and for us. They already have the power to capture and concentrate our attention.[19]

Active Participation through Dreams

All dream symbols—frightening images, conquering figures, helpers, victims—are aspects of the dreamer. Unfortunately, most dreamers have not recognized the strength of their abilities to mobilize positive resources to cope with the negative elements within themselves. We can become our own shaman, confronting our malevolent spirit with our own positive forces, invoking help when necessary and exorcising the evil spirit inside us.

By picturing the battle _within_ us, especially in our dreams, whether it represents physical breakdown or emotional disturbance, we can begin the process of coping. We can confront. We can fight. We can get help. We can overcome. We can become whole. We can learn to use our body's own mechanism for self-healing. We can enhance our entire well-being.

Isn't this faith-healing? Of course. But the fact is that a picture held vividly in the mind over time can produce physiological effects. Expectation has powerful repercussions. Prisoners of war who believed they would be free by Christmas time died off in excessive numbers after Christmas arrived and they were still imprisoned.[20] Cancer patients who have an optimistic outlook and a desire to live have spontaneous recoveries, whereas their equally ill "colleagues" who feel pessimistic die as predicted.[21]

I am not suggesting that we should stop medical treatment or substitute dream imagery (or waking visualization) for medical care. I am suggesting that we become cooperative partners in our healing, active coworkers in the process. Eat well, sleep well, exercise regularly, follow indicated medical treatment. But take your picture pill three times a day until cured. Use your power to visualize to enhance the treatment. Direct your mind to cooperate with your body.

People can take responsibility for their well-being. We can read the messages in our dreams and be guided to prevent illness and to enhance our general health. We can help ourselves to become radiantly healthy on every level.

The lotus of the Eastern mystics that symbolizes illumination and the sweet gardenia that unfurled that sunny day on the porch are not so far apart. The whole flower, dazzling white, with its deep fragrant center, is symbolic of a wholeness of self: a mandala to carry in the mind's eye, an image to focus on, awake or asleep, that may one day bring a unity of personness.

Notes

1. Patricia L. Garfield, *Creative Dreaming* (New York: Simon & Schuster, 1974).
2. Raymond De Becker, *The Understanding of Dreams* (London: George Allen & Unwin, 1968).
3. Ibid.
4. Ibid.
5. Ibid.
6. Mike Samuels and Nancy Samuels, *Seeing With the Mind's Eye* (New York and Berkeley: Random House, 1975).
7. Ibid.
8. Patricia L. Garfield, op. cit.

9. Maxwell Maltz, *Psycho-Cybernetics* (Englewood Cliffs, N.J.: Prentice-Hall, 1960).

10. Ibid.

11. Ibid.

12. Tim Gallwey, *The Inner Game of Tennis*, described in *Powers of Mind* by Adam Smith (New York: Random House, 1975).

13. Carolyn Winget and Frederic Kapp, "The Relationship of the Manifest Content of Dreams to Duration of Childbirth in Primiparae," *Psychosomatic Medicine* 34 (1972): 313–20.

14. Aldous Huxley, "Visionary Experience," in *The Highest State of Consciousness*, ed. John White (Garden City, N.Y.: Doubleday, 1972).

15. Roger Wescott, as described by John White in *The Highest State of Consciousness*, ed. John White (Garden City, N.Y.: Doubleday, 1972).

16. Richard Wilhelm, "Death and Renewal," in *The Highest State of Consciousness*, ed. John White (Garden City, N.Y.: Doubleday, 1972).

17. C. G. Jung, *Modern Man in Search of a Soul* (New York: Harcourt, Brace, 1933).

18. Ibid.

19. Richard Wilhelm, op. cit.

20. Viktor E. Frankl, *Man's Search for Meaning: An Introduction to Logotherapy*, 8th ed. (Boston: Beacon Press, 1969).

21. Mike Samuels and Nancy Samuels, op. cit.

Bibliography

Arnold-Forster, Mary. *Studies in Dreams*. New York: Macmillan, 1921. Charming account of adventures in dream control.

De Becker, Raymond. *The Understanding of Dreams*. London: Allen & Unwin, 1968. Scholarly overview.

Faraday, Ann. *Dream Power*. New York: Coward, McCann & Geoghegan, 1972. Presents Gestalt view.

Garfield, Patricia. *Creative Dreaming*. New York: Simon & Schuster, 1974; paperback. New York: Ballantine, 1976. Presents methods for changing dreams.

Jung, C. G. *Modern Man in Search of a Soul*. New York: Harcourt, Brace and Company, 1933. Classic.

MacKenzie, Norman. *Dreams and Dreaming*. London: Aldus Books, 1965.
Popular and well-illustrated overview.

Martin, P. W. *Experiment in Depth*. London: Routledge & Kegan Paul, 1955.
Popular presentation of Jungian view.

Rossi, Ernest. *Dreams and the Growth of Personality*. New York: Pergamon
Press, 1971. Expansion on concept of idiosyncratic dream images.

Samuels, Mike, and Samuels, Nancy. *Seeing with the Mind's Eye*. New York:
Random House, 1975. Visualization techniques.

18

Victor M. Margutti

Homoeopathy, Homoeotherapeutics, and Wholistic Healing

TODAY, DRUG proliferation in disease treatment is raging rampant. Some drugs *are* wonder drugs, but their number alone causes confabulation and confusion—unavoidable with valid observation, excellent ideation, and conflicting conclusions.

This problem is compounded, yet simplified, by the growing awareness of the Oneness of all life, the uniqueness of the individuality of man (indicated by the permanent personality of the fingerprints), and the importance of health on a wholistic basis. This treatment of the totality of Being as a wholistic person has been emphasized for over one hundred and fifty years by homoeopathy, which as a methodology is ancillary to all care, yet panacea to none: that extra arrow in the therapeutic quiver that may work when all else fails!

Definition and History

Homoeopathy, the basis of homoeotherapeutics, is a term derived from the Greek *homoios* ("like," "similar"), and *pathos* ("feeling," "suffering").[1] As a scientific methodology, homoeopathy employs specific substances ("remedies") that cause certain signs and symptoms in "healthy" people. The remedies are administered to those who in their illness exhibit similar signs and symptoms and resultingly relieve them of these signs and symptoms. This principle was illustrated by Samuel Hahnemann, the founder of homoeopathy—that revival of paracelsian principles rooting deep in antiquity—in his own experiences with "Jesuit" or "Peruvian" bark, the cinchona bark of the Incas.

Hahnemann was master of fourteen languages, including Latin, Greek and Hebrew, and also had a great knowledge of botany, chemistry, and physics, as well as the medicine of his day. In his translating of Cullen's *Materia Medica*,[2] he became interested in the reports on cinchona, and being an avid experimenter (and his own best subject), after six years of intensive study concluded that the toxology of the bark generated all the classical signs and symptoms of the "ague" then prevalent in Europe. He then showed that, when concoctions of this bark were given to "ague" patients, their syndrome of symptoms was relieved. From these observations and the results of other careful studies, he formulated the principle of *Similia Similibus Curentur*, or "Like Cures Like"—that is, the toxic signs and symptoms of substances as determined by use in the "well" can indicate the clinical use of these substances in the "sick": when properly used, the symptom-producing substances alleviate these selfsame signs and symptoms.

Chemistry and Physics of Preparation

In developing homoeotherapeutics, it was found not only that any substance could be used, but that succussion (the vigorous shaking of the dilutions) added specific qualitative factors to the remedial actions of the substances so treated. This qualitative-quantitative character, or the combination of dilution factor and development, in time became post-Avogadrian in nature. [Post-Avogadrian, according to Dr. Margutti, means remedial actions of the substances in which no physical particle of the original substance can be found, in a dilution of 1×10^{-23}.]

The combination of a homoeopathic solvent and solute in a microdilution succussion often contains less than the gram-molecular weight of certain substances. Thus, classically, there is no particle mass of these substances to have any effect, yet homoeopathic microdilutions of 30, 50, 900, 1,000, etc., each in its own particular way, have clinically benefited patients. (Thus the order of magnitude of minimal dosage becomes important, but we have to look for a mechanism other than that of direct proportionality.) As Mock states,

The first study examined the effect of "microdoses" of mercuric chloride upon the rate of starch hydrolysis by malt diastase. Because the dilutions of mercuric chloride in distilled water used were in the order of 10^{-61} to 10^{-71}, the term "microdoses" seems almost gross, for in terms of contemporary physical thought, not a single molecule of the mercuric chloride should be present in the test solutions. Nonetheless, the introduction of these extraordinarily high dilutions induced a paradoxical acceleration of the starch hydrolysis by the diastase rather than invoking the expected inhibition which regularly occurs with lower concentrations (10^{-6} and below). But the crux of the issue in this experiment is the degree to which the active agent ($HgCl_2$) was attenuated and still delivered its effect with a striking validity ($P=<0.001$) when compared with samples of distilled water.[3]

A mechanism allowing for the disproportionate quantitative effect of the minimal amount of solute, or "microdosage," on the solvent could be a sudden shift of electromagnetic energy frequency in direct proportion to intimate differences in molecular structure. Thus a sudden discharge of electrical energies, with concomitant ionization changes causing oxidative-reductive changes, could accomplish the very rapid responses often noted with the application of the properly selected remedy.

Boericke and Smith (and later Smith), working with succussed high dilution beyond 10^{-24} (at which point and beyond, any solute in a chemical dilution disappears), showed that by using nuclear magnetic resonance techniques (NMR), ultrasonics produced serial dilution effects similar to those of succussed solutions.[4] It is opined that there are physical-spatial changes on the OH solvent radical (possibly the "fingerprints" of hydrogen?),[5] so that the solute imprints "on" the solvent so that the latter bears the "stamp of approval" for therapeutic action, and that this phenomenon extends to as yet unknown stages of dilution-succussion. (For those interested in the specifics of these principles, there is an excellent summary in *Journal of the American Institute of Homeopathy*, 60: 159 ff.)

Lawrence showed not only that a "transfer" principle exists, but that (for human use) "the human is the best, perhaps the only, experimental animal that could be used."[6] These observations in man didn't fit with the results other workers had obtained in experimental animals. Just recently it seems to have dawned on everyone that the animal studies were extremely difficult to reproduce and that the human is the best—perhaps the only—experimental animal that could be used. (These conclusions were based upon the injection of live white blood cells from subjects immune to tuberculosis into tuberculin-negatives. The results showed that tuberculin hypersensitivity had been passively transferred. Small volumes of cells could provoke an immunity lasting a long time.) Lawrence asserted,

> My view has been that you can't quarrel with nature. You have to take the results as they come. Perhaps nature was trying to reveal something new that experience and theory had not prepared us to understand. In any event, the facts will remain the same. It's our interpretations that may vary as our factual knowledge and understanding enlarge.[7]

Particularistically oriented scientists are often given to subjective rejection on purely theoretical grounds, rather than by objective experimental examination (just as Cardinal Bellarmine's representatives found nothing in Holy Writ to allow for the existence of moons around Jupiter, and so they believed it unnecessary to look through Galileo's telescope). That is, such scientists have a compulsion to "concern themselves only with experimentally derived data which suit existing theory."[8] Fortunately, the physical eye can "see" the moons, but the mind has to "eye" many abstract ideas before they can be "seen" and comprehended, and due to the uncomfortable strain of trying to comprehend the "new," it too may suffer from the refusal to consider anything not in "sacred scientific scripture."

Immunity Factors

Life per se, as we know of it, cannot exist without the power of immunity, that ability of a living organism to resist and overcome infection. This basically is an antibody stimulus-response complex, (probably) determined by amino acid antigen spatial linkage in the DNA molecule,[9] so that form would be a primary factor. Reaction may be largely a surface absorptive transfer phenomenon requiring the presence of an electrolyte.

Nuclear-cytoplasmic separation is by a dielectric semipermeable membrane, an extremely thin, possibly monomolecular, oil film with a capacitator reaction directly proportional to its thinness. Thus the sudden impact of a change in electrical potential, activated by a minimal homoeopathic and/or antigen dosage, could be telegraphically shocked throughout the appropriate system by means of central nervous system nuclei selective sieving, with possible resulting changes in solvent molecular structure and an end result in physical phenomena.

Antigens may be so highly diluted in the bloodstream that structure (such as amino acid linkage and atomic-molecular spatial arrangement) and threshold exposure may be of basic importance. Human immune-globulin type molecules are apparently multiple rather than single polypeptic molecular chains, either "light" or "heavy," and may be held together by disulfide bonds, hydrophoid bonds, and electrostatic force.[10] The area of variability within the molecule allows for a vast number of specific reactions. Apparently, not only do separated halves spontaneously recombine at neutral ph to form complete molecules, but removal of blocking agents allows the re-formation of disulfide bonds native to the molecule. This indicates within the H chain architecture the presence of an inherent ability, an organizer so to speak, for precise combinations. This could be accomplished by spatial pattern preferentiality, as may be illustrated by the fact that (apparently) the amino acid sequence determines the "folded character of a protein chain of 400 or more amino acids."[11]

The Association of Function and Structures

Nisonaff's studies support the importance of studying structure as an indication of function.[12] His work indicated that somehow the genetic DNA-RNA mechanisms are stimulated to form protein antibodies complementarily configurative to antigenic determiners.

Thus processes in vivo are pyramided complex chemical actions and reactions, which in turn are based upon subcomplex chemical actions and reactions, and these in turn are based upon patterned arrangement, rearrangement, and subsequent motion of electrons and atomic nuclei. These in turn are based upon electromagnetic field interactions characteristic of each elementary particle, and all takes place in weakly conducting electrolytes, therefore being difficult to obtain in strong electromagnetic fields.[13]

All earth life exists in a geomagnetic field of low minimalike intensity of around 0.5 Oe; and as Schuster and Wilson indicated, evidently even most celestial bodies have magnetic moments proportional to their angular moments so that life as we know it may be impossible without electromagnetism.[14] Man, as a small, circumscribed, discrete energy force-field unit, inescapably meshed in the *vis-a-terge* of living with fellow creatures and creations, irrevocably dependent on drawing energy from surrounding force-fields, must establish a reciprocal relationship with his environment. Thus life, as we know of it, is immutably bound by universal and planetary magnetic laws, and the warp and woof of the life process at all levels involves constant dynamic exchange and balancing of surrounding force-field energies (probably) as surface phenomena at all levels: energy manifests only by action. Biologically, on the cellular level, the alkaline cytoplasm is separated from the acid nucleus by a semipermeable colloidal membrane.[15] Electromagnetic potential differences concomitant to cellular oxidation and reduction are in direct relationship to detailed differences in molecular atomic patterned structure, each with its own characteristic ionization and accumulation of electrical energies. Protoplasm en masse may be thought of as a micro and millimicro, many sided, surface energy, transferring and transforming system.

Thus chemical structural information at times may have a greater role than chemical mass, e.g., the chemical, in forming a template for polymerization of the solvent. In passing its structural information content to pure configuration entropy of the solvent, the substance may have served its purpose. However, material doses may give reactions proportional to ionic concentrations in dealing with end products of disease and thus present attendant dangers of iatrogenicity. Goodman and Gilman prophetically stated that

> The actions of drugs are intimately related to their chemical structure. . . . Indeed, the structural requirements for biological activity may be so exacting that a drug may be a competitive antagonist to its optical isomers . . . . At the present time it is impossible to choose between the various theories of drug action . . . . Unfortunately, the primary actions of drugs have been elucidated in only a very few cases.[16]

This ancient Pythagorean principle of form determining function is also supported by Selye's observation that "glass objects regularly produce cancer when implanted under the skin of a rat. They fail to do so unless they have a certain shape." He has no explanation for this at this time.[17]

Spatial Concepts of Molecular Chemistry

As Barnard and Stephenson state,

> the concept that space is the formative matrix which gestates matter is both ancient and widespread, that in pre-Einsteinian science, spatial view of sensate matter shifted from a two to a three dimensional concept. Pasteur introduced space into chemistry with the description of levo and dextro-optical isomers of tartaric acid, each with different formulas, different properties, and different rotations of light. The spatial concepts of Watson and Crick developed the helical deoxyribonucleic acid (D.N.A.) as one of the vital genetic building blocks of biological life, a genetic formative force in its own essence. Thus protein specificity is the resultant of the exact order of amino acids in the polypeptide chain, that in drugs of similar chemical structure, minute changes in spatial arrangement can alter toxicity. Thus we return to the Pythagorean concept that the reality of things lie more in their form than in their materiality.[18]

The Vedas express a concept that the Real animates sensate reality in their concept of aether (Akasa) underlying and determining space; in their pondering of What is the origin of this World? "Aether . . . for all these beings take their rise from the aether only, and return into the aether. Aether is greater than these, aether is their rest."[19] This is also seen in the yin and yang of the ancient Orientalists, expressed through the "five element" theory in acupuncture.

Barnard and Stephenson point out that the spatial molecular chemistry of Pasteur was ancestral to the concept of helical DNA—in its own essence a genetic generative force with qualities attributable to the spatial formative essences of the ancients—the archetypal forms, so to speak.[20] Thus the DNA double helix could be an expression of "cosmic field energy" geometrizing in the precipitation of form. This may be seen in meiotic cell division with the arranging of chromosomes into helices, and also when the spindle lattices connect the centrosomes to the centrospheres. Burr summarizes these principles in his statement that the Universe in which we find ourselves and from which we cannot be separated is a place of Law and Order. It is not an accident, nor chaos. It is organized and maintained by an Electro-dynamic Field capable of determining the position and movement of all charged particles.

For nearly half a century the logical consequences of this theory have been subjected to rigorously controlled experimental conditions and met no contradictions.[21]

Conceptual Variations of "Dis-Ease"

Allopathic Occidental medicine considers disease as being the result of organic morphological changes, whereas Oriental (acupuncture) medicine, like homoeopathy, considers disease largely as the "dis-eased" balance of the body which functions as a whole unit, dynamically adjusting and balancing to stress throughout its body fluids, tendons, and ligaments by the reflex adjustments of the autonomic nervous system.[22]

Biddle gives an excellent summary of the body mechanics of stress:

> The point at which the integrity of a substance begins to be interrupted marks the beginning of strain. It need not manifest its tearing or injury so that we can see it, but *it feels!* The body acts and reacts at all times and opposite is not always discernible since it opposes [mechanical] force with a living force and [is] capable of bringing support to a part in need so that weight may be balanced by energy instead of by weight alone . . . . This is why the body is constantly in reaction or play to universal forces without it being noticed.[23]

A drug ultimately "cures" only through the sensitivity of the immunological system, dependent on cell surface membrane processes based upon micro and millimicro molecular exchanges involved in aqueous and crystalloid polymers.[24] Any action and/or reaction is an accumulation and a culmination of a genetic code affected by a lifetime of experience; a response to a chain of events as ecological excesses, deprivations, and traumas both physical and psychological; and reaching back through birth into prebirth. (So "exact" animal analogues, the precise allocation of responsibility for response among countless factors, recent and remote, are not only unreasonable but impossible to expect.)

Thus the prophetic reemphasis by Hahnemann of ancient Hermetic wisdoms in the principle of the minima in catalyzing the inherent defense mechanisms of the patient as an individual; his *"Personna of Illness,"* a principle clinically substantiated for well over 100 years, universally applicable in all cases due to the presence of low-intensity natural electromagnetic force on and within the body—for all life exists in a geomagnetic field of low minimalike intensity of around 0.5 Oe.

Energy-Life Fields and Homoeotherapeutics

To understand homoeopathy, it is essential to understand the concept that the space we live in is, and contains, a formative matrix, a vast eonic universal energy field perpetually gestating all matter. Burr, in his studies of over forty-three years, indicated the presence of electrodynamic fields of the body that mold and maintain its shape, regardless of any material poured into it and regardless of how often the material may be changed.[25] Thus the bread, beans, cabbages, and "stuff" mysteriously become "us." He called these fields "life fields," or "L" fields; they control all molecules, which are largely space, so that cells are rebuilt as before and maintain the same overall pattern. The chemistry provides the energy, but the electrical phenomena of the electrodynamic field determines the pattern.

Russell points out the statement of Dodd that "when one contrasts the great complexity of the protein molecule with the fact that millions of these substances are constantly being built up and disintegrated in the human body, and moreover built to precisely the same structure, one cannot help but speculate about the controlling mechanism, . . . where even a single amino-acid must not be out of place if the hormone is to have its activity or the antibody its potency."[26] (Hoagland estimates that there are about 60,000 billion cells in the human body and of these, 500 billion cells of some type die every day and are replaced by new ones.[27]) Russell refers to Sherrington's statement that "the brain is, of course, a corporeal thing and composed like other body organs of just physico-chemical stuff, which break down finally into waste products."[28] On the other end of the scale, according to the National Institutes of Health, "bone, once thought to be completely inert, actually wears out and is replaced constantly in the normal human skeleton. This turnover is similar to the continual replacement of the body's skin."[29] Thus, as Russell points out, all constituents of living matter, functional or structural, are in a steady state of rapid flux; furthermore, all living forms possess and are controlled by electromagnetic fields, . . . the organizing mechaniques, the "Life" or "L" Fields of Burr, that "keep all living forms in shape and that build, maintain and repair them through constant changes of material," which the genes and DNA are subordinate to.[30]

Voltage gradients in the "L" fields are pure, direct current potentials and accompany fundamental biological activity, as was demonstrated by showing that the moment of ovulation can be determined electrically,[31] and by Ravitz, who through the use of a voltmeter objectively measured the depth of hypnosis,[32] thus indicating the presence of what Russell calls "T," or "Thought Fields" as specific identities that yet intermingle and work with the "L" fields. The two kinds of fields form the "warp and woof" of the psyche and soma in the matrix of life.

The presence of the "L" fields and "T" fields as common to all life as we know it is indicated by the work of Vogel with philodendrons. He repeatedly demonstrated the effect of thought ("T" fields) on these plants' "T" and "L" fields, even over great distances.[33]

Man as a Physical Creature

"Man lives not on an island alone, but must be in constant contact with his environment or perish."[34] Enveloped in a dermal coat sensorially communicative with the surrounding media of pressure, gases, liquids, solids, heat and cold, electromagnetic gravitation, he is in reciprocal balance and exchange with internal-external-energy-force fields, which are autocratic in nature.

The cerebrospinal nervous system roots the mechanism of the conscious mind. Man, as Mind, may be considered as an inner force field energy, mediating with external force fields through the pia mater, brain, and nervous system and the interlocking endocrine and exocrine systems and the osseous-muscular ligamentous structures, all enclosed in a dermal coat. Thus man as man may be considered as a circumscribed, individualized energy complex in which pure spirit and grossest matter are joined by mind.

Man as Mind

Psychological energy, like all energy, is both centripetal and centrifugal, for mind and body can only function when work is done, and work is done only in response to a stimulus regardless of its source. Thus the life process is basically a balancing of energy field patterns between body, emotions, and mind.

It is of deepest concern today that the increase in scientific knowledge, hence power, is not paralleled by a coincident rise and development of human wisdom. Man in general is still an emotionally sensate creature. From the cradle to the grave, man craves rewards, enjoyments of sensations, praise, and gratifications of passions; he feels thwarted and deeply frustrated when he thinks that he has missed one iota of that which is "rightfully his." It is too easily forgotten, or deliberately ignored, that there are no rights or privileges in life. Everything must be earned. As we earn we generally learn, and as we learn we may get to "know." "True knowing" is the result of being and is universal and eternal in character, whereas "truth knowing" is a matter of semantics and time living. With the development of forebrain consciousness comes the capacity to select. With selection there develops the problem of the "good" vs. the "bad," and the latter leads to the development of guilt when the "bad" is repressed. With guilt comes conflict and duality.

The Somatic Basis of Medicine

Accepting the "good" into the conscious mind and pushing the "bad" into the unconscious does not cause the latter to cease to exist, for the energy of the "bad" always reappears in another reaction of equivalent energy value (generally an unconscious somatic action pattern), for psychological energy, like all energy, is subject to the laws of conservation, and within these alterations, the remanifestation of suppressed energy in another somatic pattern, lies the heart of all medicine.

Man's soma inherently is rooted in chemical and physical laws originating from the primordial mire. Thus material substances not only nurture the body but may also influence alterations in the living organism and so disturb its normal order of rhythm. The life process ultimately depends on surface membrane transfer processes, a primordial persistence of cellular individuality allowing pattern change responses to minute quantities, and so it is also basically qualitative in character. This correlative quality in turn often resembles a disease syndrome with all its mental and physical characteristics. This was noticed by Hippocrates in the fourth century B.C. and still earlier by Ayruvedic medicine; it was reemphasized by Hahnemann, who stressed the mentals of the case, then the physical signs and symptoms from the head down and from within out. Actually the doer, the act, and the environment are inseparable.

Again, there are no rights or privileges in life; all have to be earned. One can do whatever one wishes, but one must pay the price. This is the inexorable rule of life. This is the only way learning can be accomplished. Thus, as the world changes, the self will grow, and the only security lies within the self. Diseases are the self-created penalties proclaiming the frailties of the flesh and the will. The basic wholistics of homoeotherapeutics were well expressed by Kent, who stated that "mind is the key to Man, and Man consists of what he thinks and what he loves, and there is nothing else in Man. If these two grand parts of Man, the will and the understanding be separated, it means insanity, disorder, and death. Nothing exists without a cause. The sick man is prior to the sick body."[35]

Notes

1. *Webster's New Twentieth Century Dictionary*, unabridged, 2nd ed., s. v. "Homeopathy."

2. T. L. Bradford, *The Life and Letters of Dr. Samuel Hahnemann* (Philadelphia: Boericke and Tafel, 1895): 16.

3. D. Mock, "What's Going On Here Anyway?—A Review of Boyd's Biochemical and Biological Evidence of the Activity of High Potencies," *J.A.I.H.* 62 (1969): 197–98.

4. R. Smith and G. Boericke, "Modern Instrumentation For the Evaluation of Homeopathic Drug Structure," *J.A.I.H.* (1966): 263–65.

5. R. Smith and G. Boericke, "Changes Caused by Succussion on N.M.R. Patterns and Bioassay of Bradykinin Triacetate (B.K.T.A.) Succussions," *J.A.I.H.* 61 (1968): 197–200.

6. S. H. Lawrence, "Our Cells Learn Sensitivities—And Transfer Them," *Modern Medicine* (March 15, 1976): 78.

7. Ibid.

8. G. P. Barnard and J. A. Stephenson, "Fresh Evidence for a Biological Field," *J.A.I.H.* 62 (1969): 75.

9. V. M. Margutti, "Immunology and Homeopathy. A Review of Immunological Mechanisms and the Actions of Homeopathic Medicines," *J.A.I.H.* 60 (1967): 287–300.

10. V. M. Margutti, "The Minima Principle's Universality As Illustrated in Physiotherapy. A Research Study," *J.A.I.H.* 63 (1970): 143.

11. V. M. Margutti, "Minima Principle," p. 143.

12. Alfred Nisonoff, "Molecules of Immunity," *Hospital Practice*, 2 (1967): 19.

13. M. F. Barnothy, *Biological Effects of Magnetic Fields*, vol. II (New York and London: Plenum, 1969), Introduction XI.

14. Ibid.

15. V. M. Margutti, "Minima Principle," p. 149.

16. L. S. Goodman, and A. Gilman, *The Pharmacological Basis of Therapeutics* (New York: Macmillan, 1941): 17–21.

17. H. Selye, "Clinical Implications of the Stress Complex," *The Osteopathic Magazine* (March, 1970): 23.

18. G. P. Barnard and J. A. Stephenson, op. cit., pp. 73–74.

19. Ibid., pp. 23–24.

20. Ibid.

21. H. S. Burr, *Blueprint for Immortality* (London: Neville Spearman, 1972): 13.

22. V. M. Margutti, "Acupuncture in Treatment and Rehabilitation: Some Practical Points," *J.A.I.H.* 69 (1976): 27.

23. V. M. Margutti, "Minima Principle," p. 147.

24. V. M. Margutti, "The Minima, Man, and Biomagnetism: Some Contemporary Concepts," *J.A.I.H.* 65 (1972): 107.

25. H. S. Burr, op. cit., p. 13.

26. E. R. Russell, *Design for Destiny* (London: Neville Spearman, 1971): 23–24.

27. Ibid., p. 25.

28. Ibid.

29. Ibid., pp. 23–25.

30. Ibid.

31. Ibid., pp. 30–31.

32. Ibid., p. 31.
33. P. Tompkins and C. Bird, *The Secret Life of Plants* (New York: Harper and Row, 1973): 16.
34. V. M. Margutti, "The Value of Homeopathic Mentals in Relation to Psychiatry and Psychotherapy," *J.A.I.H.* 61 (1968): 21–27.
35. J. T. Kent, *Lectures on Homoeopathic Philosophy*, 4th ed. (Chicago: Ehrhart and Karl, 1937), pp. 13–15.

Bibliography

Barnothy, M. F. *Biological Effects of Magnetic Fields.* Vol. II. Plenum, New York and London: 1969.

Bradford, T. L. *The Life and Letters of Dr. Samuel Hahnemann.* Philadelphia: Boericke and Tafel, 1895.

Burr, H. S. *Blueprint For Immortality.* London: Neville Spearman, 1972.

Goodman, L. S., and Gilman, A. *The Pharmacological Basis of Therapeutics.* New York: Macmillan, 1941.

Journal of the American Institute of Homeopathy. Suite 506, 6231 Leesburg Pike, Falls Church, VA 22044.

Kent, J. T. *Lectures on Homeopathic Philosophy.* 4th ed. Chicago: Ehrhart and Karl, 1937.

Russell, E. R. *Design For Destiny.* London: Neville Spearman, 1971.

Tompkins, P., and Bird, C. *The Secret Life of Plants.* New York: Harper and Row, 1973.

19
Dolores Krieger

Therapeutic Touch and Contemporary Applications

THE LAYING ON of hands has been all but ignored in the West as a serious contender for scientific consideration. Our culture still suffers from the rigid social perspectives of the Victorian era, so that, in spite of the social revolutions of the 1960s, we are still largely a no-touch culture. A notable exception to the tight strictures of this code of behavior is nursing. Touch, one might say, is almost a badge of the nursing profession, its imprimatur, so to speak. We are allowed to touch, we allow intimacies that no other group in our culture is permitted under formal circumstances. Consequently I, as a nurse, have found *therapeutic touch*—a name I have coined for treatment by the laying on of hands—to be a very meaningful experience. I call this type of personalized interaction therapeutic touch simply because the term appears to be more acceptable to curriculum committees and other institutional bulwarks of today's society. However, in its long and ancient history, it has more descriptively been called the *laying on of hands*. It is a mode of therapeutic intervention that seems to have been extant, according to histories of many literate cultures, throughout the world; however, because of its subjective nature, it has been given little credence in modern technological society, whose scientific methodologies have been so deeply based on empirical evidence.[1] In looking back at my previous experiences, I had come to realize that patients remember your touch long after they have forgotten your face. Because of my strong conviction that this was important to the contemporary development of nursing theory at this rather unique

297

time in our cultural history, I felt it important to offer myself as a sort of research guinea pig, or more properly, a guinea pig researcher willing to try to bring some theoretical meaning to an area of human experience that has heretofore been veiled by a thick cloak of fearful awe and superstition.

Touch, as we well know, is not the sole province of nursing but is a subtle though universal signal among men for expression of empathy, of compassion, of friendliness. We have all had this experience of touch, if from no one else, then certainly from our mothers and fathers, those others significantly close to us at some stage of our becoming, our friends, and our guides. Nobody who has undergone any experiences of self with any degree of intimacy escapes knowledge of how important can be the touch of another.

Touch, of course, is probably one of the most primitive of sensations. Neurologically, touch and pain—two factors one is very much involved with when helping ill people—depend on the two central nervous system nerve tracts that are myelynized most early in the human neonate. During the time of labor and subsequent delivery through the birth canal, among the first sensations that the baby has is that of cutaneous stimulation. From the moment of birth, beginning while the baby is *en utero*, there is a whole evolution of touch experiences, from hand-mouth explorations of the environment to the hand-eye coordination that brings the environment to the individual, and these are built into the very fiber of human growth and development.

It is perhaps because touch is so primitive that it is so powerful as a fundamental therapeutic tool. All persons, whether nurse or doctor, therapist or friend, can look back upon times when touch was extremely meaningful in a personal way, either to themselves or to those they sought to help. Currently I have on file over 100 first-person accounts from nurses who have used touch quite unknowingly, or rather unknowledgeably, in a spontaneous manner during their nursing intervention with patients. These reports state that the encounter frequently resulted in unusual therapeutic changes that came as a surprise to themselves as well as to other members of the health team. In addition, I have had perhaps three dozen other communications from medical doctors, therapists, ministers, and laymen telling me of similar experiences that occurred when they were helping others. For the most part, however, therapeutic, comforting effects via touch are such a common occurrence that most of us become all but indifferent to the experience, and we are unaware that something, anything, has happened except in retrospect. We rarely, in other words, give its significance cognizance.

Nurses use healing by the laying on of hands quite naturally, I think, in responding with an empathetic touch to the person who is frightened or in pain, or a comforting touch for a primapara during her first birth experience, or in a quieting touch for a psychotic in frenzy. The use of touch as a therapeutic tool should be acknowledged.

I developed my own interest in touch as a therapeutic tool as a nurse and continue it as a nurse. Both the Grad studies and the studies of Sister M. Justa Smith at Roswell Research Park in Buffalo challenged my interest as a nurse practitioner, teacher, and researcher;[2,3,4] however, because I am a nurse my concern is with the effect on the total human being, rather than on the dissociated enzyme, or plants or animals, and I set as my goal *in vivo* human studies that would help clarify the process through which the effect of the laying on of hands is made known.

For several years it happened that I had an opportunity to make use of my nursing abilities during the few weeks when Oskar Estabany (the "Mr. E." of Grad's and Sister Justa's studies) annually visited the United States to set up a healing clinic with a well known investigator of paranormal healing, Dora Kunz.[5,6] During these times I would take case histories, check vital signs, and in general carry out the role of nurse as the need arose. Many of the patients came to these sessions from diverse parts of the country, and I had an opportunity to observe their interactions with the healer quite closely. What I saw was not startling. The atmosphere was friendly and quiet, and conversation, when it occurred, was natural and spontaneous, although subdued. Estebany's touch was light and relaxed, with no unusual passes or maneuvers. To a casual observer it might seem that nothing was happening. At the end of the session, I was involved in the follow-up of these patients' conditions. As the returns came in (many of these patients had been medically referred), I was astonished to find upon analysis of the data that a significant proportion of these patients got better or actually became symptom free, and this on the basis of verified case histories. Nothing in my previous education or experience had prepared me for these kinds of findings, and so I decided to study this phenomenon in considerable depth, particularly since the obvious independent variable was touch, a therapeutic modality very familiar to nurses. A quite thorough search of the literature from Western countries, however, did not prove fruitful in eliciting a clue to the modus operandi of this healing process. I have a considerable background in the study of comparative religion, particularly the Eastern religions, and so my next search was directed towards the East, rereading material I had come upon several years before for clues that might guide my search.

In the East, the interaction between healer and subject is thought to occur by means of a state of matter for which we in the West have neither the word nor the concept. It is called *prana* in Sanskrit; the nearest translation we have would be "vitality" or "vigor"—i.e., that which lies behind the animation we recognize as the life process. The literature states that the healthy person has an overabundance of prana, and that the ill person has a deficit; indeed, the deficit is the illness. This prana can be activated by will and can be transferred to another person, if one has the intent to do so. The literature also states that prana comes from the sun and is intrinsic in what we in the West call the oxygen molecule.

As I began to put the pieces together, the research findings from the West and the literature from the East, I realized that the test object I sought within the person being treated by the laying on of hands might well be hemoglobin.[7,8,9] Hemoglobin is that component of the red blood cells that is highly sensitive to oxygen uptake and its deliverance to the tissues. In his study of barley seeds, Grad had reported an increase in chlorophyll in the sample irrigated by water that had been held by Estebany. Both chlorophyll and hemoglobin are tetrapyrroles and have exceedingly similar stereochemical structure, the major difference being that the chlorophyll molecule focuses around an atom of magnesium while hemoglobin centers around an atom of iron. Moreover, Sister Justa's study on enzymes also pointed to hemoglobin, for in both its biosynthesis and its functioning, hemoglobin is deeply involved in many enzyme activities. By synthesizing this knowledge with other information of a hematological nature, I concluded that hemoglobin would be a valid choice for a test object through which to study the effect of the laying on of hands on human beings.

The conceptualization that I began to develop from all of the above ran something like this: I realized that my basic assumption was that human beings are open systems, that they appear indeed to be a nexus for all fields of which life partakes—inorganic, organic, psychic, and conceptual, the electrodynamic being only one part of the whole—and as such they are exquisitely sensitive to wave phenomena, i.e., energy. The healer I saw as an individual whose health gave him or her access to an overabundance of prana (health indicating a highly efficient interaction with the significant field forces), and whose strong sense of commitment gave the healer a certain control over the projection of this vital energy for the well-being of another. The act of healing, therefore, would entail the channeling of this energy flow by the healer for the supplementation of that of the ill individual. I felt this occurs on the physical level by electron transfer resonance. The resonance would act in the service of the ill person to reestablish the vitality of the flow in this open system, to restore, as it were, unimpeded communication with the environment—for given this, all literature agrees, the patient really heals himself. Further analysis of this paradigm suggested the hypothesis that if the healee were able to sustain this threshold, e.g., if his or her own recuperation powers were activated, the individual would go on to full recovery. However, if the integrity of his system were too fragmented to fully respond, recovery would be relatively less, or after an initial spurt he or she might relapse, or there might be no apparent effect.[10]

In 1971 I carried out a pilot study, which supported the hypothesis that the hemoglobin of persons being treated by the laying on of hands would change post treatment, whereas there would be no significant change in the hemoglobin values of comparable persons who had no such treatment over a similar period of time.[11] The following year, I ran a full-scale study with forty-three patients in the experimental group (those who were treated by the laying on of hands) and thirty-three patients in the control group.[12] In 1973 the study was replicated with forty-six patients in the experimental group and twenty-nine patients in the control group.[13] In both studies my hypotheses were confirmed at a confidence level of 0.001 (student t test for correlated and uncorrelated samples). This meant that there was only one chance in a thousand that the findings were random in nature. Estebany acted as healer in all the studies noted above, and I controlled for the following variables: age, sex, medication, diet, smoking (re: carboxyhemoglobin), recent surgery, strenuous exercise, certain biorhythms, breathing exercises, and meditation in both the experimental and the control groups.

While these studies were going on, I was taught the technique of laying on of hands by Kunz, noted above, and found in time that I got results with patients that were similar to results described in the literature. Specifically, the patients felt heat distinctly and locally over the diseased areas of their bodies when I placed my hands on those areas; they felt relaxed and in a state of well-being following treatments; and their hemoglobin values changed posttreatment. I therefore realized that one need not be a chosen person to do therapeutic touch; rather it seemed to me that *therapeutic touch is a naturally human potential that can be actualized by those who have a fairly healthy body* (so there is an overabundance of prana), and *a strong intent to help or to heal ill persons, and who are educable*—this last because, although therapeutic touch looks like a simple act, in reality it is quite complex to do in a conscious manner.

In 1974, I designed a research study to test out this hunch. This study utilized registered nurses under my direction in hospitals and other health facilities in the metropolitan New York area.[14] In its final form, the study included thirty-two registered nurses and sixty-four patients in an experimental-control, before-after research design. Because of the nature of the study and the opportunity for highly controlled conditions, the following delimitations were included in addition to the controls noted above: I requested that each of the participating nurses, whether in the control or the experimental group, abide by the Patients' Bill of Rights, that is, each patient had to give informed consent; but I also asked that the patients not be told whether they were in the experimental or the control group. I further asked that each nurse obtain the cooperation as well as the consent of each patient's medical doctor, as well as the cooperation and consent of the Department of Nursing in the health facility. Where there was a Board of Research Review, I asked that a formal request for approval to use the facilities be instituted, and appropriate materials were made up for presentation. To reduce possible bias, it was stipulated that the laboratory technicians at the health facility not be told that a study was in progress, and data were only included in the analyses on hemoglobin values where the same type of blood analysis equipment was used (Coulter). Hematocrits were also done as a check on the hemoglobin readings.

The hypotheses were essentially similar to those of the previous studies—specifically, that the hemoglobin values of patients in the experimental group, that is, whose nurses treated them by therapeutic touch, would undergo significant change, whereas the hemoglobin values of comparable patients in the control groups would not change significantly after a similar period of time. This proved to be the case, the level of confidence being 0.001.

Since the above-noted study, I have completed other research; however, the results are not ready at the time of this writing. The sum total of all my investigation of this very ancient mode of healing has engendered a hearty respect for the power of this personalized interaction. The universality of its use among people of diverse cultures throughout the world seems to me to indicate its key position as a clue to natural laws that underlie the manner in which man may act therapeutically and humanely to man. This is a quest worthy of genuinely strenuous efforts in research, and I welcome those who would pick up the challenge.

Notes

1. Dolores Krieger, "Therapeutic Touch and Healing Energies From the Laying on of Hands," *Journal of Holistic Health* (San Diego: The Mandala Society, 1975–76): 24.

2. G. Grad, "A Telekinetic Effect on Plant Growth, Part 2. Experiments Involving Treatment of Saline in Stoppered Bottles," *International Journal of Parapsychology* 6:473–98.

3. B. Grad et al., "The Influence of an Unorthodox Method of Treatment on Wound Healing in Mice," *International Journal of Parapsychology* 3:5–24.

4. Sister M. Justa Smith, "Paranormal Effects on Enzyme Activity," *Human Dimensions* 1 (1972): 15–19.

5. D. M. Rorvik, "The Healing Hand of Mr. E.," *Esquire*, 81 (February, 1974): 70, 154, 156, 159–160.

6. Shafika Karagulla, *Breakthrough to Creativity* (Los Angeles: De Voss, 1967): 123–46.

7. M. F. Perutz, "The Structures of the Hemoglobin Molecule," *Nature* 228 (1970): 726–39.

8. S. Sassa, et al., "Effects of Lead and Genetic Factors on Heme Biosynthesis in the Human Blood Cell," *Annals of the New York Academy of Science* 244:419.

9. L. G. Israls, et al., "Heme Binding and Its Possible Significance in Heme Movement and Availability in the Cell," *Annals of the New York Academy of Science* 144:639.

10. Dolores Krieger, op. cit., p. 27.

11. ———, "The Response of In-Vivo Human Hemoglobin to an Active Healing Therapy by the Laying-on of Hands," *Human Dimensions* 1 (1972): 12–15.

12. ———, "The Relationship of Touch with Intent to Help or to Heal, to Subjects' In-Vivo Hemoglobin Values: A Study in Personalized Interaction," *American Nurses Association Ninth Nursing Research Conf. Proceedings* (Kansas City: American Nurses Association, 1973): 39–51.

13. ———, "Healing by the Laying-On of Hands as a Facilitator of Bioenergetic Change: The Response of In-Vivo Hemoglobin," *International Journal of Psychoenergetic Systems* 1 (1976): 121.

14. ———, "Therapeutic Touch: The Imprimatur of Nursing," *American Journal of Nursing* 75: (1975): 784–87.

Bibliography

Blofeld, John. *The Tantric Mysticism of Tibet*. New York: E. P. Dutton, 1970.

Caasi, P. I., Hawswerth, J. W., and Nair, P. P. "Biosynthesis of Heme in Vitamin C Deficiency." *Annals of the New York Academy of Sciences* 203:94.

Eliade, Nurcea. *Yoga: Immortality and Freedom*. Translated by Will R. Trask. Bollinger Series 56. Princeton, N.J.: Princeton University Press, 1969.

Evans-Wentz, W. Y. *Tibetan Yoga*. London: Oxford University Press, 1967.

Grad, B. "A Telekinetic Effect on Plant Growth. II: Experiments Involving Treatment of Saline in Stoppered Bottles." *International Journal of Parapsychology* 6: 473–98.

Krieger, Dolores. "The Relationship of Touch, with Intent to Help or to Heal, to Subjects' In-Vivo Hemoglobin Values: A Study in Personalized Interaction." In *American Nurses Association Ninth Nursing Research Conference Proceedings*. Kansas City: American Nurses Association, 1973.

Lehninger, A. L. "Molecular Biology: The Theme of Conformation." In *The Neurosciences*, edited by G. C. Quarton, T. Melnechuk, and F. O. Schmitt. New York: Rockefeller University Press, 1967.

Maslow, A. H. *Motivation and Personality*, New York: Harper, 1954.

Mundakopanishad [The 13th Principal]. Translated by Robert Ernest Hume. Upanishads. London: Oxford University Press, 1921.

Rorvik, D. M. "The Healing Hand of Mr. E." *Esquire*, February 1974, pp. 70, 154, 156, 159–60.

Seiverd, C. E. *Hematology for Medical Technologists*. Philadelphia: Lea and Febiger, 1968.

Shostrum, E. L. *Personal Orientation Inventory Manual*. San Diego: San Diego Educational and Industrial Testing Service, 1966.

Smith, M. Justa, Sister. "Paranormal Effects on Enzyme Activity." *Human Dimension* 1 (1971): 12–15.

Wallace, R. K. "The Physiological Effects of TM." Ph.D. dissertation, University of California at Los Angeles, 1970.

Watson, H. C., and Kendrew, J. D. "The Structure of the Hemoglobin Molecule." *Nature* 190 (1961): 670.

20
David Goodman

Ultrasonics and Holography: Use in Clinical Diagnosis and Wholistic Healing

She stood in tears amid the alien corn,
The same that oft-times hath
Charmed magic casements, opening on the foam
Of perilous seas, in faery lands forlorn.

John Keats, "Ode to a Nightingale"

Introduction

THE VISITOR, an intelligent woman of thirty-two, carefully lowers her body into a 300-gallon immersion tank kept warm at 75°F. Not quite ten feet away, her obstetrician, eyes turned towards a video monitor, begins the ultrasonholographic examination of his patient. Seated comfortably, she slowly begins to rotate her hips on command. For a moment all is dark on the television screen and quiet save for the routine hum of machinery. Then suddenly, the image of another human being hoves into view. With growing excitement, obstetrician and patient observe their happy discovery: a little human being of thirty-five weeks who turns his face in their direction, arches his back, and kicks his mother.

Is this vignette reality today? Is it possible for an expectant mother to view her child in real time while it is still inside her womb? An affirmative answer to both these questions is possible as a result of the synergistic convergence of two new medical technologies of the last ten years: (1) ultrasonics, or "seeing with sound"—the ability to form images of living tissue *in vivo* without disturbing the body surface; and (2) holography, a lensless photographic technique for viewing objects in three dimensions. The conjunction of these two technologies, so important to the future of medicine, is called ultrasonic holography or, as it will be called in this paper, ultrasonholography. Because we reasonably expect that the technique will become increasingly used in the next decade, it is important for professionals and interested citizens alike to have a working knowledge of how ultrasonholography will be used in clinical diagnosis and wholistic healing.

The paper begins with the uses of the technique in clinical diagnosis—specifically, ultrasonholography in obstetrics, orthopedics, mammography, and oncology—then shifts to its possible uses in healing and in visualization of the whole body. The wide range of present applications includes direct visualization of the fetus possibly as early as the fourteenth week—its form and often its physiology; also orientation—breech or vertex—of the fetus in the womb. In orthopedics and clinical diagnosis, the technique permits direct visualization of the soft tissue of the extremities—muscles, muscle fascia, tendons, ligaments, and blood vessels. In mammography and oncology, it aids the search for cysts, abscesses, clots, and tumorous masses. Additional applications possible in the future with modified technique include imaging of the parenchymal viscera, including liver, pancreas, kidney, and spleen. Eventually, scarcely an organ of the entire body will escape the "penetrating gaze" of ultrasonholography.

Ultrasonics and Holography

What are these ultrasonics and holography so useful in clinical evaluation? A brief description of each of these useful technologies seems in order:

Ultrasonics

First, what is ultrasonics? We know that the upper limit of audibility of sound waves is between 17,000 and 20,000 cycles per second (17 to 20 kHz.). Above this frequency, sound waves are inaudible to humans.

Ultrasonic waves are sound waves whose vibrational energy is beyond the range of ordinary hearing: ultrasound varies from a low useful frequency of approximately 40,000 cycles (40 kHz.) up to ten million (10 MHz.). Frequencies of 1 to 7 MHz. are frequently used in clinical medicine. Typically, these high-frequency waves are released in bursts or pulses lasting no longer than thousandths or millionths of a second. In customary ultrasonics—the so-called B and C scans and echocardiography—short bursts of very-high-frequency sound are used to explore the inside of the body; images formed are in two dimensions.

These high-frequency sound waves have an interesting property that makes them especially useful in clinical medicine. Unlike light waves, which are absorbed and reflected by surfaces, sound waves pass through the skin. It is this ability to penetrate into the body that is utilized in the clinic for laboratory investigations of functioning organs inside the body. Although the skin is relatively transparent to sound waves, the same cannot be said for tissues and organs inside the body. Their differential absorption, reflection, and transmission form the basis for acoustic imaging. For example, in actual practice ultrasonic technicians know that bone has different sound conduction properties than placenta or tissue such as the breast. It is this difference of tissue properties regarding sound waves that forms the basis for the technique: waves passing through the body are slowed, diverted, and generally deflected in such ways that images of various internal structures can be formed on a sensitive detector. By selecting the optimal frequency of the ultrasonic probe, the physician can choose the tissue he wishes to image. A lower frequency might be used to image muscle, while a higher frequency—3 or 7 MHz.—may be used to "see" inside a fluid-filled cavity such as the uterus, as in the example that begins this article.

Holography

Holography used as a form of lensless photography and as visual display is probably quite familiar to the educated adult, who by now knows it was invented by Dennis Gabor in 1948 and that it is a technique for recording all the information of a scene—phase as well as intensity. The hologram is a recording of intensity information (as in a photograph) and depth (three-dimensionality) as well. Since 1962 and the work of Leith and Upatnieks, laser light holograms have been recognized as an improved method of visual display and information storage. However, what many viewers of laser holograms do not know is that holograms are formed by the interference of energy waves of any kind. When waves in space collide (interfere) and the interference pattern is captured on a sensitive recording medium, the result is a hologram including all the information of the original waves. Under appropriate playback conditions, these original waves can be reconstructed. In holograms formed by light waves from a laser, the viewer sees waves exactly like those reflected from the surface of the original object. But holograms can be formed from energy waves of any kind, ranging from tiny electron waves and microwaves (radar) all the way up to the vibrational energy waves of inaudible and audible sound. These sound waves penetrate the surface; hence playback of a sound hologram reveals the hidden side of the observed object, the inside.

This "inside" story of the human body—possible since Dennis Gabor and Pal Greguss joined ultrasound and holography—is a very recent scientific discovery. Although in 1967 Suckling and Moody had proposed use of ultrasonholography for imaging biological structures, not until 1969, with the development of the "holosonic" imager by Byron Brendon, were clinical investigators able to demonstrate its feasibility in examination and diagnosis. Brendon, who began study in 1964 of ultrasonholography for industrial applications, was inventor of the Holosonic Model 100 imager that was used by Dr. David Holbrooke to image the fetus of thirty-two-year-old Susan. Requiring a 300-gallon imaging tank, the Model 100 was for four years the standard ultrasonholographic machine. More recently, the Holosonic Model 300 and the Actron/McDonnell Douglas sound holography system that dispense with the water tank have become popular.

Applications of Ultrasonholography in Clinical Diagnosis

The most successful applications of ultrasonholography have been in the areas of obstetrics and orthopedics. More recently, it has been used in mammography and for the detection of soft-tissue tumors. For historical reasons, we begin with an examination of Dr. Holbrooke's patient Susan.[1]

Obstetrics

Holosonics Model 100 "Acoustic" Holography unit, shown in Fig. 20.1, presents a real-time through transmission image on a viewing screen. Imaging frequencies are 3, 5 and 7 MHz. delivered in bursts of from 30 to 120 millionths of a second. The patient sits in the immersion tank with her abdomen transverse to the acoustic sound source. Ultrasound passes through her body, through acoustical lenses, off a reflector to the water surface. Interference of this beam with a second acoustic beam forms a hologram at the liquid surface. A laser and special optics are used to project this image onto the viewing screen or television monitor.

An image of a gravid human uterus viewed on a screen, television receiver or videotape monitor shows, not only the fetus, but also soft tissue surrounding the placenta, including muscles and blood vessels. The real-time sound hologram of a fetus turning and kicking in the living womb is best appreciated on videotape film. Early holosonic films of the fetus *in vivo*—fetal head above the cervical canal, heart beating, limbs in motion—still pack a tremendous emotional impact on the viewer. Subsequent improvements, possible with the Model 300 and with the Actron system developed by Alex Metherell, show not only fetal head and body contours and motion inside the uterine walls, but internal structures of the fetus as well.

David Holbrooke, at Children's Hospital San Francisco, and Alex Metherell, at the University of California Irvine Medical College, have both reported this ability to clearly image specific fetal structures, including spine, pelvis, abdominal wall, buttocks, lower extremities, upper arms; the cranium, the jaw bones, and the soft tissues of the face. Fascinating cinepictures reveal ribs, developing bones of the arms; the fetal liver and umbilicus; even the brain inside the fetal skull. In one memorable instance, Metherell reports on a fetal calcified cranium *in vivo* that displayed the brain including structures thought to be "gyri and sulchi of the frontal, parietal, occipital and temporal lobes."[2]

Orthopedics

Beyond obstetrics, ultrasonholography is of excellent use in imaging the internal structure of the extremities. The skin of arms and legs is transparent before the ultrasonic beam: blood vessels, tendons, ligaments, muscles, and muscle fascia leap into view. At the Holosonics

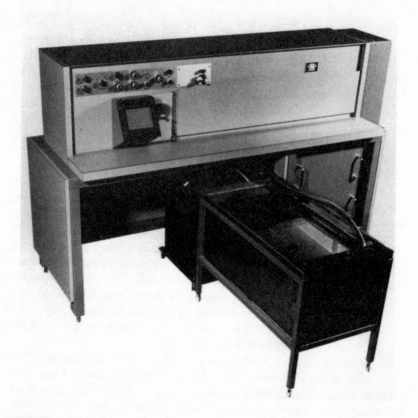

Fig. 20.1 A Holosonics Model 100 Liquid Surface Acoustic Holography Machine. *On the right* is the heated 300-gallon imaging tank. *On the left* is the video viewing screen with three-dimensional information. This is the traditional immersion holograph used by Brendon and Holbrooke.

immersion imager, visiting scientists frequently plunge hands and arms into the tank. Arteries throb and pulse before the eye; tendons and ligaments as threads and cables branch to the fascia; muscles dynamically change size on being contracted.

Fig. 20.2, from a report by Byron Brendon, illustrates the power of ultrasonholography in imaging of the extremities. Branched venous

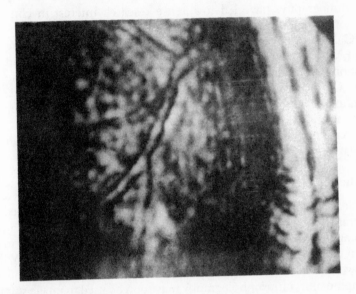

Fig. 20.2 Acoustic image of vascular structures of the biceps of the arm. Note branching of the blood vessel. Inset shows region of the arm shown in the acoustic hologram.

structures are visible running along the surface of the biceps muscle. In similar pictures, tendons and pulsating arteries are visible as well as certain large nerves. Familiarity with the physiological well-being of the arm allows the physician to identify malfunction or disruption of normal body processes. Pursuing this line of reasoning, David Holbrooke has used ultrasonics to diagnose pathology not visible to X ray or thermographic probe.[3]

Mammography

Ultrasonholography, since Brendon's pioneering work in 1967, has been used for the examination of normal and pathological tissue in the female breast. As a result of his careful work, using ultrasonic scan and immersion imaging, it may soon be possible to differentiate breast glandular tissue and fat from fluid-filled cysts and hard tumorous masses.[4] The promise of this technique and improving technology, along with doubts expressed about the safety of traditional X ray

mammography, have led to intense research interest in clinical ultrasonics mammography.

Gabor's ultrasonic body scans—based on the success of some forms
of EMI X ray body scans—may have, in the future, widespread application as a method for examining breast tissue of asymptomatic wom-
en. Closer to immediate clinical application for the present is the
technique reported by Baum and Stroke, in which two-dimensional
ultrasound scans are converted, holographically, into three-
dimensional images. Their report, in late 1975, of the technique for
breast scanning has been well received by colleagues.[5]

Other applications

Scarcely a decade since its first application to clinical medicine,
ultrasonholography, limited as recently as 1972 to the immersion
holograph, is presently undergoing a tremendous upsurge of interest
that promises additional applications to clinical medicine. With the
newer, nonimmersion Holosonics 300 and Metherell's Actron holographic unit, ultrasonholography may soon be used to image soft tissue
of the visceral parenchyma, including liver, spleen, pancreas, kidney,
and possible tumors in these organs.

The imaginative Baum and Stroke approach to ultrasonics and
holography and a related technique of Pal Greguss and H. J. Caulfield
may allow visualization of head and neck structures and organs of the
chest.[6] The brain, enclosed by bony cranium, and the heart, within
the thorax, may also be imaged in the years ahead. These successes
would extend the range of ultrasonholography to all the structures of
the body.

Prognosis: The Role of Ultrasonholography
in Clinical Medicine

Some advantages of ultrasonics and holography are evident even to
the casual observer: using safe, low-level sound, the physician can scan
body organs without pain or discomfort to the patient.[7] The technique
extends the concept of *in vivo* imaging to include soft tissue as well as
bone, now visualized with X rays. In addition, "seeing with sound"
allows real-time internal examination without the need for multiple
roentgenal exposures, the swallowing by the patient of potentially

dangerous substances and the injection of chemical dyes whose side effects may not show up for years.

Ultrasonholography also allows the physician to see inside the body without exploratory surgery that entails cutting through integument, subcutaneous tissue, and muscle, which, in the least, interrupts normal energy flow; at worst, the incisions may be slow to heal or become infected. Even to the casual observer, these advantages of the technique represent an obvious improvement over traditional methods.

A still more positive future is promised by sophisticated "one-shot" ultrasonholographic techniques that further lessen the exposure of patients to ultrasound. For example, the system developed by Metherell at Actron requires pulses lasting only millionths of a second. In that one exposure, the physician stores on film a comprehensive image of much of the body cavity. Retakes are unnecessary, because holography, being lensless photography, captures the whole of the scene; only afterwards, after the film has been developed, does the viewer focus on a specific organ. It is impossible for the exposure to be out of focus. Additionally, with four frames shot a second, the physician has motion pictures of dynamic organ action in the viscera. A sitting in which the visitor sees a Metherell film of parenchymal tissue, or more commonly, the interior of the hand or arm or a fetus kicking in the womb is adequate to excite our imagination for the positive future of ultrasonholography in clinical medicine.[8]

Applications of Ultrasonholography to Wholistic Healing

Wholistic Introduction

Susan, whom we've observed in the opening vignette of this article, is an affable trend setter whose concern and interest in her unborn son will introduce the reader to a new age of ultrasonholography in the service of clinical medicine. By now the reader may want to get to know her as she wants to know her unborn son. By her willingness to immerse herself in the holosonic bath, she is leading us to baptism in a wholistic world of the future. The ultrasound that penetrates her womb passes deep into our awareness. Mother and son have begun an active nurturing, caring relationship—a mutual interawareness. The child, of course, senses his mother and her moods. Now Susan is aware of her son. He is alive and kicking at his walls as if to pound his message home. And what is the message? No drugs during our pregnancy. Natural childbirth. Synergy and symbiosis, then the birth process: a child entering a new age. The water in the tank as the water in the womb reminds us of the emergent Aquarian age.

Wholistic Awareness

If clinical obstetrics beacons in a wholistic age, consider the metaphorical meaning of clinical orthopedics. To see inside the arm. To see inside the body. The meaning of it all: to see our arteries pounding inside the body; to see our muscles inside the cavity that is us. Can we, really, use ultrasonholography to "get in touch with ourselves"? What is the status of the symbionts that share our body—muscles, bones, blood vessels? Are they functionally well? What is their nutritional status? For the first time in our lives, we might see muscles as "real." Previously the declivities and hollows of our own body, for all their familiarity, might have occupied the surface of Mars. Cut off from light, perception, and feeling, remote from conscious awareness except when in pain or touched by the surgeon's knife, one's own body interior remained the last terra incognita. Before ultrasonics and holography, one accepted on faith that the body's outside had an inside. Now we see it as another world to explore.

Biofeedback: if we see something intrapersonal, can we alter its function? Does not this new form of biofeedback go the Eastern Yogis two better? Biofeedback I of the early 1970s: wired like astronauts, we dared convert inner space to outer space. But it was through a cockpit. Dials and digital readouts, flashing lights in colors. This was us, wasn't it? Numbers meant heartbeats; lights were brain waves. But with biofeedback II, ultrasonholographic biofeedback, we crash through to a new dimension, a third direction. We see, as no Yogi or astronaut ever did, an artery pounding and a muscle contracting. On concentration, the blood flow slows or speeds up; the muscle relaxes and changes size.

As long as we explore the body wholistically, why not a leap to another dimension, a fourth dimension: what's the wholistic meaning of viewing the breast with holography and ultrasound? To see the breast healthy, and if not, perchance to see a small tumorous mass. Then, day by day, to use a mental imaging technique such as the one used by the Simontons, to actively fight its growth.[9] With ultrason-

holography, we might add another dimension in the fight for life—
the emergence, perhaps, of a healing wholography in the service of
wholistic medicine.

Ultrasonholography: Two Routes into the Future

In this article, I have tried to introduce the reader to the two routes
to the future of a promising new technology—ultrasonholography—
that is the conjunction of ultrasonics ("seeing with sound") and holography (lensless three-dimensional photography). It has been my objective to survey a fifteen-year period beginning in 1967, when holography
and sound were first used for the imaging of biological structures.
More than merely writing a review article on the present status of
ultrasonics and holography, I have attempted, as applied scientist, to
present the human side of an exciting new technology.

From where we stand, two roads of ultrasonholography lead into the
future: one, ultrasonholography in clinical diagnosis; the other, ultrasonwholography in wholistic healing. The intelligent society sends
its researchers down both these routes.

David Holbrooke, in clinical and emergency medicine, pursues the
route of clinical diagnostic ultrasound: immersion and the new
nonimmersion holographs for his practice. In obstetrics, to distinguish
a vertex from a breech birth by examination *in utero*. Or, to distinguish
single from multiple implantations; eventually, to ascertain additional
prenatal parameters. Moving ahead to orthopedics: the hobbled
athlete to be examined: a muscle stretched? ligament pulled? tendon
popped? No way to image soft tissue is known save ultrasonholography. And lastly, a new mammography, without X rays, to survey the
breast masses with gentle ultrasound, a technology that has already
defined its clinical role in the routine screening of healthy and viable
tissue. This is clinical ultrasonholography and its role in the present
and near-term future; perhaps in as few as five, no more than ten years,
we acquire the ability to image all the soft tissues in the body. With this
chance of success, this is an important road to the future.

A second road, that slopes upward to the reaches of imagination—
that's another route to the future worth taking. Rising sun–watchers,
we advance to a world of wholistic thought: to see ourselves as we really
are. This is the route selected by the Aquarian transpersonal soul in

San Francisco, sitting and waiting for the fetal image to appear. She is Susan. Our thoughts fly forward to future ultrasonholographic applications: dynamic visualization of the body and its organs; seeing the body as a whole physiological system; real-time biofeedback; direct visualization for tumor and wound healing. It's all waiting for us and Susan if we but show the inclination. The image of this future is ultrasonwholography, and it's half the image of the future, as real to the foreseeing mind as the right brain is to the left. The future belongs to Susan as it does to David, and we are all the godparents of a new age. Welcome us to a wonderful world of tomorrow . . . and ultrasonholography . . . and ultrasonwholography.

Notes

1. D. R. Holbrooke, E. E. McCurry, and V. Richards, "Medical Uses of Acoustic Holography," in *Acoustic Holography*, vol. 5, ed. P. S. Green (New York: Plenum, 1974).

2. K. R. Erikson, et al., "Through-Transmission Acoustical Holography for Medical Imaging: A Status Report," in *Acoustic Holography*, vol. 6, ed. N. Booth (New York: Plenum, 1975).

3. D. R. Holbrooke et al., "Acoustic Holography for Surgical Diagnosis," *Annals of Surgery* 178 (1973): 547–58.

4. B. Brendon, "Ultrasonic Holography: A Practical System," in *Ultrasonic Imaging and Holography: Medical, Sonar and Optical Applications*, ed. G. W. Stroke et al. (New York: Plenum, 1975).

5. G. Baum and G. W. Stroke, "Optical Holographic Three-Dimensional Ultrasonography," *Science* 189 (1975): 994–95.

6. P. Greguss, and H. J. Caulfield, "Multiplexing Wave Fronts by Holography," *Science* 177 (1972): 422–24.

7. Wells, P. N. T., "Absorption and Dispersion of Ultrasound in Biological Tissue," Dennis White, ed. *Ultrasound in Medicine and Biology*, vol. 1 (New York: Plenum, 1975): 369–76.

8. K. R. Erikson et al., op. cit. See also, for similar findings, "Through-Transmission Ultrasonic Imaging of Intrauterine and Fetal Structures Using Acoustic Holography" by D. R. Holbrooke et al., in *Ultrasonics in Medicine*, ed. M. de Vlieger, D. N. White, and V. R. McCready (Amsterdam: Excerpta Medica, 1973).

9. O. Carl Simonton and S. S. Simonton, "Belief Systems and Management of the Emotional Aspects of Malignancy," *Journal of Transpersonal Psychology* 7 (1975): 39–47.

Bibliography

Booth, N. *Acoustic Holography*. Vol. 6. New York: Plenum, 1975.

Brendon, B. "Imaging Capabilities of the Liquid Surface System." In *Holography in Medicine*, edited by P. Greguss. London: IPC, 1975.

Gabor, D. "A Project in Ultrasonic Tomography." In *Ultrasonic Imaging and Holography: Medical, Sonar and Optical Applications*, edited by G. W. Stroke; W. E. Kock; Y. Kikuchi; and J. Tsujiuchi. New York: Plenum, 1975.

Green, P. S. *Acoustic Holography*. Vol. 5. New York: Plenum, 1974.

Greguss, P. "Acoustic Holography." *Physics Today*, October, 1974, 238–48.

Greguss, P. and Galin, M. A. "Holography." *Annals of Ophthalmology* 4 (1972): 817–20.

Holbrooke, D. R., Richards, V., and Pitt, William L. "Medical Acoustic Holography." *Annals of the New York Academy of Sciences* 267 (1976): 295–311.

Jones, E. D. "Ultrasonic Imaging at Stanford Research Institute." In *Ultrasonic Imaging and Holography: Medical, Sonar and Optical Applications*, edited by G. W. Stroke; W. E. Kock; Y. Kikuchi; and J. Tsujiuchi. New York: Plenum, 1975.

Kock, W. E. "Sound Visualization and Holography." *The Physics Teacher* 15 (1975), 14–21.

Korpel, A. "Acoustic Imaging and Holography." *IEEE Spectrum* 5, pt. 3, October, 1968, 45–52.

Metherell, A. F. "Acoustic Holography." *Scientific American*, October, 1969, 36–44.

Metherell, A. F. *Acoustic Holography*. Vol 3. New York: Plenum, 1971.

Metherell, A. F., El-Sum, H. M. A., and Larmore, L. *Acoustic Holography*. Vol. 1. New York: Plenum, 1969.

Metherell, A. F. and Larmore, L. *Acoustic Holography*. Vol. 2. New York: Plenum, 1970.

Mueller, R. K. "Acoustic Holography." *Proceedings of the IEEE* 59 (1971): 1319–35.

Sikov, M. R., Pimmel, R. L., Reich, F. R., and Deichman, J. L. "Visualization of Soft Tissue by Ultrasonic Holography." *Radiology* 102: 191–92.

Varshavskii, Yu. I., Braginskaya, K. C., Kruglyakova, K. E., and Dudasher, R. S. "Use of Ultrasonic Holography for Visualizing Biological Objects." *Akademiia Navk SSR Doklady: Biological Sciences Section* 212 (1974): 719–21.

Wade, G. *Acoustic Holography*. Vol 4. New York: Plenum, 1972.

21

William A. McGarey

Edgar Cayce's Contribution to Holistic Medicine*

Introduction

MORE THAN eighty years ago, a boy by the name of Edgar Cayce astounded his father by reading, clairvoyantly, a spelling book held in his father's hand. Perhaps it was the threat of a spanking that sparked the ability into reality. It may have been the voice that spoke to him inside his head and gently advised him to lie down with his head on the book for a few moments. Whatever the cause, Cayce slept on the book—moments later handed the book to his father and was able to read the words at a distance for his unbelieving parent, spell them correctly, and thus avoid the threatened damage to his posterior.

Cayce didn't finish school, moved from being a book salesman to an X ray technician to a career as a photographer, trying to avoid a destiny that seemed to be forcing itself upon him. He finally succumbed to this inner insistent urging and began a very unusual forty years as a seer, a psychic who has been acknowledged as the most accurate clairvoyant of the twentieth century, certainly the most studied and the most documented, a man who became known to millions of people all over the world as the Sleeping Prophet.[1]

Edgar Cayce gave nearly fifteen thousand readings (psychic discourses) during those last forty years of his life. He died at the age of

* *Edgar Cayce Readings,* © 1971 Edgar Cayce Foundation. Reprinted courtesy of the Edgar Cayce Foundation.

sixty-seven in 1945. But he lived long enough to see the good that his work had brought to thousands of individuals. Two-thirds of his work was directed toward people who were ill, who were seeking help for their physical or mental problems that had not been solved by the doctors of his day. He saw spiritual difficulties entwined with the sickness of the physical body, and his diagnoses of one's problem seemed frequently to be closely aligned with a concept often repeated in his readings, that "the Spirit is the Life, the Mind is the Builder and the Physical is the result."

In giving a reading, Cayce simply lay down on a couch after removing his shoes and unloosening his collar; he closed his eyes and his hands were clasped over his forehead. After a few moments, he moved his hands down over his solar plexus and his eyelids fluttered. At that point, he was given a suggestion, and shortly he started talking. In this state of extended consciousness, his mind would reach out and contact the unconscious mind of the person for whom he was giving the information, and the two minds would communicate. Since it is the unconscious mind of any physical body that directs the physiological functioning of the entire body, it is not surprising that Cayce's words would describe the activity going on inside that body, the manner in which that activity was balanced or incoordinant, and the substances that were lacking, the needs of the ailing body.

Cayce's work in the field of what might be called physiological diagnoses, and his suggestions in the realm of therapy for correction of those abnormalities of function, became the basis of a library, for they were carefully recorded and are readily available for study, carefully indexed, and open to the professions and to the public in Virginia Beach, Virginia.[2]

The physical readings (those dealing with illnesses of the human being) have a scope that is surprising—for example, individual readings on just the common cold were obtained; one complete reading came about because of a physician's questions about multiple sclerosis, and Cayce insisted the cause of this disease was a lack of gold in the system, an assimilative defect in the body. Cayce gave information about arthritis, cancer, gallbladder disease, appendicitis, fractures of various extremities, and problems such as colitis, myasthenia gravis, Hodgkins disease, tonsillitis and amyotrophic lateral sclerosis. He suggested rehabilitative techniques for stroke, cardiac disease, tuberculosis, baldness, schizophrenia, ingrown toenails, and warts. There seemed to be no lack of knowledge within the minds of the persons he contacted in regard to causation of disease, and his unconscious mind would reach out into what he called the akasha—what has been called the total stream of consciousness for information about therapy.

Cayce's mind sought out the forgotten portions of dreams for certain close friends as he helped them in dream interpretation, and his understanding of the total scheme of things led to an obvious conclusion that help of a physical nature can be found in the dream content, suggestions that can be and are often helpful. His reaching out for assistance often took the listener into the understanding of life as being a continuous thing, extending into a limitless future and back through a series of incarnations in the earth—all of them having some meaning in one's present experience.

The philosophical concepts emerging out of the Cayce material, made available by the Edgar Cayce Foundation in the A.R.E. Library, describe man as a spiritual entity, created in a spiritual sphere by the Creator of all things. Man lives an adventure in materiality, in the earth plane, what we call a physical existence, but returns to his natural habitat when he dies—taking his consciousness with him as a part of his total being. Cayce's first biographer describes these philosophical concepts in detail and puts substance behind the idea of man as a spirit-mind-body being.[3]

The Concept of Holism

The concept of wholistic medicine certainly has its roots in the wholeness of the human being. For Cayce, this always meant body-mind-spirit wholeness. My experience with these readings dates only back to 1955, some ten years after Cayce died. Never having talked with him or having observed a reading myself, I was left with the task of studying the material produced by this seemingly boundless unconscious mind. And the bulk of the information available to study defines very clearly that Cayce was not a medium, but rather reached out with his own mind at a level of consciousness we find it hard to understand, gaining information that was often unique, always interesting. In the process, Cayce demonstrated that the human mind is indeed capable of amazing abilities—for the documentation obtained has proved that his information is accurate and that his suggestions produce results when applied in the human body.

My background led me to understand and accept a philosophy that the only reasonable therapy for an illness of the body had to be a multi-level approach that reaches not only the body, but the mind and the spiritual being itself. This is not a simple thing when first identified as a goal. But the details begin to fit in as the answers are sought in the very nature of the human body.

Dr. James Windsor, president of Christopher Newport College of the College of Newport News, Virginia, named what we were trying to do in a paper he presented at the Second Annual Medical Symposium sponsored in Phoenix by the Edgar Cayce Foundation.[4] Entitled "A Holistic Theory of Mental Illness," Windsor's thesis was based in Cayce's viewpoint of a person "as a whole, with mind, body and spirit as a single unit, all so closely tied that it was not possible for one aspect to be diseased, either physically or mentally, without the whole person suffering the consequences. . . ." This point of view is expressed in the following statement from one of the readings:

> For, the body-physical becomes that which it assimilates from material nature. The body-mental becomes that which it assimilates from both the physical-mental and the spiritual. The soul is all of that the entity is, has been, or may be.[5]

Cayce saw the relationship of mind and body constantly at work, and it becomes quickly evident in this material that the mind builds conditions in the body in a variety of ways. Cayce's own words from another reading are specific in the manner that he spoke during the readings:

> And thus the nerve forces for the body, this body as any body, any individual, who makes destructive thought in the body, condemning self for this or that, will bring, unless there are proper reactions, dissociation or lack of coordination between the sympathetic and cerebrospinal system, and it may develop any condition which may be purely physical by deterioration of mental processes and their effect upon organs of the body.[6]

Windsor went on to describe how, in mental illness, the causation seen in the Cayce readings is physical, mental or spiritual imbalance. Regardless, however, of the precipitating factor, all aspects are affected adversely. The person is a complete unit which can only function as a whole.

Similarly, in treatment, the whole person is involved. Cayce suggested provisions for the building of nerve tissue, the cleansing of the system, the stimulation of the glands and circulatory system, proper diet, sympathetic attendants, and also a time for meditation and prayer.

Windsor's paper was the first published article defining the concepts in the Cayce readings as a wholistic approach to medical care of the individual, but it is a title used frequently in our efforts to apply this information to the healing of the human body.

Holistic Healing—The Total Person

The A.R.E. Clinic, Inc., in Phoenix, Arizona, was established to research the material in the Cayce readings and bring it into a relationship with the practice of medicine as the latter has developed over the centuries. The merging of the two then is utilized in treatment of the ills of those who come to the clinic for care. The problem is major in its nature, for it involves the changing of a deeply ingrained concept in the practice of medicine—a concept that is not spoken, but rather has evolved over the past sixty years as teaching of medicine has gone from the doctor-preceptorship relationship to the science of the large universities.

Gradually, physicians have moved their cumulative attention from the patient to the disease. The patient, you see, is a multifaceted creature—understood at a subconscious level as spirit-mind-body. One does not readily understand or scientifically study a being with so many unpredictable nuances. Double-blind studies are not easily adapted to the human being, with his mind that so wonderfully flits here and there, even when it is held down tightly by the thinker.

The disease, on the other hand, is wonderfully adapted to study. It can be controlled, measured, named, identified by texts, often put into a test tube, and generally is of such a nature that it can be documented, studied in double-blind or even triple-blind situations. Statistics can be evolved about the diseases and significance of a statistical nature can be attained or denied. Diseases are simple and clear, wonderfully adapted to the accepted scientific method for study, when compared to the multiplicity of the nature of the human body, for man is indeed wonderfully made and unlike anything else in all of creation.

The problem, then, it seems, is that the attention of the physician has been lured away from the originally intended recipient of that attention, the patient, and turned—almost imperceptibly, but without question—to bear, almost without exception, on that consciously un-invited guest, the disease.

When the doctor pays attention to the disease, the person is finally completely forgotten in the excitement of the conquest. The love and patient concern that might be given is forgotten, the worry that ravages the patient's mind and emotions is swept aside as the fight with the disease continues. The end result is often a loss of the patient-doctor relationship that used to be the cornerstone of therapy, and often the only instrument needed to repair an ill body-mind-spirit.

Another problem pointed up by our study of man in the concepts developed by the Cayce material is that found when one considers that it may be that the mind is the builder—not only of ideas but the diseases that exist in the body. If this information is correct, then we are faced with the reality that, through disruption of physiological activities, the groundwork is laid for any given disease. Through some confluence of conditions that we sometimes cannot fully understand, all the elements of a disease process are brought together in the body through the activity of the mind, and a disease is born. The illness is apart from the normal of the human body, and, given the proper thought patterns, beliefs, and activities of the body, it would not exist. It has, in fact, little if any reality.

Research, then, about the disease process or the disease itself, be it organism or destructive reality in the body, cannot bring about any understanding of the nature of the body itself. This is fact if, indeed, man is body-mind-spirit in nature. It is perhaps like looking at the rim of a wheel to understand what the hub is like.

If a disease is not to be studied, then, what would one study? How heal the body, if one does not rid it of the disease? The obvious answer to the latter question is that one must indeed often attack the disease to let the body regain health or at least a reasonable degree of homeosta-sis. In other instances, however, a restoration of balance, according to these readings, will cure the body and let the person establish healthy living once again. It would seem reasonable, if there is a balance of functions that is important to health, to help the patient toward this balance, even if the disease needs to be destroyed. Otherwise one might, and then again might not, regain a healthy status. The disease may be gone, but the body may remain sick in the inadequacy of its body balance.

What should be studied, if not the disease? Perhaps a start might be made in simply recognizing certain facts and making other assumptions. Cayce talked about healing in many places, but the following reading gives us certain ideas.

> For, all healing comes from the one source. And whether there is the application of foods, exercise, medicine, or even the knife—it is to bring the consciousness of the forces within the body that aid in reproducing themselves—the awareness of Creative or God forces.[7]

In our approach to healing, whether the problem is colitis or hypertension, we involve the physician, the patient and Creative Forces in a cooperative effort. We regard illness as an adventure in consciousness—an opportunity for spiritual development as well as physical improvement, and an activity of the mind that is helpful. Healing is not merely a structural repair process, but rather a happening that should lead toward the redirection of the entire person, providing a new vision of wholeness and health toward which each of us can strive.

Perhaps wholistic medicine is not only recognizing the patient coming to us with his problems and illnesses as a oneness of body, mind and spirit, but going one step further in treating him as such. This would mean communication, meeting the patient as one friend would meet another, as one soul is intended to meet another: Recognition. The patient is a veritable storehouse of wonderful information and fascinating events that deal with the wholeness of that person. The physician should be honored to participate in that information.

A sixty-seven-year-old woman became a patient at our clinic because, as she put it, she had to make a decision, and she thought we could help her. She had been diagnosed as having cancer of the uterus for the past year and had been bleeding profusely for almost the entire period of time. She refused her physician's pleas to enter the hospital for surgery. Three years before, her husband had died. She remembered that, as a small child, she answered questions concerning what she wanted to do when she grew up with the words, "I want to be of service." Always, "I want to be of service." When she was eighteen, she was seriously ill, and she died. She was pronounced dead, and she told us that she was outside her body, watching the doctors working furiously on her thin, debilitated, sorry-looking physical body. Standing behind her at her right shoulder was a being whom she did not see well, but who was talking to her. "You must decide whether you are going back there or staying here," she was told.

"I can't decide that," she argued—she saw the wonderful things that surrounded her there on the plane she was then experiencing. And, she thought, her parents would soon get over her death. But "I just can't decide, Lord," she repeated. And, in an instant, she was back in her body.

Her life straightened out, she was subsequently married, had eight children and a wonderful life until her husband died. She remembered how she had talked her ankle into healing itself when she was just a young mother and she knew she was needed at home.

And now, at sixty-seven, she knew that perhaps she should be really learning just how she did that earlier healing process. She knew her decision would let her stay here or move on.

A dream she experienced a week before coming to the clinic was of a round white dog, lying on its back, asleep, with its paws outstretched. At each of its forepaws was a little round puppy, also asleep. She was told that such an arrangement looked much like the uterus and the two ovaries, and this would be saying that the cancer had not spread, but was asleep.

Her decision? Not important except to her. But the point is that she, like every other human being, is a world unto herself, with a world of wonderful experiences that need to be shared by those who hope to bring her help in achieving the healing, whether death is the healer or not.

Wholistic medicine may also consist of simply recognizing that the body is really pure energy and treating the patient who sits in front of us as if that person were indeed pure energy. The body is constructed of cells, the cells are made up of molecules, and the molecules are formed of atoms. The atoms are pure energy. The body is pure energy. Energy is a form of electricity. I recall another of the Cayce readings—this one having to do with electricity:

As we may see in a functioning physical organism, electricity in its incipiency or lowest form is the nearest vibration in a physical sense to Life itself; for it is the nucleus about each atom of active force or principle set by the atomic activity of blood pulsation itself, that begins from the very union of the plasm that creates life itself in a physical organism.[8]

Electricity, moving through any conductor—including the human body—produces an electromagnetic field. There are energy patterns formed and energy movements. For example, we do not yet know the full meaning of the acupuncture procedure and its healing potential in the body. Over the centuries, people have seen the aura. One of my patients sat recently in my examining room and described my aura for me—evidence that that particular individual had a wealth of other experiences that we do not ordinarily see. Evidence also that recognition of these energies in the human body will bring not only better communication, better rapport, but also a fuller understanding of how to help that person to a fuller experience of health.

Wholistic medicine may perhaps be simply a recognition that energy transfer from one person to another is possible—and touching the patient with whom we work as if this were true. I remember visiting Gerard Croiset in Holland and watching him "treat" a hemiplegic poststroke patient. He moved his hands up and down, on each side of the paralyzed leg, not touching it, but holding the palms of his hands perhaps a couple of inches from the skin itself. Gradually, as he "warmed up," the paralyzed leg began to twitch; the leg began to jerk with movement as Croiset continued his work. An energy was passing from his hands to that leg, evidence of the same thing that is now being taught nurses,[9] and the same kind of energy that many physicians consciously pass on to their patients as they work with them. Not a laying on of hands, so to speak, for the doctor, but rather a recognition that when his hands are placed on the patient, there is a transfer of energy that is of a healing nature, from him to the patient.

Perhaps wholistic medicine is the recognition and application of the concept that simple patience, persistence, and consistency are spiritual qualities; used by the physician, they aid in the patient's movement toward health. Instructed as a prescription for the patient to use as he applies any given modality of therapy, they become a spiritual aid in healing the patient. The mind listens, the body applies, and the spirit is mobilized as the individual with an illness applies simply a persistence in therapy.

Perhaps, finally, wholistic medicine is simply recognizing that all healing comes from within that person who is ill—the physician sometimes being only the instrument to make the patient aware that such is the fact.

Conclusion

Edgar Cayce has been dead for over thirty years, but his work is recorded, its authenticity is documented in a variety of ways. The excitement of the concepts contained in his readings is evidenced by literally dozens of books published in many languages dealing with experiences, work, and research founded on his information. His work overlaps into the field of medicine, psychology and religion as his suggestions to individuals paint patterns of thinking and believing in the minds of men. Perhaps the following extract from one of his readings expresses best the heart of the concept that allows one to think in terms of wholistic healing, of wholistic medicine. It is based on the assumed facts that man is a spiritual being created by God; that each person has a spiritual nature, a spiritual origin, and a spiritual destiny; and that these conditions affect his physical and his mental being.

> Know that all healing forces must be within, *not* without! The applications from without are to create within a coordinating mental and spiritual force. Set the mind to believe in SOMETHING, and let that be creative—and as we find, as we have indicated, it must be of a spiritual nature.[10]

Notes

1. Jess Stearn, *Edgar Cayce, The Sleeping Prophet* (New York: Doubleday, 1967).
2. The Association for Research and Enlightenment, Library/Conference Center, 67th and Atlantic, Virginia Beach, VA 23451.
3. Thomas Sugrue, *There Is a River: The Story of Edgar Cayce* (New York: Holt, 1942).

4. James Windsor, "A Holistic Theory of Mental Illness," *Proceedings of the Second Annual Medical Symposium of the A.R.E. Clinic and the Edgar Cayce Foundation* (Phoenix: 1969).

5. Papers of Edgar Cayce, 2475-1, Association for Research and Enlightenment, Virginia Beach, Va.

6. Papers of Edgar Cayce, 5380-1, Association for Research and Enlightenment, Virginia Beach, Va.

7. Papers of Edgar Cayce, 2696-1, Association for Research and Enlightenment, Virginia Beach, Va.

8. Papers of Edgar Cayce, 3950-1, Association for Research and Enlightenment, Virginia Beach, Va.

9. Dolores Krieger, "Therapeutic Touch: the Imprimatur of Nursing," *American Journal of Nursing* 75 (1975): 784–87.

10. Papers of Edgar Cayce, 1196-7, Association for Research and Enlightenment, Virginia Beach, Va.

22

Alfred A. Barrios and William S. Kroger

Psychological Variables and the Immunological Response: A New Approach to the Treatment of Cancer*

THERE IS A large body of evidence that psychological variables can predispose one to cancer. If so, it would seem a logical conclusion that by controlling the psychological factors we might possibly be able to aid in preventing and even reversing the cancerous process. The purpose of the paper is to present a case for investigating this hypothesis. It is felt that there are two basic reasons why we have not gone sufficiently in this direction before, both of which are no longer felt to be valid. First, we hesitated lest we be labeled as charlatans; there just did not seem to be any rational explanation for how one could possibly affect an organic disease such as cancer by "merely working on the mind." But now such an explanation is available. The "mind" or a person's mental state could play a part by affecting the body's natural defenses against cancer. And if we had some means of eliminating the psychological interference, we could revive the natural defenses and reject the cancer. Which brings us to the second previous stumbling block—the fact that heretofore medicine has not had an effective enough means for dealing with the interfering mental state. Psychoanalysis, which has dominated psychiatry for most of this century, just was not an effective enough tool. But now we do have more effective modes of therapy. To be specific, the paper proposes that hypnotherapy would be one such effective means. Evidence, both

* Reprinted by permission from *Journal of Holistic Health* and by permission from the authors, Alfred A. Barrios, Ph.D., and William S. Kroger, M.D.

direct and indirect, already available in support of this hypothesis is presented, including the studies of Hedge and Simonton. There is a discussion of how the latter studies might be improved, including the use of more effective hypnotic induction methods (where, among other things, bio-feedback is used for reinforcement purposes) as well as a more comprehensive use of the hypnosis (with the aim of helping the patient towards self-actualization). And finally, a simple study is proposed to further test the hypothesis following these new lines, using the hypnotherapy in conjunction with whatever medical treatment the patient is receiving for the cancer.

The following was taken from the concluding remarks of the president of the American Cancer Society in his presidential address several years ago:

> Now, finally, I would like to leave you with a thought that is very near to my heart. Anyone who has had an extensive experience in the treatment of cancer is aware that there are great differences among patients. . . . I personally have observed cancer patients who have undergone successful treatment and were living and well for years. Then an emotional stress, such as a death of a son in World War II, the infidelity of a daughter-in-law, or the burden of long unemployment, seem to have been precipitating factors in the reactivation of their disease which resulted in death. . . . There is solid evidence that the course of disease in general is affected by emotional distress. . . . Thus, we as doctors may begin to emphasize *treatment of the patient as a whole* as well as the disease from which the patient is suffering. We may learn how to influence general body systems and through them modify the neoplasm which resides within the body.
>
> As we go forward in this unrelenting pursuit of truth to stamp out cancer . . . searching for new means of controlling growth both within the cell and through systematic influences, it is my sincere hope that we can widen the quest to include the distinct possibility that within one's mind is a power capable of exerting forces which can either enhance or inhibit the progress of this disease. (Pendergrass, 1959, 1961)

The year was 1959, sixteen years ago, when Dr. Pendergrass expressed his hope. Why did this plea for increasing emphasis on the psychological approach seem to fall on deaf ears? Was it because there was no real evidence that psychological variables can influence the course of cancer? No. Even by 1959 a considerable amount of evidence had already accumulated in support of this contention. In a review of the area, Kroger (1963) made note of a number of studies already pointing in this direction by 1959 (Trunnell, 1952; Blumberg *et al.*, 1954; Greene, 1954; LeShan and Worthington, 1955; LeShan and Gassman, 1958; LeShan, 1959).

Since then the evidence has continued to grow. This evidence, thus far, can best be summarized (Bahnson, 1971) as indicating that the psychological factors most likely to predispose an individual to cancer are: object loss, despair, depression, and hopelessness, such factors being present *prior to* as well as during the disease (Schmale and Iker, 1964; Greene, 1966; Greene and Swisher, 1969; LeShan, 1966; and Hagnell, 1966). This is especially so when these factors are present in an individual who tends to deal with stressful or traumatic life events with such maladaptive coping mechanisms as denial and repression (Henderson *et al.*, 1958; Cobb, 1959; Kissen, 1966; Henderson, 1966; Bahnson, 1966; Kissen, 1969; Katz, 1969; Bahnson, 1969).

If psychological variables are playing a major role, then, it would seem logical that by controlling the psychological factors we just might be able to prevent and *even reverse* the cancerous process, as implied in Dr. Pendergrass' address. Why then haven't the medical and psychological professions followed through on this?

In the past, there have been two basic obstacles holding back any advance along these lines, both of which, however, are no longer felt to be valid. First, those who do believe this might be one approach to cancer have hesitated to promulgate it lest they be labelled as charlatans. Both present authors have communicated with a number of doctors who have privately confided that they have brought about relatively permanent cures of cancer through hypnosis, but who would not make such claims public because they feared the reaction of their peers.

We realize it is human nature to reject that which seems to defy reason and that, heretofore, there just didn't seem to be any rational explanation for how one could possibly cure an organic disease such as cancer by "merely working on the mind." However, this is no longer the case. Thanks to the tremendous advances in the immunological approach to cancer, we now know the probable mechanism by which "the mind" or a person's mental state can affect cancer.

Evidence that the body has a natural defense mechanism against cancer has actually been available for years. In a paper investigating the possibility for curing cancer through hypnosis, written twelve years ago (Barrios, 1961), a number of such enlightening studies were mentioned. Perhaps the most interesting was that of West (1954) where he observed:

> Mass surveys which have been conducted for the detection of early cancer of the uterine cervix have produced some very enlightening information. A large group of women in whom carcinoma *in situ* was detected by the Papanicolaou technique and later confirmed by Punch biopsy were followed. In only 20% of these did the malignant cells invade the basement membrane and become Grade One carcinomas requiring treatment. In the remainder, this growth disturbance was *self controlled and vanished.* Thus, we are confronted with the very likely possibility that all of us may have had, have, or will have, some form of cancer. But because of *inherent natural control* of the neoplastic process, we will never know it and will, in all probability, die of unrelated causes.

More recent advances in the immunological approach as discussed in a recent review of the area (Stoler, 1973) now seem to confirm that the body does indeed have natural defenses against cancer.

Now, if this is true, isn't it just possible that psychological variables could somehow interfere with the body's natural defenses and, in this way, affect the cancerous process? A number of current researches at the first and second conferences on psycho-physiological aspects of cancer (Bahnson & Kissen, 1966; Bahnson, 1969) seem to think so (Bennett, 1969; Friedman, *et al.*, 1969; Solomon, 1969; Adler, 1965). See also Kroger (1962, 1963). Dr. Claus Bahnson, summing up this evidence, concluded as follows: "Thus, hard-nosed data from the Neurological and Endocrinological fields corroborate the notion that psychological events mediated by the nervous system may influence endocrine and immune reactions related to malignancies" (Bahnson, 1971).

If such is the case then it seems a logical conclusion that if we had some effective tool for reversing these negative psychological factors, we should in turn revive the defense mechanism. This, in turn, would lead to the body's natural rejection of the cancer. Thus, we should no longer fear proposing the hypothesis that one means of facilitating the cure of cancer may very well be through "the mind."

However, as mentioned, there has been a second major factor holding back progress in this area. And that is the fact that medicine has not been provided with an effective enough tool with which to deal with the psychological variables. Psychoanalysis, which has dominated the field of psychiatry for most of this century, has just not been sufficient to meet the needs, in terms of effectiveness, time and cost.[1]

Fortunately, there are other more effective forms of psychotherapy available now. One such approach is hypnotherapy. In a 1970 paper, "Hypnotherapy: A Reappraisal," Barrios (1970) pointed out that the clinical evidence indicated that hypnotherapy as currently practiced was considerably more effective than psychoanalysis and even more effective than behavior therpay:

> For the studies compared, it was found that for psychoanalysis one can expect a recovery rate of 38% after approximately 600 sessions. For Wolpe's behavior therapy we can expect a recovery rate of 72% after an average of 22 sessions and for hypnotherapy we can expect a recovery rate of 93% after an average of 6 sessions.
>
> The experienced therapist should really not be surprised at the effectiveness of hypnosis in facilitating therapy. Hypnotic induction can be looked upon as a technique for establishing a very strong rapport, for establishing a greater confidence, and a greater belief in the therapist, whereby the latter's words will be much more effective. As Sundberg and Tyler (1962) point out, one of the common features among all methods of psychotherapy is the attempt to 'create a strong personal relationship that can be used as a vehicle for constructive change.'

Let us now go over some of the additional evidence, both direct and indirect, that hypnosis would be an effective tool in reviving a person's natural defenses against cancer.

First, if we are investigating the possibility of influencing the host of defenses through hypnosis, we might ask the question of whether there is any evidence that other physiological mechanisms have been controlled through hypnosis. The answer is yes. Hypnosis has been used to control a host of physiological mechanisms including: cardiac function (Schneck, 1959), changes in basal metabolism, control of blood sugar level, regulation of leucocytes, water metabolism, temperature regulation (Platinov, 1959), regulation of enzyme production and gastric acidity (Weitzenhoffer, 1953), etc.

For those who cannot see how "mere words" can influence physiological responses, for those who still suffer from the mind-body dichotomy syndrome, there is a simple explanation. Words and, therefore, thoughts have the ability to produce physiological responses because of their previous association either with such responses or with stimuli provoking such responses. That is to say, words can come to act as conditioned stimuli. Or to quote Pavlov (1927): "Speech on account of the whole preceding life of an adult is connected up with all the internal and external stimuli which can reach the cortex, signalling all of them and replacing all of them, and, therefore, it can call forth all those reactions of the organism which are normally determined by actual stimuli themselves." The word or thought "steak" with its attendant mouth-watering response is a good example of this.

Next, there is the evidence that hypnosis has been used to effect cures of other organic diseases. This includes tuberculosis as well as a number of different skin diseases such as red flat ringworm and warts (Platinov, 1959) as well as diabetes, glaucoma, and rhinitis (Kroger, 1963). With regard to warts, it is interesting to note that in a recent study where hypnosis was used to cure warts (Surman, *et al.*, 1973), which can be classified as a type of tumor produced by a virus (Kroger, 1951), one explanation proposed was that the hypnosis somehow bolstered the patient's immune response to the virus.

Finally, there is the more direct evidence of at least two studies where hypnosis or some facsimile of it has been used as a means of attempting to cure cancer.

One of the first studies was published by A. R. Hedge in 1960. The following excerpt from his report gives you an idea of the procedure followed and the results obtained.

> The series included patients with metastatic breast cancer, with advanced bowel cancer, ovarian cancer, cervical cancer, bronchogenic cancer, and one with Hodgkin's.
>
> In the general discussion with these patients, it was pointed out that many people appear to have a natural immunity to cancer, and they often may live for several years without apparent progression. For this reason, it was assumed that the apparent immunity was something that could be developed and under hypnosis it was suggested that their antibody reaction would become greatly increased and the biochemistry of the cellular growth could be altered so as to revert to a more mature phase. The picture of the physiological and chemical changes expected was verbally painted for them and, amazingly enough, that appeared to be exactly what was taking place in their tissues.

All cases showed a marked improvement and in some there was *actual tumor regression*. Two of them who had been bedridden were able to perform light chores or housework. One woman with breast cancer had multiple tumor nodules over the surface of her chest. Yet, she later showed a complete disappearance of these metastatic growths (without any hormone therapy, X ray or adrenalectomy).

The experiment is still in progress although three of the patients have already succumbed. Those remaining may or may not continue with us for a lengthy time, but they have already long passed the period when one would have normally expected their demise.

The shortcomings of Hedge's study, as pointed out by Barrios (1961) were: (1) He seemed to use only one standard hypnotic induction. More effective and varied hypnotic induction techniques it seems would increase the effectiveness of the hypnotherapy. (2) He did not make full use of the hypnosis. Hypnosis is a tool, and what you get out of it depends on how you use it. Apparently, Hedge used it primarily to instill a positive attitude regarding one's own ability to fight off this disease. This is *definitely* an important part of the therapy, but, in addition, we must also permanently eliminate whatever negative attitudes, beliefs, and habits were precipitating factors in causing the host's natural defenses to malfunction. A systematic holistic approach must be followed, one that will insure that the patient uses more adaptive means for coping with stress and depression, one that will insure more joy and happiness as opposed to despair and hopelessness (see Wittkower and Lipowski, 1966).

A more recent and currently on-going study seems to be more in this direction. Simonton (1972, 1973, Simonton and Tatera, 1972) has incorporated certain techniques for improving mental attitude in his radiation therapy patients. In addition to pointing out to the patient that the body has natural defenses against cancer in a manner similar to Hedge, Simonton has also incorporated techniques aimed at instilling a positive attitude toward life and bolstering the will to live. His basic tool seems to be a simple form of meditation or self-hypnosis exercise (suggesting relaxation to oneself with every breath exhaled) which he uses to give the patient greater control over the ability to relax. He also shows the patient how to use it for instilling positive suggestions via positive imagery. One might say his approach is similar to such positive thinking approaches as Psycho-Cybernetics or Mind Dynamics.

So far, the results are quite encouraging. In a study involving 50 patients, he reports local control of the disease in 48 of the patients with no local recurrence. The period covered by the report (Simonton, 1973 a), however, is only October '71 to May '72; so we cannot say yet what the long term effect will be. However, also of interest was the fact that Simonton found a strong correlation between positive mental attitude and control of the disease.

A major shortcoming of the Simonton approach is the same as that of positive thinking approaches in general. A program like Psycho-Cybernetics can be extremely beneficial if a person truly believes in it. But this is where the problem lies—getting the person to really believe in it. As Simonton himself points out, "Positive thinking is very easy to say and very hard to do" (Simonton, 1973 b).

This shortcoming is similar to the one mentioned in regard to Hedge's study—that is, that only one standard form of hypnotic induction was used. By using more varied and more effective induction techniques, you can increase the belief factor which is so important if you want your words to really get through to the patient. You can have the best program in the world, but if it doesn't get through to the person, it is worthless for him.

One such program that is felt to have many of the necessary ingredients for the purpose at hand is called Self-Programmed Control (Barrios, 1973 a & b). This program has two major components: First, there are the SPC techniques, seven highly effective self-hypnosis techniques (although the term hypnosis is not usually referred to because of all the misconceptions and negative connotations often associated with it) which in combination with the use of biofeedback as a reinforcer give a person greater control over his involuntary side— habits, attitudes, emotions, tensions, etc.—and make the possibility of a positive change really believable. This, in turn, opens a person's mind to the second component of the program—the positive philosophy of Psycho-Cybernetics (Maltz, 1960) which helps the individual to develop new positive attitudes towards life and oneself, and provides the answers to many questions and solutions to many personal problems plaguing the average person.

The combination of these two components is, we feel, very effective for eliminating the negative psychological factors interfering with the natural defenses of the body. It is especially effective for opening the patient to greater satisfaction from life, thereby eliminating the feeling of despair which has been felt by many to be the major culprit.[2]

The program has many advantages. To mention a few: It is simply structured and easy to teach to doctors and paramedics as well as patients. As with most forms of hypnotherapy, it takes considerably less time than conventional forms of therapy. It was designed specifically for working with groups, thereby also cutting down on costs. And since the techniques are aimed at self-control, there is much less of a dependency factor created.

To test the hypothesis that such an approach can improve a person's ability to raise host resistance to cancer (and we would like to stress the fact that at the present time it is still just a hypothesis), we propose the following initial study: The use of SPC in conjunction with any ongoing medical therapy being applied (surgery, radiation therapy, chemotherapy, immunotherapy, etc.).[3] As comparison controls, we can use statistical expectations or, if necessary, a matched control group. Tests for the immunological response (Twomey, *et al.*, 1974) as well as measurement of mental attitudes can be run concurrently to also test the hypothesis that these factors are all correlated with the course of the disease.

It should be stressed as pointed out by Sacerdote (1966) that in any such study it is important to convince anyone in contact with the patient of the feasibility of the program, especially attending physicians and nurses. For any negative attitude can adversely affect the patient. Also, the study should not be done using only terminal cancer patients.

Notes

1. This is not to say that a modified form of psychoanalysis would be completely ineffective for cancer patients. In one of the first attempts at using psychotherapy with cancer patients, LeShan obtained some rather encouraging results with a modified version of psychoanalysis (LeShan, 1958) leading him to conclude: "It is the author's strong *impression* that psychotherapy considerably slowed the development of the neoplasm, but no definitive proof can be given at the present time." (LeShan, 1966)

2. This is not to say that psychological variables are the only factor to be dealt with. As much as possible, any carcinogenic agents present should also be eliminated—such as excessive smoking, X rays, asbestos fibers, cancer-

producing viruses and carcinogenic chemicals, etc. The body's natural defenses may be able to handle a certain amount of such carcinogens, but only up to a point.

3. If at all possible, it would be best if the SPC treatment preceded the medical treatment, thus hopefully lessening the amount of the latter needed. This is suggested in light of a current study by Penn (1974) who concludes: "There is also much circumstantial evidence suggesting that cancer chemotherapy, while allowing control of one cancer, may permit or induce the growth of a second neoplasm. These findings have important implications for the management of patients with malignancies, as other forms of cancer treatment such as radical surgical procedures and radiotherapy may also impair the host's resistance to cancer."

References

Abse, D. W.; Wilkins, M. M.; Kirschner, G.; Weston, R. S.; Buston, W. D. "Self-Frustration, Nighttime Smoking and Lung Cancer." *Psychosomatic Medicine* 34 (1972): 395–403.

Adler, R., and Friedman, S. B. "Social Factors Affecting Emotionality and Resistance to Disease in Animals; V. Early Separation from the Mother and Response to a Transplanted Tumor in the rat." *Psychosomatic Medicine* 27 (1965): 119–22.

Bahnson, Claus B. "Second Conference on Psychophysiological Aspects of Cancer." *Annals of the New York Academy of Sciences* 164 (1969).

Bahnson, Claus B. "The Psychological Aspects of Cancer." Paper presented at the American Cancer Society's 13th Science Writer's Seminar, 1971.

Bahnson, Claus B. "A Psychologic Study of Cancer Patients." Paper presented at American Psychosomatic Society Meeting, 1971.

Bahnson, C. B., and Bahnson, Marjorie B. "Role of the Ego Defenses: Denial and Repression in the Etiology of Malignant Neoplasm." *Annals of the New York Academy of Sciences* 125 (1966), 277–86.

Bahnson, M. B., and Bahnson, C. B. "Ego Defenses in Cancer Patients." *Annals of the New York Academy of Sciences* 165 (1969), 546–59.

Bahnson, C. B., and Kissen, David M. "Psychophysiological Aspects of Cancer." *Annals of the New York Academy of Sciences* 125 (1966).

Barrios, Alfred A. "Hypnosis as a Possible Means of Curing Cancer." Unpublished manuscript, 1961.

Barrios, Alfred A. "Hypnotherapy: A Reappraisal." *Psychotherapy: Theory, Research, and Practice* 7 (1970): 2–7.

Barrios, Alfred A. *Self-Programmed Control Manual and Kit.* P.O. Box 49939, Los Angeles, 1973.

Bennett, Graham. "Psychic and Cellular Aspects of Isolation and Identity Impairment in Cancer: A Dialectic of Alienation." *Annals of the New York Academy of Sciences* 164, pp. 352–64.

Blumberg, E. T., West, P. M., and Ellis, F. W. "A Possible Relationship between Psychological Factors and Human Cancer." *Psychosomatic Medicine* 16 (1954): 277–86.

Cobb, Beatrix. "Emotional Problems of Adult Cancer Patients." *Journal of the American Geriatrics Society* 1 (1959): 274–85.

Friedman, S. B., Glasgow, L. A., and Adler, R. "Psychosocial Factors Modifying Host Resistance to Experimental Infections." *Annals of the New York Academy of Sciences* 164 (1969): 381–92.

Greene, W. A., Jr. "Psychological Factors and Reticuloendothelial Disease: I. Preliminary Observations on a Group of Males with Lymphomas and Leukemias." *Psychosomatic Medicine* 16 (1954): 22–230.

Greene, W. A. "The Psychosocial Setting of the Development of Leukemia and Lymphoma." *Annals of the New York Academy of Sciences* 125 (1966): 794–801.

Greene, W. A., and Swisher, S. N. "Psychological and Somatic Variables Associated with the Development and Course of Monozygotic Twins Discordant for Leukemia." *Annals of the New York Academy of Sciences* 164 (1969): 394–408.

Hagnell, O. "The Premorbid Personality of Persons Who Develop Cancer in a Total Population Investigated in 1947 and 1957." *Annals of the New York Academy of Sciences* 125 (1966): 846–55.

Hedge, A. R. "Hypnosis in Cancer." *British Journal of Hypnotism* 12 (1960): 2–5.

Henderson, J. G. "Denial and Repression as Factors in the Delay of Patients with Cancer Presenting Themselves to the Physician." *Annals of the New York Academy of Sciences* 125 (1966): 856–64.

Henderson, J. G., Wittkower, E. D., and Longheed, M. N. "A Psychiatric Investigation of the Delay Factor in Patient to Doctor Presentation in Cancer." *Journal of Psychosomatic Research* 3 (1958): 27.

Katz, J.; Gallagher, T.; Hellman, L.; Sachar, E.; and Weiner, H. "Psychoendocrine Considerations in Cancer of the Breast." *Annals of the New York Academy of Sciences* 164 (1969): 509–16.

Kavetsky, R. E., Turkevich, N. M., and Balitsky, K. P. "On the Psychophysiological Mechanisms of the Organism's Resistance to Tumor

Growth." *Annals of the New York Academy of Sciences* 125 (1966): 933–45.

Kissen, D. M. "The Significance of Personality in Lung Cancer in Men." *Annals of the New York Academy of Sciences* 125 (1966): 830–26.

Kissen, D. M., Brown, R. I. F., and Kissen, Margaret. "A Further Report on Personality and Psychosocial Factors in Lung Cancer." *Annals of the New York Academy of Sciences* 164 (1969): 535–45.

Kowel, S. J. "Emotions as a Cause of Cancer." *Psychoanalytic Review* 42 (1955): 217–27.

Kroger, W. S. *Psychosomatic Gynecology*. Philadelphia: W. B. Saunders, 1951.

Kroger, W.S. *Psychosomatic Obstetrics, Gynecology and Endocrinology*. Springfield, Ill.: Charles C. Thomas, 1962.

Kroger, W. S. *Clinical and Experimental Hypnosis*. Philadelphia: Lippincott, 1963.

LeShan, Lawrence. "Some Observations on Psychotherapy with Patients Suffering from Neoplastic Disease." *American Journal of Psychotherapy* 12 (1958): 723–34.

LeShan, L. "Psychological States as Factors in the Development of Malignant Disease: A Critical Review." *Journal of the National Cancer Institute* 22 (1959): 1–19.

LeShan, Lawrence. "An Emotional Life History Pattern Associated with Neoplastic Disease." *Annals of the New York Academy of Sciences* 125 (1966): 780–93.

LeShan, L., and Worthington, R. E. "Some Psychologic Correlates of Neoplastic Disease: A Preliminary Report." *Journal of Clinical and Experimental Psychopathology* 16 (1955): 281–88.

Maltz, M. *Psycho-Cybernetics*. Englewood Cliffs, N.J.: Prentice-Hall, 1960.

Neerloo, J. A. M. "Psychological Implications of Malignant Growth: A Survey of Hypotheses." *British Journal of Medical Psychology* 27 (1954): 210–15.

Pavlov, I. P. *Conditioned Reflexes*. New York: Dover, 1960.

Pendergrass, Eugene P. Presidential Address to American Cancer Society Meeting, 1959.

Pendergrass, Eugene P. "Host Resistance and Other Intangibles in the Treatment of Cancer." *American Journal of Roentgenology* 85 (1961): 891–96.

Penn, I. "Occurrence of Cancer in Immune Deficiencies." *Cancer* 34 (1974): 858–66

Platinov, K. I. *The Word as a Physiological and Therapeutic Factor*. Foreign Languages Publishing House, 1959.

Sacerdote, Paul. "The Uses of Hypnosis in Cancer Patients." *Annals of the New York Academy of Sciences* 125 (1966): 1011–12.

Schmale, A. H., Jr., and Iker, H. P. "The Effect of Hopelessness in the Development of Cancer. I. The Prediction of Uterine Cervical Cancer in Women with Atypical Cytology." *Psychosomatic Medicine* 26 (1964): 634–35.

Schneck, J. M. *Hypnosis in Modern Medicine*. Springfield, Ill.: Charles C. Thomas, 1959.

Simonton, O. Carl. "The Role of the Mind in Cancer Therapy." *The Dimensions of Healing: A Symposium*. Palo Alto, Calif.: Academy of Parapsychology and Medicine, 1972.

Simonton, O. Carl. "Meditation and Cancer." Tape of Science of Mind Symposium: Scientific Approach to Spiritual Healing. *Science of Mind Magazine*, 1973.

Simonton, O. Carl, and Tatera, Bernard S. "The Role of Increased Fractionation and Patient Attitude in Radiation Therapy." Unpublished report, Air Force Base Medical Center, California, 1973.

Solomon, George F. "Emotions, Stress, the Central Nervous System and Immunity." *Annals of the New York Academy of Sciences* 164 (1969): 335–43.

Stephenson, J. H., and Grace, W. J. "Life Stress and Cancer of the Cervix." *Psychosomatic Medicine* 16 (1954): 287–94.

Stoler, Peter. "Toward Cancer Control." Cover story, *Time*, March 19, 1973.

Sundberg, N. D., and Tyler, L. E. *Clinical Psychology*. New York: Appleton-Century-Crofts, 1962.

Surman, O. S.; Gotlieb, J. K.; Hochet, T. P.; and Silverberg, E. L. "Hypnosis in the Treatment of Warts." *Archives of General Psychotherapy* 28 (1973): 439–41.

Trunnell, J. E. "Second Report on Institutional Research Grants of the American Cancer Society." New York: American Cancer Society, 1952.

Twomey, P. L., Catalona, W. V., and Chreten, P. B. "Cellular Immunity in Cured Cancer Patients." *Cancer* 33 (1974): 435–43.

Weitzenhoffer, A. M. *Hypnotism: An Objection Study in Suggestibility*. New York: John Wiley and Sons, 1953.

West, Phillip M. "Origin and Development of the Psychological Approach to the Cancer Problems." *The Psychological Variables in Human Cancer*. Berkeley and Los Angeles: University of California Press, 1954.

Wittkower, E. D., and Lipowski, A. J. "Recent Developments in Psychosomatic Medicine." *Psychosomatic Medicine* 28 (1966): 722–37.

23

James W. Knight

A Physician's Use of Healing Energies

Philosophical Preface

SOME SCIENTISTS have recently speculated that many of the moral, ethical, and spiritual values of man are intrinsically part of the universe. Through their observations and experiences, these philosophical individuals have formed personal religions, beliefs, and practices that incorporate a scientific approach to life based on universal spiritual laws.

Science and religion have often been regarded as two ends of a life view continuum. And yet, the very definition for the religious core word, *spiritual*, derives from the Latin root *spirare*, "breathing," or the life energy. Energy is equally regarded in the realm of religion and that of science.

The building blocks of the universe are the elementary particles of the hydrogen atom. These particles are brought into being by the organizational capability of the cosmic imagination and will. They combine to form the trinity space, time, and energy (or matter). There exists an equivalency between matter and energy which is described by Einstein's theory of relativity. In fact, Einstein himself defined the term "cosmic religion" as the relationship of matter to the cosmic field of energy: the reciprocal conversion of matter and energy. This is one of the major pieces of knowledge that help explain the persistence of elementary particles and the imminent evolution of matter systems into higher forms with greater organization.

A basic philosophical precept is that the universal power of energy and its law have been in existence from the beginning of time and being. They are imminent in all that is seen in the universe. It is the ability of the human being to live in harmony with this power of energy and its laws that brings about a state of health and well-being. Ignorance of the laws or disregard for them leads to the disease processes of our physical body. By continued disharmony with the perfect laws of energy, chaos, confusion, pain, suffering, and death result. This is true not only for the individual, but also for the collective.

The existence of disharmonic aspects of the life process necessitates a creative healing process. It must consist of methodologies and techniques that bring about a state of health for the individual and the collective. If the state of disease exists, the healing should bring about a recreative process that reconstitutes the trinity of Being as space, time, and energy in matter.

Healing must be both an intuitive and a cognitive process in the life of the individual—a process aimed at attaining and maintaining a state of health. The individual is the master of fate, the creator of the self-life process, the emancipator of self from slavery and ignorance, and the liberator of self into the harmony of the universal laws of energy and matter.

Principles of Wholistic Healing

The wholistic healing concept is both ancient and modern in scope. Embodying values and truths from the past and utilizing modern scientific advances, the core of the wholistic approach rests with the totality of the individual. In addition to viewing the individual as a total being, wholistic healing challenges the individual to assume responsibility for the healing process. Through the learning and the awakening of consciousness, the individual becomes aware of the many aspects of himself/herself and then becomes at one with the healing process. The healing process is a part of the health process, even before an illness takes place.

The most fundamental principle of wholistic healing recognizes man as spirit, mind, emotion, energy, and physical being. Wholistic healing is concerned with the obstructive forces within the individual that interfere with the soul energy–life energy flow through all levels of spiritual, mental, emotional, and physical being. Not only are the elements of spirit, mind, emotion, energy, and physical being interrelated in the individual, but the individual interrelates with family, community, society, and the world. By this same point of view, the collective individualities are responsible for the healing process in our society and world.

Methodologies of Healing

In order to elicit the optimal healing forces within the individual, the physician healer employs a variety of energies, disciplines and methodologies. In his book *Healing: The Divine Art*, Manley P. Hall suggests that healing methodologies can be classified into five basic groupings: physical healing, mental healing, magnetic healing, occultism, and mystical healing.[1]

Physical Healing

This area of healing is concerned with the physical body of man. It alludes to the natural causes of disease: malnutrition, bacteria, environmental factors, trauma, and biochemical abnormalities. The practitioners in this field range from herbalists, nutritionists, and homeopaths to the modern scientific physician and surgeon. Current scientific instrumentations and methodologies for dealing with physical ills are included in this category.

Mental Healing

The mental and psychological factors involved in the healing process are ancient in origin. Manley Hall defines the mentalist approach as teaching that

> . . . various phenomena of life are of mental origin, that the universe itself is a creation in mind, that the laws of nature originated in the world of thought, and are administered by cosmic intelligence, and that God is the mental or Intellectual Principle that rules all things, and not a spiritual Being.[2]

Mental healing is any form of spiritual-psychological therapy that operates on the principle that the mind can correct the evils of sickness and disease, and restore health by conditioning the mental outlook.

Psychology and psychosomatic medicine are two fields that are concerned with mental healing. Hypnotism, psychotherapy, religious science, psychosynthesis, guided imagery, and meditation are some of the mental healing techniques.

Magnetic Healing

Magnetic healing is an ancient as well as a modern healing method. Perhaps one of the most noted magnetic healers was Anton Mesmer, whose contribution to this area of healing is alluded to by Dr. Bernard Grad in Chapter 12 of this book. Magnetic healing aims to mobilize the electromagnetic life energies and healing forces in the individual through a variety of techniques. Some mesmerists, as magnetic healers have come to be called, use various instruments; others use only the magnetic energies of their own body. Dolores Krieger, who contributed Chapter 19 of this book, is actively engaged in practicing and teaching the "laying on of hands" modality in the field of nursing. Walter J. Kilner has contributed much to the development of the field of magnetic healing energies. Harold Saxton Burr has devoted a lifetime of work to the area of electrodynamic fields of energy that are visible and tangible. Through his "L" field theory, he has explained much about the electromagnetic energy flow in the human body during periods of health and disease.

The practice of the Yogis comes within the area of magnetic healing. Meditations, mantras, Hindu hymns, and Kundalini Yoga exemplify some of the magnetic practices designed to mobilize the electromagnetic life energies. The study of aura or magnetic emanations to diagnose and treat disease also falls under this classification.

Occultism

This is the ancient science that, according to Hall,

> . . . deals with the hidden forces of nature, the laws governing them, and the means by which such forces can be brought under the control of the enlightened human mind.[3]

The most important of the occult sciences are magic, demonism, spiritualism, alchemy, exorcism, astrology, Cabala, and the currently popular modality of extrasensory perception. Occult practitioners have ranged from saviors, prophets, and seers to initiated philosophers, astrologers, and metaphysicians. Jesus, Buddha, Pythagoras of Samos, Dr. William Lilly of England, and Dr. Henry Cooley practiced occultism. The most modern example of an occultist is Dr. Carl Jung.

Mystical Healing

> Mystical healing may be academically defined as the belief that the direct knowledge of God and Truth is possible to man through an extension of his spiritual insight toward union with the substance and essence of Divinity.[4]

Formal religious theology is rejected by mystics because they believe that God must be approached through personal devotion and by contemplation of universal and divine truths. However, examples of mystical healing can be seen in Christianity, Hinduism, and the Buddhaic mystical cultures. The shrine at Lourdes represents a Roman Catholic mystical entity. Kathryn Kuhlman and Oral Roberts are examples of two contemporary mystics of faith healing.

Personal Development and the Wholistic Healing Concept

Wholistic healing integrates knowledge and practices of all the above-mentioned methodologies. With its emphasis on the total person and the individual's responsibility for the healing process, wholistic healing encourages a more active participation by the patient, and in order to elicit the greatest amount of awareness possible, techniques are not limited in the healing process. Many physicians down through the ages have used wholistic techniques in their practice. An outstanding current example is Robert Leichtman, M.D., an internist practicing in Maryland.[5] Dr. Leichtman has worked with Norman Shealey, M.D., a neurosurgeon, in the area of psychic diagnosis. Currently, Dr. Leichtman is a practitioner and lecturer in psychic diagnosis and other healing modalities. In combining healing methodologies, he and other physicians have broadened the healing process in their practices.

In establishing a wholistic treatment plan, it may be necessary for the physician-healer to initially present wholistic concepts on subtle, nonverbal, or more orthodox levels. This aids in acceptance of the wholistic framework and guards against alienating the patient toward the healing process. Once rapport and acceptance are established between the patient and the physician-healer, a variety of methodologies and additional healing individuals can be utilized in the treatment plan. *This process of wholistic healing is evolutionary, not revolutionary*. Its purpose is to aid the individual to grow and develop awareness; the process seeks to bring about health through healing of an illness and through maintenance practices for continued health. It is not a process that relies on parlor and party techniques. Rather, it incorporates a multitude of healing modalities.

In my own practice of the wholistic healing process, I have worked with a variety of individuals and techniques. Further, my practice will evolve into an increasingly wholistic-oriented one as more and more techniques become known to me. The multifaceted approach to healing that wholistic healing offers relies on aid from individuals in many fields and on continued learning for the physician.

I have worked with psychics—Kay Beck, Myra Fairbanks, and Joseph Martinez—over the past two years. At various times, they have expanded the healing process with several of my patients. Jack Schwarz, N.D., also a psychic, has aided me in the diagnostic process with some of my patients. Dr. Schwarz is an aural reader and is noted for his ability in controlling his internal states. Currently, he is conducting annual seminars at the University of California in San Francisco. Rev. Wayne Cook, whose specialty over the past seventeen years has been a method of dowsing of the human body, has worked with me. His method involves measuring energy fields and doing a particular technique of psychotherapy and healing that is rather dramatic in its full operation. Acupuncture has been used in our own practice in cooperation with local internists, Fred Smith, M.D., and Hector Prestera, M.D. I have studied with Christopher Hills from the University of the Trees in Boulder Creek, California, to gain knowledge of pendulums and supersensonics as therapeutic tools. In the near future I hope to be involved in research with Mr. Hill in this area.

The wholistic healing process invites physicians to explore healing modalities in many fields. The psychological modalities of psychosynthesis, guided imagery, meditation, the Intensive Journal,[6] and Autogenic Training are areas in which I hope to extend my knowledge. These along with allopathic medicine,[7] nutrition, homeopathy, herbology, ayurvedic medicine, Tai Chi, Yoga, music, dance, art, gestalt awareness, and the body of esoteric healing as taught by Alice Bailey and Vitvan, I hope to integrate into my practice. The areas of energy, electromagnetic energy, and psychosomography[8] represent research fields I intend to explore.

To date, many of the above-mentioned techniques have not been fully documented and evaluated as to their effectiveness and relatedness to patient treatment, though some information has filtered down from antiquity regarding the techniques themselves. Scientific information is available regarding allopathic medicine. This modality remains a superb tool for dealing with the crisis of disease in the patient. Unfortunately, it has been limited in scope to this area. I am hopeful that it will begin to cooperate more fully with the wholistic framework in the future and encompass a greater arena in the healing movement.

Wholistic healing remains, then, a total approach involving a variety of methodologies. The physician who is involved in the wholistic healing process extends his accrued knowledge and techniques continually and works with individuals in many fields to provide expanded patient care.

The Practice of Wholistic Healing

A firm conviction that the psychological and spiritual aspects of the individual are as significant as the physical aspects can greatly influence the physician as diagnostician and healer. Renewed health is derived from a cooperative effort between patient and physician. An essential first step in establishing such cooperation is the creation of trust that is based on intuitive understanding; this takes place when the physician and patient have established rapport. Through quiet and constructive discussion of the signs and symptoms of the disease process, the physician-healer can gain insights into the patient's state of mind. With mutual acceptance, the consciousnesses of physician and patient interact on various levels, often nonverbally. Through intuitive communication, the physician-healer may then perceive the patient's depth of awareness, the degree of progress, and any mental or emotional obstructions that interfere with renewed health. This "tuning in" also allows the physician to recognize specific disease states and the organ systems that they affect.

Understanding is essential for the healing process. If the patient cannot comprehend the physician's approach, he or she will not be able to cooperate in the healing. The physician-patient relationship must begin in a comfortable manner for both parties. Through ongoing interaction that elicits trust, the physician is able to instruct the patient in methods of healing. By educating the patient, the physician brings the individual to a full understanding of his or her responsibility for effecting an improvement in health. Once patients become aware of their role in the healing process, changes may be rapid and dramatic. Sometimes, weeks, months, or even years of slow, steady improvement are necessary. In other instances, the disease process has become so entrenched that concentration must be centered on developing new life meanings and conscious awareness by the individual in order for living to be as harmonic as possible.

The following five cases from my files illustrate the concepts of healing and living in harmony with disease. They were chosen as examples of the wholistic healing process from the viewpoint of both the physician-healer and the patient.

Case One

A mother and son, both with a long history of respiratory disease, came to me simultaneously for treatment.

The mother was in a terminal state of cardiopulmonary failure. Her condition was characterized by severe edema and liver enlargement, and at the time of the initial physical examination, her pulse rate was 140 beats per minute. Obesity and a two-pack-a-day cigarette habit further deterred from a positive state of health.

When the mother was confronted with the seriousness of her condition and her failure to cooperate in overcoming the disease, she indicated a desire to alter the fatal course she was pursuing. She became aware of the habits that were contributing to the severity of her condition. Through involvement in the healing program, she became aware of the positive alternatives to her illness. This patient worked cooperatively with the medical regime established for her. She experienced immediate reversals of the disease process and continued her efforts in understanding the purposes and effects of her treatment. Ultimately, she was encouraged to imagine the healing action of the dietary and medical therapy on her body. Through a combination of medical and self-healing actions, this female patient recovered to a remarkable degree. She resumed her role as wife and mother, and for the first time in seven years, she was able to go on a vacation with her family.

Several years later, a diagnosis of pancreatic cancer profoundly depressed this patient. No longer was she able to maintain positive attitudes toward life and health. Her condition deteriorated, including her respiratory health. Two months after the diagnosis, she succumbed to acute respiratory failure.

The son of this patient came to me after many years of severe asthmatic attacks. He had a history of repeated hospitalizations (an average of three each month) for treatment of respiratory distress. Since beginning a program of medical care prescribed for him, this young patient has pursued a positive course. The use of self-healing imagery has been extremely important in his therapy. In eight years, he has only been hospitalized once. This was for a head injury.

Case Two

A patient who has either healed a cancer or lived with it for over ten years is a fifty-nine-year-old male whom I first saw and diagnosed as having a carcinoma of the stomach at the junction with the esophagus. An operation was performed to remove the diseased segments. At operation, the lymph nodes in the region of the pancreas were positive for carcinoma but were not removed. The patient refused any chemotherapy or radiation treatment. He did, however, enroll in a program of guided imagery and self-healing. By cooperating with this program, he was able to maintain his body free from any evidence of cancer and returned to a full and productive life, supporting wife and twelve children.

Approximately eight and a half years after the initial diagnosis, the patient returned to me. He was depressed over deep-seated family problems. Over several months' time he had experienced guilt and profound depression. Examination revealed a metastatic tumor of the liver that measured approximately 9 cm. in diameter. At that point, the patient, his wife, and their children all enrolled in a healing program. The patient received counseling and this, together with family cooperation, aided in his understanding of the situation. He was then able to free himself from negative feelings and again involved himself in the process of living. Within two and a half months, the liver tumor was no longer palpable on physical examination. Five months after the initial liver scan, a repeat study showed only a small (1–2 cm.) scar. This patient has continued to do well for an additional two years and is at present free from any evidence of generalized carcinomatosis or localized spread of the disease.

The following two case studies represent examples of intuitive knowledge on the part of the physician-healer.

Case Three

A fifty-four-year-old female whose medical history was unknown to me came to my office for a scheduled appointment. As I approached the examining room where she was waiting, I suddenly had an intuitive knowledge that her illness involved an atypical blood clot in the right iliac artery. At that moment, I was aware of the course the disease would follow. I envisioned the surgical intervention that would be employed and the progressive clotting that would ultimately result in kidney failure and death. For the ensuing three months, I had the traumatic experience of witnessing the entire sequence of events as I had envisioned them. Fortunately, the outcome is usually not as dramatic or traumatic as this. But whatever the consequences of the disease state, the fact of the disease and its probable outcome can be known to the physician-healer in many instances.

Case Four

On another occasion, an experience of intuitive knowledge strongly influenced my decision to see a new patient. I had been told by a third party that a woman who had been suffering from shortness of breath would be calling my office for an appointment. At 3:30 one afternoon, I overheard my receptionist explaining to a caller on the phone that an appointment for a new patient would be impossible to arrange for two weeks. At that moment I had an intuitive experience—an image of this new patient and of an X ray that showed a complete pleural effusion of the right chest. Following these images, I experienced yet another one. This was of a carcinoma in the body of the pancreas measuring approximately 2 cm. in diameter and overlying the aorta. I quickly told the receptionist to inform the caller that we would see his wife, the new patient, at 5:30 that afternoon. Before the patient arrived I shared my experience with the office staff. I included a description of the patient's appearance, although I had yet to meet the woman. I explained the image of the X ray and the findings from it. (While I also shared my experience of knowing the diagnosis, I did not relate my conviction that the outcome of this particular case would be fatal.)

The patient arrived at my office at 5:30. X rays were taken, and the patient and I went to the consultation room, where I took her history. She looked just as I had seen her in the earlier intuitive encounter. During the ensuing physical examination, I suspected the presence of pleural effusion. Later, with the office personnel present, I reviewed the X rays, which demonstrated a total right pleural effusion.

The patient was subsequently admitted to the hospital where 1,600 cc. (3 ½ pints) of pleural fluid were extracted from the chest cavity by needle aspiration. Laboratory analysis confirmed the presence of cancerous cells in the fluid. Additional studies, including gallbladder series, gastrointestinal series, barium X rays, kidney X rays, and liver and pancreatic scans failed to reveal the primary disease site. The patient then underwent exploratory abdominal surgery. When the area of the pancreas was palpated and visualized, a nodule of 2 cm. in diameter was observed. Biopsy of this mass confirmed adenocarcinoma of the body of the pancreas, a finding consistent with an analysis of the cancer cells in the pleural fluid.

Despite an aggressive course of treatment, the patient's condition deteriorated rapidly. She underwent radiation therapy and became involved in the healing process through healing imagery. Later, however, a metastatic tumor of the brain was detected. Further radiation therapy and chemotherapy were necessary. The patient succumbed within five months of the original diagnosis.

Case Five

This case history represents an example of the healing process allowing the patient to achieve greater harmony in life.

A female patient was diagnosed as having cancer of the right lung. The size and extent of the tumor defied surgical removal. For more than twelve years, repeated bronchoscopic examinations revealed the presence of cancer cells. The patient continuously refused radiation therapy and medical treatment for this condition, but she was deeply involved in promoting her own healing through a program of imagery. This process focuses the patient on living and on having control over, or living in balance with, the disease. The patient was unable to create an image of herself as being healthy and totally free from cancer. But she continued in harmony with the disease for ten years.

Suddenly she became depressed. Two rib tumors appeared on the chest wall. At my suggestion, this patient returned to the community of her childhood and on that visit she encountered a friend from earlier years. An old romance was rekindled between them, and sparked by this new emotional attachment, the patient focused on a renewed positive living process. Once again she mobilized her energies toward healing imagery. The results were dramatic: within two months, three 1 ½-inch cancerous tumors on her chest wall were no longer detectable. The patient lived an additional two years. Ultimately, death was caused by the disseminated carcinoma, but the patient had lived a full and positive life with that potential outcome for twelve years.

I do not believe that such dramatic changes in health and attitudes are solely the result of any miraculous healing energies. I do, however, strongly contend that, when patients themselves come to the realization of their self-help potential in overcoming disease, their lives do change. Further, dealing with the negative impact of disease on their lives does bring patients to a more harmonic state of living.

Through a program of self-healing and the technique of guided imagery, afflicted individuals bring into awareness the positive qualities of living. These, of course, contribute mightily to the person's healing process. When the diseased state is advanced and may run its fatal course, healing energies may bring individuals into potential harmony with their living process instead of their disease.

At the Center for Wholistic Healing, the program which we have developed involves all of our personnel.[9] All staff members are trained to encourage positive attitudes in all clients and in all aspects of a person's care. Only in this way can each individual seeking medical care also encounter attitudes that lead toward assumption of responsibility for his or her own well-being. This positive approach is also conducive to the channeling of an individual's particular energies. It creates and maintains stable human relationships and preserves the person's financial responsibility. Through the coordinated program offered by the Center, we believe our clients are provided with total care that engenders feelings of self-worth: of being uniquely valuable individuals who seek to take a positive course of action in healthy, harmonious relationship with their total life process.

Notes

1. Manley P. Hall, *Healing: The Divine Art* (Los Angeles: Philosophical Research Society, 1971).
2. Ibid., p. 176.
3. Ibid., p. 158.
4. Ibid., p. 169.
5. A discussion of Dr. Leichtman and his work may be found in Robert Neubert's article "Profiles: Dr. Robert Leichtman, M.D.," *Psychic* (January/February, 1976).
6. Ira Progoff, Ph.D., *Intensive Journal* (New York: Dialogue House Library, 1975).
7. Allopathic Medicine is the contemporary, orthodox system of techniques used to treat the physical ills of mankind.
8. *Psychosomagraphy* is a term coined from the root origins *psycho*, "soul," "spirit;" *soma*, "body" (of any organism); and *graphy*, "a recorded description." The term depicts a futuristic technique used to describe mind-body energy through photography.
9. The Center for Wholistic Healing, 212 San Jose Street, Salinas, CA 93901, was established in July, 1976, for the purpose of expanding the concepts of healing to self-care techniques and lifestyle modifications that complement contemporary medicine, and promote a healing of the whole person.

Bibliography

Bailey, Alice. *Esoteric Healing*. New York: Lucis, 1953.

Burr, Harold Saxton. *Blueprint for Immortality*. London: Neville Spearman, 1972.

Day, Langston, and De La Warr, George. *New Worlds beyond the Atom*. London: Vincent Stewart, 1956.

Edwards, Harry. *The Healing Intelligence*. New York: Hawthorn, 1965.

Einstein, Albert, and Infeld, Leopold. *The Evolution of Physics: The Growth of Ideas from Early Concepts to Relativity and Quanta*. New York: Simon & Schuster, 1938.

Gallimore, J. G. *Unified Field Theory Research Book: Using Subjective Response to Psi-plasma for Analysis of Properties of Neutral Charge Plasma Fields.* Mokelumne Hill: Health Research, 1974.

Hills, Christopher. *Supersonics: The Spiritual Physics of All Vibrations from Zero to Infinity.* Boulder Creek, Calif.: University of the Trees Press, 1975.

Kervran, Louis C. *Biological Transmutations.* Binghamton, N.Y.: Swan House, 1972.

LeShan, Lawrence. *The Medium, the Mystic, and the Physicist.* New York: Viking, 1974.

McCamy, John C. *Human Life Styling: Keeping Whole in the 20th Century.* New York: Harper and Row, 1975.

Motoyama, Hiroshi. *The Non-Physical in the Correlation between Mind and Body.* Tokyo: The Institute for Religious Psychology, 1972.

Russell, Edward W. *Design for Destiny.* New York: Ballantine, 1970.

Turner, Gordon. *An Outline of Spiritual Healing.* New York: Warner, 1972.

Vitvan. *Teachings for the New Age: Healing Technic.* Baker, Nevada: School of the Natural Order, 1946.

Worrall, Ambrose, and Worrall, Olga. *The Gift of Healing.* New York: Harper and Row, 1965.

A Course in Miracles. New York: Foundation for Inner Peace, 1975.

24

Carl D. Levett

Utilization of a Transpersonal
Approach in Psychotherapy

IN THE PAST, psychotherapists have provided specialized treatment services in dealing with disturbances of mind and body, internalized emotional conflicts, and interpersonal breakdowns. They have also offered therapeutic guidance for those seeking greater fulfillment in regard to love, sex, work, and communication. The thrust of such efforts has been to strengthen the identity of the personal self, to free individual capacities, and to help in the resolution of humanistic goals.

The recent emergence of Transpersonal Therapy has expanded the dimensions of psychotherapy, holding forth considerable promise in furthering human actualization.

Sutich has given us a workable definition of Transpersonal Therapy:

> At the present time it may be described as that therapy which is directly or indirectly concerned with the recognition, acceptance and realization of ultimate states. As such, it is not "new," but perhaps the oldest of all therapeutic approaches. It has a vital part of most, if not all, of the systems throughout history that have been concerned with the realization of ultimate states.[1]

Ultimate states are levels or spaces of consciousness that traverse the boundaries of ordinary awareness, beyond a reliance on processing consciousness solely to serve the desires of a personal self. Ultimate states become known through direct experience, where intuition and openness to impression of pure, vibrational energy flow abound.

Ultimate states, however, are byways to the ultimate—to cosmic union. Those who have surrendered to the inner reaches of ultimate consciousness suggest that the essence of oneness represents the source of all that is. Meher Baba depicts the source as "the state which prevails beyond the beginning of the beginning of creation."[2] Yet, how can we identify a condition that is in advance of any-thing?

Knowing the source registers for us vibrationally, as transcendental knowing, as "The Void—the universe in its unmanifested form,"[3] "beyond time and space, beyond any change, and beyond polarities such as good and evil, light and darkness, stability and motion, agony and ecstasy."[4]

Man is capable of joining with the *potential* of phenomena, that field of energy and vital force in advance of form, behind the spectrum of mundane impressions, emotions, sensations, and thoughts that ordinary consciousness processes and records. The productions of creation can be described as content manifestations, aspects of a wholistic "void-source." By turning consciousness back to an iden-tification with that original, predivisional, predualistic, preconflictual condition, we connect with an ultimate resource for serving man's fuller harmony and integration.

In earlier transpersonal work, I found that patients were capable of contacting this underlying source of essence by drawing on my energy field for such transcendence.[5]

Carter-Haar has arrived at a similar conclusion:

> This fundamental reorientation of our awareness becomes perfectly natural, and also extremely simple—once we realize how to do it and practice it. Some people have found out gradually, on their own, how to achieve it. Others are able to do it, but don't practice it because they do not know that it *can* be practiced, or do not recognize the value of doing so. . . . In other words, for many people it is a matter of understanding *what* to do rather than *developing the capacity* to do it.[6]

This is in line with other research—that the desire to alter con-sciousness is an innate psychological drive.[7]

Turning consciousness back to the source generally proceeds along graded levels of depth and breadth rather than in one heroic leap. Each involutional stage increases the availability of undifferentiated life-force potential. Patients characterize this pure vibrational base as flawless, absolutely trustworthy, the essence of perfection, free of problems, a presence that is always there.

In retrospect, the principal purposes for reversing consciousness are—

1. To connect with the potential of undifferentiated consciousness at the void-source.
2. To utilize the grounding source potential as a purifying agent for resolving inner and interpersonal conflict.
3. To free consciousness from overidentification with the personal self as the singular instrument for processing awareness.
4. To harmonize disparate phenomenal life as part of a wholistic renaissance of consciousness.

Space does not allow for a detailed discussion of the steps involved in gaining access to consciousness at the source. I have dealt with this in recent writing.[8] In general, the initial stage involves opening to a clear, flawless field of awareness beyond the personal conceptions, images, ideas, emotions, sensations that ordinary consciousness conveys. The second phase launches experience as pure vibration, indescribable from the standpoint of rational, logical definitions but recognized as valid to the nervous system. The third segment of consciousness transcends both the open field of awareness and the pure vibrational realms and merges with the potential of creation at the source.

Access to the void-source does not follow a precise route. The sequence of the essence-development process in depth and breadth has a certain disorder as well as order, with gaps and overlappings of consciousness spheres quite commonplace. Nevertheless, each reentry permits fuller utilization of the essence potential as a resource for dissolving and clearing out impacted pockets of mental, emotional, and bodily disturbance.

The patient's essence connection also provides a core of security for utilizing a procedure that I have designated the Living Theater. Patients focus on the entire spectrum of fears, aversions, conflicts, hopes, and desires in exposing themselves to internal Living Theater processing. Once the flow of content material is underway, the patient is encouraged to let the drama run free, without control, to a point of climax. At this juncture, two broad channels of consciousness encounter one another—the content of mental, emotional, and physical impressions as phenomena in flux, and the changeless, flawless presence of essence awareness. As the internal, acting-out process of the Living Theater intensifies, so does the struggle for a reconciliation, reconstruction, and resynthesis of consciousness.

An example of a Living Theater episode can be gleaned from Pamela, a young divorcée, who was given brief instructions regarding her impulse to cry:

> Now that you have made an essence connection, let the channel of mental activity, emotional stirrings and body sensation within your field turn on . . . let your flow of awareness go with the energy involved in the crying impulse; let it pick up anything that appears vital, is sensed as poignant, or that might produce considerable release for you if lived out.

Here is Pamela's description of her Living Theater experience:

> The crying began to build up in the back of my throat. There was pressure way up at the top, back where the tonsils are. The tension was so strong, it began to hurt. The whole area was one big spasm and clamp. The hurting became so tremendous, I thought I would die if I didn't cry. But I still resisted crying. I had the thought that I didn't want my mascara smeared. While that was going on, I thought to myself, "That must be why people get sore throats."
> In trying to explain what happened, it just doesn't come out as strong as I felt it. It was so tremendously strong; there was so much more involved. Finally the clamp went further than the tonsils—way up into my head. But I still didn't give in to the crying, even though the pressure kept mounting more and more.
> But then I gave in to it. It was a totally new experience for me. There have been times when I wanted to cry, but I would control it. The impulse was probably as strong those other times. But I would shift my awareness away from letting go. The physical experience this time was so tremendous. It had the intensity of being on the verge of giving birth and having a baby. Then when I let go and began to cry just a little, the whole thing turned to relief, a real contentment about it.
> I finally cried as a way of knowing what was and is, rather than living in the dark about things, living a medium gray, a preference to know and feel what's true rather than to act polite, making my feelings feel polite. By the time I got finished squeezing myself into that nice, comfy

space, I realized I wasn't anywhere with myself. This was a direct way of experiencing things. Even so, I'm scared of opening up too much. What a stupid thing! But that must be everybody's problem.

Repeating Living Theater dramas permits fuller clearing of long-standing, suppressed material. Witness Pamela's follow-up Living Theater excursion:

What happened physically was that I felt the pain in my forehead. Last time I felt it up my throat as I described, with much more pain then. I also didn't mind your seeing me this way, something I would not have wanted to happen before.

This time there was a voice saying, "You can't really live in an open way, connected to the fullest degree of essence. You're not supposed to have this for yourself."

Then I related all of this to my breathing, equating my breathing to the essence connection. As I allowed the breathing and the flow of essence to widen, the stress and pain in my forehead just cleared out. But it didn't involve any intellectualizations; that was the interesting part. I didn't do any serious thinking about it for that to happen. It just seemed to result from letting the flow of activity do whatever it wanted to do.

But there was something that happened before that. I sensed that it might be all right to breathe fully within myself now—not like before, when I felt I couldn't in the presence of another person. That was the fear and the clinker. I knew at that moment what I was crying about. I realized I wasn't supposed to live. That was my mother's script—that I really shouldn't have been born. I had actually been told this by her, that I was a real inconvenience. I knew then that that hang-up was producing the crying. The narrowing of the breathing was in relation to my going along with this, that I wasn't supposed to have this for myself. But then I started to move toward a fuller measure of the breathing—connected to essence again. It was a quick thing. But I chose life because that's what I felt was coming to me. I didn't spend any more time on the question of life or death once I decided in favor of life.

Then I started to breathe in a lustful way; I guess it was just natural breathing, deeper breaths which I kept experiencing. I could feel the air going through my nostrils, like it is doing in going up my nose right now. It has a viscosity and substance to it. It isn't just air. It seems to have opened me up. I'm trying to describe the details because it is such a new experience for me. Yet I'm saying more than that. Maybe that's how animals breathe. After a time I guess a person gets used to breathing this fully. Maybe then it won't be such a high to breathe this way.

The release of such areas of distress not only enhances Living Theater operations but allows expanding realms of essence potential to serve as a unifying and integrating resource.

Mrs. D, a homemaker in her mid-thirties, had undergone psychotherapy in another part of the country before turning to me. She expressed positive feelings about having been helped with her marriage and in her role as mother of two young girls.

She continued to have a strong need to involve herself in psychic phenomena as a means of finding more relevance to her life. However, Mrs. D had had some disturbing experiences recently, apparently precipitated by a number of group sessions offered by a local organization for the purpose of developing paranormal powers.

Mrs. D's initial Living Theater revelations were fairly typical, featuring the release of uncleared, stressful material from earlier years. With deeper attunement to the essence potential, she began to explore realms of consciousness beyond the dependency needs of her coping adjustment.

> I guess I've struggled with this dependence-independence thing all of my life, particularly in relation to other people. The Living Theater brought this out even more. During the first scene I went with the dependence, letting everybody take care of me. I was a baby, being looked after completely. Then I began to see all kinds of bindings—being controlled by the other person, how I was being demanding of them. It became a trap, a form of suffocation and strangulation, like a death grip.
>
> After a time, I thought, "All I have to do is rely on what is within me." That seemed to be a logical outcome of all that I was going through. When I went back into the drama, I began to experience a stronger pull of the essence within me. As soon as I reconnected at the source, there was no longer any struggle or conflict around dependence. I could even visualize being out on the ocean alone, in a violent storm or confronted with death. Yet nothing like that bothered me once I felt the return of essence.
>
> Then the dependence-independence stuff just became garbage. It

erased the nonsense before there was any pain. Pictures of how I had been with other people reappeared, how I would depend on them to give me something, and how I was supposed to give to them in return. Seeing that again wasn't startling since I had been fighting with myself over that for so many years.

But what I got from the living theater experience was the reassurance that I didn't have to be afraid of my dependent needs anymore. All I had to do was to connect at the source of essence within myself at the essence level and I was there—with essence—me taking care of me.

All through the drama, part of me was watching the other parts of me while I was connected to essence. I could be objective and didn't have to do anything other than just let essence consciousness look after things. Then the drama became boring, like watching a TV show and knowing beforehand what the outcome would be.

Once the patient is able to establish an essence connection based on choice, there is increasing interest in testing out Living Theater programs at home. Such experimentation expands the patient's role in the therapeutic relationship beyond dependency on the doctor-patient relationship. Greater patient responsibility not only provides integration of effort outside the office but also reinforces positive attitudes toward the essence process. This is epitomized by one person's statement:

Being able to dive into the Living Theater experiences on my own is like being in one of those fancy restaurants with their extravagant menus, describing a great assortment of dishes. It came to me that I have so much to pick from in choosing which Living Theater drama I might want to try today, tomorrow, or next week.

Essence viability does not proceed without struggle, strain, and suffering. Countless minicrises occur to test the mettle of inner commitment to fuller growth and resolution. This is clearly evident in the ploys ego uses in attempting to maintain its consciousness preserve. Nevertheless, the essence connection provides the life force for working through such resistances, as evidenced once again by Mrs. D:

During the week I could feel all the problems in my life—especially the feeling sorry for myself bit. I didn't fight it; I just listened to what was going on. Then I realized, "Oh, well! That's the ego part laying

itself on me again." I just watched it while I laughed. It let go as soon as
I didn't judge it any longer.

So I merely lived it and lived with it. It made me realize that all of the
personal fears are just ego trips, a lot of wasted motion. There was the
sense of letting it go and learning from it as it did. It's difficult to talk
about since it encompasses so much beyond my intelligence. It might
sound mushy or even phony if I try to say any more.

Mrs. D's later revelations offer further clarification:

The heavy stuff of ego has dissolved to an extent. The bindings that
remain somehow feel different, as if they are no longer serious
problems in the way I have felt previously. I'm not saying I've achieved
any great thing; it's just that I'm at a much quieter, calmer, more
peaceful place within myself. For the most part, I don't get hung up in
the real sticky stuff of ego. The unraveling is still awkward and a
sputtering thing, but I don't mind that now. In fact I enjoy it as being
part of the flow and in a flow with it.

Although patients are unable to define the essence connection in
categorical terms, they do equate its power to a tool of dynamic
precision transcending ordinary consciousness. This potential is experienced as innately and inherently wholistic, to be relied upon in
spearheading and in expanding the dimensions of awareness to full
capacity.

Mrs. D furnishes us with further insight into this in her search for
completeness, through a Living Theater episode that she lived out by
herself at home:

I had this strong urge to live out the experience of being a man. I
must say that the Living Theater really gave me the freedom to do that
in a way I would never have thought possible. So I just followed that
feeling and let it build up. I could see that the feminine part of me
didn't allow any acceptance of virility or strength—things that would be
associated with maleness. I saw myself with a penis and with many
other masculine characteristics, along with the sense of being manly. I
must say I enjoyed experiencing the whole scene.

I remembered I had bought a piece of jewelry, a carving of two
monkeylike figures, each having breasts and penises. I realized more of
the meaning of that symbolism for myself, in being more whole, a kind
of universal unity around love and sex.

But the dispensing of greater assertiveness, power, and maleness in the drama was really startling. It was definitely aggressive, something which has been quite alien to my way of functioning. Yet, living it was really fun. I thought, "Gee! I've got to do more of that."

I can see where it is possible to repeat this in all sorts of ways. There was no judging, no hassling to it. Being connected to essence gave me great security and freedom from fear in living out that flow of consciousness. That didn't mean I didn't evaluate what had happened. I did that afterwards, like going back over things after sitting through the entire show. But that kind of judgment is different. It can be very objective, like seeing the whole thing in a new perspective.

I don't mean I got to a solution. There's no solution to something like this other than the way the essence works. But to be aware of so much afterwards is what I am referring to. In other words, I don't feel I solved the male-female issue completely within myself, but I felt feelings I had never been aware of before that experience. This told me how limited I had been in my total integration.

By feeling those feelings, I realized it was possible for me to come to see and know myself much more as a whole person. And when the curtain came down, I felt so much better. But that doesn't mean that I might not "chicken out" opening up to some deep-seated pain that might hit me in the future. I might still avoid living that out.

It was fortunate that, in continuing her Living Theater experimentations, Mrs. D was abetted by her husband, Tim, whose sensitivity and responsiveness complemented her need for consciousness expansion. This made possible a natural transfer of her consciousness explorations to her marital relationship. We can understand this more clearly from Mrs. D's report of a subsequent experience:

Something came over me. It was as if I was making love to myself, sort of soothing myself physically. Yet there was a unity, a complete sense of love I felt for him and myself—at the same time. It was all one in unity, physically, as well. I realized that in turning back to essence, the feeling just loves itself, just me loving myself.

So I just sank into it and thought, "Oh, my! It's something I've never felt before—in my entire life." It wasn't in any way like the normal way of loving myself, or trying to. As I loved myself this way, it was loving Tim. And as it was loving him, it was loving myself. The sexual part seemed to be an expression of that unity and love flow. It was just a blissful, beautiful feeling as if I was *in union with some vibrational force* within myself and with everything as well.

Such consciousness productions should not be interpreted as fantastic exploits but essentially as energy constructs in transcendence, a letting go and risking beyond previous limits of awareness. The dangers of "spacing out" to erotic extremism subside by virtue of the stabilizing base of essence. Mrs. D's reaction to the sexual encounter helps to clarify this:

> It's lovely to have sex with someone I like and care about. It helps to broaden my experience in regard to my relationship with Tim. But since I have that essence connection within my field already, it doesn't have that kind of desperate need I might have been trying to fulfill before. To that extent, you have already fulfilled the need before you encounter the other person.

The unfolding dramas lend themselves to a heightening of panoramic awareness as the coarser strains of mental and emotional configurations gradually thin out and become more subtle. But further transcendence requires that the essence potential be adapted to procedures other than Living Theater renditions.

A full review of more advanced stages of realization lies outside the scope of this paper. However, briefly stated, traditional images of self begin to fade as kinship with the pervasive force of essence quickens. Ultimately, reliance on the self as the exponent of awareness gives way, making inevitable a paroxysmal surrender to the void-source.

Suddenly we are awake! Direct experience has unveiled a hidden reality, releasing a stream of penetrating insights. Our essence is, and always was, *wholistically oriented*, in process with the harmonizing, open, and lucid dynamism of the essence process. A deepening faith in its lustral and organic integrity is self-validating.

We can *now* flow with the essence of that process.

Notes

1. Anthony J. Sutich, "Transpersonal Therapy," *The Journal of Transpersonal Psychology* 5, (November, 1975): 1-6.
2. Meher Baba, *God Speaks* (New York: Dodd, Mead, 1955).
3. Kenneth Ring, "A Transpersonal View of Consciousness: A Mapping of Farther Regions of Inner Space," *The Journal of Transpersonal Psychology* 6 (November, 1974): 125-55.

4. Stanislav Grof, "Varieties of Transpersonal Experiences: Observations from LSD Psychotherapy," *The Journal of Transpersonal Psychology* 6 (November, 1972): 45–80.
5. Carl Levett, *Crossings: A Transpersonal Approach* (Ridgefield, Conn.: Quiet Song, 1974).
6. Betsie Carter-Haar, "Identity and Personal Freedom," *Synthesis: The Realization of the Self* 1, (1975): 56–91.
7. Andrews Weil, "Man's Innate Need: Getting High," *Intellectual Digest* 2, (August, 1972): 69–71.
8. Carl Levett, *Insights to Essence Consciousness* (Ridgefield, Conn.: Quiet Song, 1976). Portions of verbatim material appearing in this article were drawn from this work.

Bibliography

Benoit, Hubert. *The Supreme Doctrine*. New York: Viking, 1955.

Blofeld, John. *Beyond the Gods*. New York: E. P. Dutton, 1974.

Huxley, Aldous. *The Perennial Philosophy*. New York: Harper Colophon Books, 1944.

Kapleau, Philip, ed. *The Three Pillars of Zen*. Boston: Beacon, 1965.

Swearer, Donald K., ed. *Secrets of the Lotus*. New York: Macmillan, 1971.

Taimni, I. K. *Self-Culture*. Wheaton, Ill.: Theosophical Publishing House, 1967.

Trungpa, Chogyam. *Cutting Through Spiritual Materialism*. Berkeley, Calif.: Shambhala, 1973.

Watts, Alan W. *Psychotherapy East and West*. New York: Ballantine, 1961.

25

Elizabeth Philipov

The Role of Suggestology in the Arts of Healing and Learning

A VISION IS hidden in our hearts since time immemorial: striving for perfect health over and in spite of any limitations, total and constant regeneration of our whole being, and eventual overcoming of death itself in a timeless as well as in the time-bound dimension of life. We have often manifested existential freedom and transcendent power in rising above or even changing psychological and somatic determinants of our existence. In the spiritual dimension of our multiple reality, we manifest freedom, assume responsibility, and become active agents of personal and social changes. Intuition of possibilities together with knowledge of psychophysical facts, of "what is," leads us to what "could be."

Consciousness is the awareness of ourselves and of the world outside of us, of what is; it is also the instrument of intuition and anticipation of what is not yet, but could become real. Consciousness is in a sense also the *Urphänomen* belonging in an existential account to the very ground of existence. In a variety of experiences, the awareness of ourselves and the world changes and becomes manifested in interrelated modes and states.

In the study of consciousness we speak of intuitive or rational-analytical modes of consciousness, depending on the kind of activity we are involved in. For example, a linear task might involve cause-effect analysis of the given, of what is. A wholistic task, on the other hand, involves a creative, intuitive, and anticipatory process where actuality and potentiality seem to merge. A new breed of scientists are exploring, by way of experience and experiments, altered states of consciousness, such as hypnagogic states, dreams, reverie states of behavior, pseudopassivity, meditation, trance, and ecstasy. In the experience and exploration of these states, hidden reserves and treasures of consciousness become revealed.

Suggestology, as the science of suggestion, studies elements of suggestive genesis in different states of consciousness and the role of suggestion as catalyst in these states. It is primarily concerned with the study of the fields of transition between conscious and unconscious processes and their effect on memory and health.

The field of our unconscious consists not only of memory of past experiences that, according to Freudian psychoanalysis, have become unconscious in an act of repression; it also contains automatized perceptions, thinking, and motor behavior and subliminal sense perceptions, which often enter the field by way of suggestion. Our unconscious has subliminal materials that have not yet reached the threshold of consciousness but influence our health, feelings, attitudes and motivations.

Suggestion works through the unconscious processes of our psyche. Many complex inner processes that result from the impact of suggestion remain to a significant extent on the unconscious level. Suggestive elements, excluded from the consciousness of the suggestively influenced person, exist in all of our person-to-person interrelations and person-environment interactions. We function in life with socially suggested norms of limitations, which are integrated in our institutions and public media of communication. We usually run through life in an inner state of tension or anxiety and in an environment of pressures, thus inhibiting our health and the actualization of our potentials. Most diseases in our time are diseases of stress. *A working knowledge of the shadows or gray zones of our consciousness, as well as of the role and function of suggestion in the arts of healing and growth of the total person, can help us to desuggest limitations and change unfavorable existential, psychological, and somatic conditions.*

History of Psychology of Suggestion

The first observations and explanations of the psychological aspect of the hypnotic phenomena were in fact also the first psychological discoveries about suggestion inducing and catalyzing these phenomena. The development of the psychology of suggestion in the very heart of the medical science was an advance over the attempts to present psychological phenomena in a purely physiological way. This development marked the beginning of psychology as an independent field of knowledge. It opened the path into the vast, but little-known, domain of our unconscious.

The psychological explanation of hypnotic phenomena was introduced by J. Braid in the mid–nineteenth century and by French investigators whose work began with the Abbé Faria in 1819 and culminated with A. Liébault, E. Coué, H. Bernheim, and Ch. Baudouin in the second half of the nineteenth century and the beginning of the twentieth century.

A. Liébault (1823–1904), who was a humble physician, used effectively curative suggestion after suggesting sleep to his patients. His work inspired H. Bernheim (1837–1919), a professor on the faculty of medicine at Nancy, who became the spokesman of the so-called Nancy School. He considered suggestibility to be a normal phenomenon and emphasized the role of suggestion for the production of hypnotic phenomena. According to Bernheim, the use of curative suggestions in medical cases was successful, except when the organic cause of disease was stronger than suggestion.[1]

The New Nancy School utilized suggestion in a wakeful state. As the spokesman of the New Nancy School, Ch. Baudouin bears the same relationship to Coué, as his theoretical exponent, that Bernheim had to Liébault. Coué was a druggist who observed the influence of waking suggestion in effecting cures when associated with the use of drugs, which were usually quite ineffective by themselves. He studied the phenomenon for a period of twenty-five years, and his work led him to abandon the trance entirely and depend wholly upon waking suggestion. In Ch. Baudouin's major work, *Suggestion and Autosuggestion*, dedicated to Coué and published first in 1920, he conceived of the role of suggestion and the working of the subconscious as a powerful and creative tool. The most important contributions of the New Nancy School were the application of suggestion for psychotherapeutic purposes without the salient features of the hypnotic state and the attribution of the most significant phenomena of suggestion to the domain of the unconscious.[2]

The well-known Parisian neurologist J. Charcot (1825–93), who established the Parisian school at Salpêtrière, as well as his followers Binet and Féré, studied suggestion in relation to phenomena of hyster-

ical cases. P. Janet, a member of the Institute of France and professor
of psychology in the College of France, was also a student of Charcot.
Like his predecessors, he derived his observations only from the abnormal, analyzing primarily the somnambulism of hystericals. He considered suggestion as one of the most fundamental stigmata of the
hysterical state.[3]

Janet observed that, in suggestion, each idea seems to develop to the
maximum, to give all it contains in the way of images, muscular
movements, and visceral phenomena. The creation by an image of a
whole dream and movement, as for example, the induction by the
word *Niagara* of the vivid visual perception of Niagara Falls, was
considered by Janet to be the evidence of an abnormal conduct. Thus
he also concluded that suggestibility is a pathological phenomenon.

The Controversy on Suggestibility

Suggestibility is an important concept in the history of psychology
and the medical science, but various authors have assigned different
meanings to the term. It has been central to the historical development
of hypnosis,[4] used to explain the placebo response in psycho-
pharmacology,[5] and employed as a measure of personality characteristics, particularly neuroticism.[6] Suggestibility has been equated
with gullibility and persuasibility.[7]

Eysenck considered suggestibility to be determined by aptitude, i.e.,
the presence or absence of ideomotor action in varying degrees in
different people, and also by attitude manifested as a controlling
mechanism. A decrease of conscious control is followed in suggestible
subjects, according to Eysenck, by an increase of suggestibility.[8]

Eysenck and Furneaux made the distinction between "primary
suggestibility of the ideo-motor kind," tested by the body-sway test, and
"secondary suggestibility of the indirection kind," measured by the
odor suggestion and the ink-blot suggestion test.[9] Evans did find that
factor analytic studies do not confirm the classification of "primary"
and "secondary" suggestibility presented by Eysenck and Furneaux.
He also noted that much more is known about the psychometric
properties of the test, which measure suggestibility as response to
standardized test suggestion, than the phenomena they measure.[10]

The study of T. X. Barber on responsiveness to test-suggestion led him to the conclusion that suggestibility is functionally related to attitudes and motives rather than to differences among individuals in enduring personality traits.[11] He finds that the three factors—attitudes, motivations, and expectancies—vary on a continuum (from negative, to neutral, to positive), and they converge and interact in complex ways to determine to what extent a subject will let himself think with and imagine those things that are suggested. The extent to which the subject thinks with and vividly imagines the suggested effects, in turn, determines his overt and subjective responses to test suggestions.[12] Barber considers responsiveness to suggestion a normal psychological phenomenon and an integral part of normal psychology.

Barber also reports experimental studies on responses of individuals to various kinds of test suggestions when no attempt is made to place them in a "hypnotic trance". Subjects who had, while awake, received brief task-motivational instruction designed to produce positive motivations, attitudes, and expectancies towards the suggestive situation were generally as responsive to the test suggestions as those who were exposed to the trance-induction procedure.[13]

Phenomena induced as a result of suggestion include: hallucinations; analgesia; amnesia; sensory-perceptual alterations, such as deafness, colorblindness, and blindness; age regression; and physiological effects such as cardiac acceleration or deceleration, improved visual acuity in some myopic subjects, inhibited or augmented allergic responses, or a reduced degree of inflammatory reaction and tissue damage produced by intense heat. When these studies included a control group that received the same suggestions as the hypnotic group, about the same number of subjects in both groups showed the suggested effects. For instance, suggestions that the heart is accelerating or decelerating, suggestions intended to produce heightened visual acuity for improving vision in myopic subjects, and suggestions intended to inhibit or augment allergic responses were as effective with a control group as with a hypnotic group in producing the desired changes.[14]

The Bulgarian School of Suggestology

G. Lozanov, the founder of the government-sponsored Institute of Suggestology in Sofia, Bulgaria, first utilized suggestion and then explored hypnotic phenomena in his medical research. According to

Lozanov, the increased suggestibility sometimes observed during hypnosis most probably originates not only from the physiological and psychological characteristics of the state of hypnosis, but also from the concealed motivation that the authority of this particular state carries with itself. The suggestive power of this motivation is probably decisive for obtaining the phenomena ascribed to hypnosis.[15] Lozanov noted that quite often hypnosis was confused with suggestion, due to the fact that hypnosis is obtained most often through suggestion. Through suggestion, he maintains, can be obtained many other changes of mental and somatic character. Their suggestive genesis does not entitle us to identify them with suggestion itself.[16]

Lozanov points out that suggestion functions by means of unconscious mental activities that exist in every condition of the mind, including sleep, hypnosis, and wakefulness. Although he researched unconscious processes in sleep and hypnosis, the emphasis in his work, as well as his most important contribution, lies in the exploration of unconscious activities and the use of suggestion in normal wakeful conditions. His main achievement consists in the utilization of unconscious activities and the application of suggestion, not only in clinical practices, but also in learning.

The Suggestological View of Unconscious Processes

We perceive, according to Lozanov, a large flow of information from our environment more or less outside the field of consciousness. There are transitory states or "shadows" outside the field of consciousness where, Lozanov hypothesizes, the unconscious processes are kept, combined, and developed.[17] Lozanov stresses the importance of the entire environment in which suggestive and rational processes occur. He maintains that rational elements in the person-environment interactions are in an indisruptable unity with suggestive elements.[18] Unconscious activities, on which suggestion is based, can play a significant role in balancing the individual with his environment. They are also an important part in all interpersonal communications, which proceed simultaneously on unconscious and conscious planes. On the unconscious plane, we receive and send without awareness all varieties of stimuli: a person radiates them unconsciously or semiconsciously through such means as gesture, diction, intonation, harmonics of the voice, and eye and facial expression. The reaction to the unconscious influence on this plane Lozanov calls *Nonspecific Psychic Reactivity* (NPR). The awareness and mastery of suggestive processes and the harmonization of the two planes of communication can lead to increase of learning and of communicative effectiveness in personal or other relations—for example, between actor and audience, teacher and student, physician and patient.

As part of the unconscious processes Lozanov also includes attitudes, desires, and motivations that have ceased to be in the center of attention, as well as automatized thinking and motor behavior. After we have learned, for example, to walk, write and read, the functions of walking, writing and reading become automatized. If they become deautomatized, we have to start learning to walk, read and write again each time we want or need to perform these functions.

Lozanov studied the ability of some persons to memorize or calculate large numbers in a matter of seconds without the help of any technical devices. These observations, among others, led him to exploration of automatized unconscious processes. He also brought attention to the ancient secret of the specially trained Brahmins of India called Stotrayas. In centuries past, they memorized their sacred writings, which contained hundreds of thousands of words.[19]

Suggestive Learning

Lozanov attempted to find the key to the ancient mystery of *hypermnesia* (heightened memory) by applying to learning in the wakeful state an enlarged study and use of the method of suggestion. After successfully using suggestion in medical and psychotherapeutic practices for prompting of unconscious processes and for desuggesting defenses and psychosomatic disorders, he used an elaborate and systematic method of suggestion applied to entire learning processes for the actualization of unconscious mental reserves and potentials.

According to Lozanov, the method produces a psychotherapeutic and psychoprophylactic impact on the learners,[20] and a significantly large volume of learning material is assimilated in a relaxed psychological state. Researchers in the Soviet Union tested the method on persons with neurosis, who learned in this way an unfamiliar language (2,200 words of vocabulary in one month without interruption of work). The outcome was typical of a successful treatment in psychotherapy. Symptoms such as headache, irritability, and depression disappeared, while the learners acquired good appetite, sound sleep, and self-confidence.[21]

The Institute of Suggestology in Sofia, established in 1966, teaches French, English, German, and Italian by the suggestopedic method (i.e., the method of suggestion used in teaching). Each language course lasts from twenty-five to thirty days, three or four hours a day. The language material consists of 1,800 to 2,200 new words for each course. All the language students are adults who carry daily their regular work. The so-called paranormal phenomenon of hypermnesia (heightened memory) becomes a typical phenomenon in the language acquisition process and manifests itself in an increased ability to learn. While performance in a relaxed state is heightened, anxiety and stress are decreased and desuggested. Learning becomes joy.

The purpose of my first experiment with the new method at the linguistics department of the University of California, San Diego, in 1973 (which was in fact the first testing of the suggestopedic method in the West) was to determine the applicability of the method to a university setting as well as its effectiveness. In less than six hours, the students learning Bulgarian mastered the Cyrillic alphabet with a suggestive technique specially created for this purpose. They pronounced correctly and wrote and spelled words using the entire alphabet, thus manifesting from the beginning a hypermnesic effect on learning.

In 120 hours of learning with the suggestopedic method, they assimilated 1,800 new words and demonstrated the phenomenon of hypermnesia with an average of ninety-one percent recall. The students also manifested higher speaking proficiency than the comparison group learning Russian with a traditional method in 360 hours. The time factor of learning was a ratio of one to three in favor of the students learning Bulgarian.

It was felt by the students that the major success in the learning process came at a time when it became apparent that they had effectively broken the restrictive, limiting conditioning from the past. *The planting of the seeds of suggestions of freedom and release from limitations was drawing forth the freeing belief that they were not limited to what was thought to be a reasonable amount or process of learning.*

In 1973–74 Lozanov initiated the application of the method to the public school system in Sofia in a pilot study with 1,400 students between eleven and seventeen years of age. The positive results of this study led to the application of the suggestopedic method on a larger scale to the Sofia public school system. For this purpose the suggestive roles of different art forms, theater, and music are explored and integrated into the learning process.

The suggestopedic method employs suggestions through such means as music, intonations, and rhythm as intrinsic parts of the teaching method. They are utilized in the presentation of specially prepared didactic materials and are designed to create a receptive inner state, as well as an outer environment of pleasant suggestive atmosphere. They also serve as a vehicle for assimilation of the material to be learned.

Subliminal Stimulation in Learning and Therapy

According to Lozanov, all means of suggestion used in this method utilize unconscious activities mainly through the use of subsensory input. Some inner mechanisms of the marginal type of subsensory perceptions are employed; i.e., part of the marginal subsensory perceptions are shifted into conscious perceptions, and part of the conscious perceptions are shifted into the field of the marginal.[22] Such shift must occur in directing attention to music when new learning material is assimilated. Thus the learning material is perceived through the audio and visual sensors while the learners become acquainted with the meaning of the written language text; in the second and main stage of the learning process, called *concert session*, only the audio sensors are employed. Music is played while the language material is artistically presented by the teacher, who uses special intonations.

One reason for using music in the learning process as a means of suggestion is to enhance the immersion of the learners into a relaxed and receptive experiential state and to create a flow for the intonational presentation of the learning material. However, its main purpose is to redirect the learner's attention from the need to memorize the language material presented by the teacher. The process of memorization is shifted into the marginal field of consciousness.

Contrary to all educational practices, concentrated attention is not required in this part of the learning process. The attention of the learners is directed to the harmonics and rhythm of the music, perceived through the tonally sensitive areas of the brain. As in meditation procedures, the attention is shifted from the abstract thought activity of an intellectual style to a receptive perceptual mode, similar to the cognitive functioning of children. The learning material is suggested; it seeps in and is absorbed, rather than being forced by the intellect. Although in the entire learning process the synthesis of the direct-intuitive and indirect-reflective approach is applied, emphasis is given to learning in an intuitive mode. The redirected attention selectively leaves the door open for the activation of unconscious processes directed toward actualization of mental potentials.

A shift must occur also in other instances, such as when the assimilated material is articulated by the learners in playful interactions and impromptu skits. Then attention is directed, not toward memorized details and on how one speaks, but spontaneously, in a childlike manner, to creative communicative acts. According to Lozanov, the means for performance of these acts, or the "how" of the communicative process, is processed and dealt with in the marginal or peripheral field of consciousness.[23]

In his recent research, Lozanov has obtained data showing an increase in long-term memory due to use of peripheral stimuli.[24] The evidence shows that peripheral information from unconscious stimuli "floats up" and enters the field of consciousness with delay. In the pilot experiments conducted by Lozanov, a so-called curve of recollection of peripheral information, as contrasted to the Ebbinghaus normal curve of forgetting, seems to become apparent.

In a different framework, Hilgard arrives at a similar view by studying of cognitive structures.[25] Some peripheral information, he maintains, is lost or dissipated, while some remains in a state of readiness for assimilation to cognitive structures. He arrives at the conclusion that the process in perception is twofold and consists of immediate assimilation of stimulus input to cognitive structure, and of unassimilated fragments that persist in time and are available for assimilation. Lozanov brings this twofold process into the study of hypermnesia (heightened memory) and long-term memory; he finds that peripheral information is directly applied to learning when various means of suggestion stimulate unconscious processes.

Peripheral stimuli (known in the Western literature also under the name of *incidental stimuli*) are perceived without awareness when a stimulus is presented above threshold for perceptual recognition but the subject's attention is diverted from it by a separate focal task. In the Western literature, the role of peripheral stimulation in perception and cognitive processes, as well as in subliminal influence on behavior, has been carefully studied. The experimental demonstration that cognition can be affected by stimuli outside of awareness promises to make possible an experimental psychology of unconscious phenomena and to provide an answer to the related issue of the contribution of consciousness to cognitive processes. [26]

The recovery of subliminal stimuli may depend on the particular state of consciousness of the subject. Studies in the West support the idea that a relaxed state enhances the probability that a wider range of thoughts, images, and cues will be activated. If at the same time there is a greater reliance on or attention to inner experience, this will tend to facilitate the incorporation and use of marginal inputs. [27] A number of studies suggest that a subliminal stimulus is more likely to be incorporated into a stream of conscious thought if it is congruent with it, i.e., if it is congruent with the already prevailing psychological set. One way of enhancing the effect of a subliminal stimulus is to prepare the subject, and by doing so, to create the needed receptive conditions. The prevailing set facilitates the subliminal effect and, at times, is a precondition for it. [28]

According to Lozanov, suggestion is the process in which a special set is brought about, mainly by means of unconscious processes. In this created set, a stimulus or carrier of useful information is used to penetrate hypertrophic antisuggestive barriers. The normal functioning of the barriers—classified as intuitive-affective, rational-logical, and ethical—Lozanov sees as a necessary protection of the individual. But the hypertrophic antisuggestive barriers prevent the healing suggestive influence and the development of mental and other potentials of the individual.

In order to penetrate and overcome such barriers, in his earlier clinical practices Lozanov used the so-called whispering method. The curative suggestions were whispered to wakeful patients in order to act as subliminal stimuli below the threshold of perceptual recognition. These suggestions were often very specific about given disorders of psychic or somatic character, and the information was always previously unknown to the patients. Experimental efforts were tape recorded in order to adjust the volume of the voice below the threshold of hearing. [29]

Indirect curative suggestion has been used in the so-called placebo therapy: remedy ineffective by itself is offered by the physician with a tone and gesture of significance. In some clinical cases, supraliminal suggestions were given to create and heighten motivation in patients or to satisfy psychological needs and anticipations. Lozanov reports positive results of treatment of ulcer, allergy, and of such "organic" diseases as diabetes.[30]

The most impressive case history of local analgesia in wakeful condition was recorded in August, 1965, in the medical school in Sofia during a fifty-minute surgical intervention for removal of ulcer. In a twenty-day period before the surgery, the fifty-year-old patient was prepared in conversations with Lozanov for a painless surgery without anesthesia or hypnosis. Immediately before surgery, suggestion was given again for local analgesia. The patient, conscious, calm, and alert, conversed with Lozanov and others present; pain was felt only for two minutes; during forty-eight minutes, a total local analgesia took place. In the postsurgical period, the patient continued to be in an excellent psychological state and had no pain.[31]

Means of Suggestion

Implicit Role of Suggestion

In the research and application of suggestion, it has become apparent that the impact of suggestion is always implicit in the relation between a helping person—for example, a therapist or physician—and the persons receiving help. This is true even when explicit means of suggestion are seldom used purposefully. Authority—a factor of suggestion recognized, studied, and used in suggestopedic learning—is also a powerful influence in such a relationship. As a result of the impact of this authority as well as of his or her psychological and physical condition, the recipient of treatment is almost always very susceptible to suggestion. Information is also sent and perceived unconsciously or semiconsciously through the facial expression and harmonics of the voice. If therapists and physicians are aware of the significance of this information, they can not only decipher the nonverbal language of their patients, but also master the suggestive power of their own means of expression.

Exponents of the humanistic trend in the medical profession have noticed that it is more important to know the patient than the disease.

They often refer to what we may call "suggested disease," known as iatrogenic or "doctor-caused" disease. They wonder to what extent a pathologist's descriptions of new pathological conditions might create the new disease by their very vividness.[32]

Imageries or fantasy play a most decisive function in the total mental and somatic structure. They link the deepest layers of the unconscious with the highest products of consciousness. Autogenic Feedback Training has shown that while the conscious processes control the voluntary physiological functions, the unconscious psychological domain corresponds to the so-called involuntary physiological domain. The gap between conscious and unconscious processes is voluntarily narrowed in a state of reverie.[33]

Suggestion, working in the domain of the unconscious, affects the involuntary physiological domain. Thus, suggestion may be seen as a *psychosomatic liaison*. By employing images and symbols, suggestion can serve not only as such a liaison, but can also link the unconscious with the higher levels of consciousness and act in this function as a *spiritual catalyst*.[34]

Suggestion is a powerful phenomenon with a definite role in psychological and somatic malfunctions; therefore it is imperative that it be used only in a positive way as an instrument for the attainment of wholistic health. Here the responsibility of the helping profession has to be emphasized again. The way a psychological or somatic condition of a patient is reported and described to this person is quite important. For example, a therapist may unintentionally create or suggest with his attitude a new problem, rather than assist in the resolution of an existing one. A physician fulfills a difficult and responsible role when he has to deliver news about a "fatal" or "terminal" disease.

Would such news lead to actualization of hidden psychosomatic potentials; to activation and mobilization of spiritual resources; to an attitude of responsibility for change in spite of limitations; and a transcendental illumination of life's meaning? Would there be a space left for intuition and anticipation of possibilities? Often unconscious processes are triggered by suggestion toward the realization of an imagined positive end; there are cases of spontaneous remissions and/or illumination of ultimate meaning even in the inevitable. Or would the concerned person become caught in the chains of physiological facticity and negative suggestion, drained by fears and anxiety?

Explicit Role of Suggestion

The implicit role of suggestion was briefly stated above. The role of suggestion can also be made explicit by the purposeful use of particular means of suggestion. Here a few means of suggestion utilized in suggestopedic learning will be mentioned again and recommended for use in clinical practices.

The use of music, rhythm, special intonation (such as a tone of significance or a whisper), and body language as means of suggestions in therapeutic and medical treatments has to be carefully designed to create an outer calm and suggestive environment, and an inner receptive, relaxed, and open attitude in the recipient of help. The suggestive atmosphere has a special, ritualistic significance. The use of classical music activates unconscious processes and contributes greatly to psychological relaxation, education of the imagination, and heightening of the intuitive mode of awareness. The rhythm of the music can have a calming effect, as listening to a heart beat does. A specific verbal suggestion can bear a potent effect when delivered with an intonation that is harmonized with the rhythm of the music. If attention is directed not to the voice but only to the music, then suggestion for mental or physical health, perceived peripherally, can surmount defenses more easily.

In my research on suggestopedic learning,[35] my teaching graduate students in clinical psychology the principles and method of suggestion, and in my consulting about the application of suggestion to learning disabilities and alcoholic rehabilitation, I have emphasized and utilized (1) the role of imagery in *symbolic suggestion* and (2) the suggestive power implicit in a process of identification. In our social, private, and professional lives, we identify with different roles and images. In cases of psychological problems and/or somatic malfunctions, a person tends to take upon himself or herself, and to identify with, the "sick role." Symbolic suggestion is the use of imageries to suggest new attitudes as well as a particular inner experience and change through symbolic metamorphosis.

These suggestions are intended to inspire transpersonal and synergetic experiences in a wakeful state or a reverie state for the purpose of desuggesting limitations and creating an open and receptive attitude toward a process of growth and healing. With the use of specially selected symbols, they act also as spiritual catalysts. Symbolic suggestions are employed together and harmonized with music and the harmonics of the voice. With the use, for example, of the image of a flower receiving abundantly the light of the sun, a receptive attitude is suggested. While a heightened awareness is further created with the flow of the music, the identification of the human being with the flower is suggested. The assumed new identity has the suggestive effect of symbolic metamorphosis and can lead to a valid inner change. Symbolic suggestions are used in learning as the direct vehicle for impartation of specific knowledge.[36]

The knowledge of the function of unconscious processes and the role of suggestion constitutes a vehicle for change and growth. We can manifest freedom and assume responsibility for a meaningful life as we increasingly become aware of the depth of the subsoil waters of our unconscious and of our ever-expanding spiritual, mental, and physical potentials.

Notes

1. H. Bernheim, *Hypnosis and Suggestion in Psychotherapy* (New York: University Books, 1964): 138.
2. Ch. Baudouin, *Suggestion and Autosuggestion* (London: Routledge, 1922): 26.
3. P. Janet, *The Major Symptoms of Hysteria* (New York: Hafner, 1965): 279.
4. A. M. Weitzenhoffer, *Hypnotism: An Objective Study in Suggestibility* (New York: Wiley, 1953): 252.
5. D. S. Trouton, "Placebos and Their Psychological Effects," *Journal of Mental Science* 103 (1957): 344–54.
6. R. B. Cattell, *Personality and Motivation Structure and Measurement* (London: Harrap, 1957): 98. H. J. Eysenck, *Dimensions of Personality* (London: Routledge & Kegan Paul, 1947): 203.
7. H. L. Abraham, "The Suggestible Personality: A Psychological Investigation of Susceptibility to Persuasion," *Acta Psychologica* 20 (1962): 167–84.
8. H. J. Eysenck, op. cit., p. 201.
9. H. J. Eysenck and W. D. Furneaux, "Primary and Secondary Suggestibility: An Experimental and Statistical Study," *Journal of Experimental Psychology* 35 (1945): 485–503.
10. F. Evans, "Suggestibility in the Normal Waking State," *Psychological Bulletin* 67 (1967): 114–29.

11. T. X. Barber, *Hypnosis: A Scientific Approach* (New York: Van Nostrand Reinhold, 1969): 180.

12. ———, *Biofeedback and Self-Control* (Chicago: Aldine, 1973): 393.

13. Ibid., p. 394.

14. T. X. Barber, "Experimental Hypnosis," in *Handbook of General Psychology*, ed. B. Wolman (Englewood Cliffs, N.J.: Prentice-Hall, 1973).

15. G. Lozanov, "Foundations of Suggestology," in *Problems of Suggestology*, Proceedings of the First International Symposium on the Problems of Suggestology (Sofia, Bulgaria: Nauka i Izkustvo, 1973).

16. Ibid., pp. 39–87.

17. Ibid., p. 265.

18. G. Lozanov, *Suggestology* (Sofia, Bulgaria: Izdatelstvo Nauka i Izkustvo, 1971): 83.

19. Ibid., p. 15.

20. G. Lozanov, "The Nature and History of the Suggestopedic System of Teaching Foreign Languages and Its Experimental Prospects," *Journal of Suggestology and Suggestopedia* 1 (1975): 5.

21. I. Z. Velvovsky, "The Ideas and Method of G. Lozanov in the Eyes of the Psychotherapist and Psychohygienist," *Journal of Suggestology and Suggestopedia* 1 (1975): 18.

22. G. Lozanov, *Suggestology*, p. 253.

23. Ibid., p. 278.

24. G. Lozanov, "The Suggestological Theory of Communication and Instruction," *Journal of Suggestology and Suggestopedia* 3: 4 (Paper presented at the First International Congress of Psychology of Consciousness and Suggestology, Los Angeles, 1975).

25. E. R. Hilgard, "What Becomes of the Input From the Stimulus?" in *Behavior and Awareness: A Symposium of Research and Interpretation*, ed. C. S. Ericksen (Durham, N.C.: Duke University Press, 1962): 46–72.

26. G. S. Klein, and R. R. Holt, "Problems and Issues in Current Studies of Subliminal Activation," in *Festschrift for Gardner Murphy*, ed. S. G. Peatman and E. L. Hartley (New York: Harper and Row, 1960): 75–93.

27. B. Lapkin, "The Relation of Primary-Process Thinking to the Recovery of Subliminal Material," *Journal of Nervous and Mental Disease* 135 (1962): 10–12.

28. D. P. Spence and B. Ehrenberg, "The Effects of Oral Deprivation on Responses to Subliminal and Supraliminal Verbal Food Stimuli," *Journal of Abnormal and Social Psychology* 69 (1964): 10–18.

29. G. Lozanov, *Suggestology*, pp. 145–46.

30. Ibid., pp. 172–73.
31. Ibid., pp. 168–69.
32. I. Oyle, *The Healing Mind* (Millbrae, Calif.: Celestial Arts, 1975): 17.
33. E. Green et al., "Voluntary Control of Internal States: Psychological and Physiological," *Journal of Transpersonal Psychology* 2 (1970): 1–26.
34. E. Philipov, "The Role of Suggestion in the Healing Arts" (Paper presented at the Physician of the Future Conference, San Diego, California, June, 1975).
35. E. Philipov, *Suggestology: The Use of Suggestion in Learning and Hypermnesia* (Ann Arbor, Mich.: University Microfilms, 1975).
36. E. Philipov, "Increased Rate of Learning a New Language with Suggestive Imagery Techniques" (Paper presented at the 27th Annual Scientific Meeting, Society for Clinical and Experimental Hypnosis, Chicago, 1975).

26

C. Norman Shealy

Wholistic Healing and the Relief of Pain

FOR THE PAST fifty years, neurosurgeons have represented the court of last resort for chronic pain patients. The beginning of this pattern of referral was initiated by the finding that destruction of the anterior quadrant of the spinal cord by a tuberculoma led to analgesia of the opposite leg. Surgical destruction of the anterior quadrants—cordotomy—was then extensively done in an attempt to control pain where primary therapy failed to relieve the symptoms. Thus, the concept of "intractable pain" arose. Such pain is that which persists after removal of the apparent cause or where the physical cause is not correctable.

Background Considerations

In the period from 1925 to 1940, most of the patients considered candidates for cordotomy were those either with cancer or with phantom limb pain after surgical or traumatic amputation. Surgical cordotomy was tried at many sites, the most common being upper neck or chest areas. The open laminectomy for performing cordotomy is a painful approach with considerable operative site pain for from one to several weeks; with all the problems of major surgery in patients, many already debilitated by their disease; and with a large number of possible complications: paralysis of leg (and possibly arm), paralysis of bladder and/or bowel, loss of sexual potency or ability to have orgasm, or development of postcordotomy dysesthesia—a new intense burning pain, far worse than that with which the patient started.

Beginning in the 1940s, and accelerating since then, a new pain syndrome appeared, that of the "failed back"—that is, pain in the back and/or leg following surgery for presumed ruptured disc. We must accept the historical fact that very few individuals became permanently crippled by back and sciatic pain prior to the discovery of the ruptured disc syndrome in 1939 by Mixter and Barr. Since that time, surgery on the back has expanded to a remarkable 50,000 to 100,000 cases each year. Unfortunately, many, perhaps most, such operations are performed on patients with discs that had "degenerated," not truly ruptured. In a review of 250 virgin operative notes, we found only 6 with clear-cut descriptions of disc herniations, 22 with "possible" ruptured discs, and 222 operations on patients who clearly did not have a ruptured disc at the first surgical procedure.

As might be expected, surgery of this type has led to a high rate of failure to relieve symptoms. "Good" series of patients are reported to have a good result about seventy percent of the time (still leaving up to 30,000 bad results per year!). And the best long-term study revealed that only thirty-nine percent of operated patients returned to work within two years (leaving possibly 60,000 still suffering each year). Surgery and the diagnostic tests leading to it cause increasing problems of scar; arachnoiditis, often involving the entire cauda equina (the nerve roots at the bottom of the spine); and total incapacitation.

By the late 1950s, patients with excruciating pain after multiple back operations began to follow the route of their cancer and phantom limb predecessors. The results were terrible. Then, in the early 1960s, a new method of spinal cord destruction was devised: percutaneous cordotomy, done with simple heating by an electrode tip, without the risks of laminectomy. This procedure then became almost as great a fad as disc surgery. Literally thousands of patients were operated over the next decade, with frequent disastrous results.

Thus, despite the neurosurgeon's role in the management of pain, relatively little impact was made. Even the addition of other destructive procedures—cutting of spinal nerve roots and frontal lobotomy—have failed to benefit a majority of those unfortunate enough to subject themselves to these procedures.

Drugs have proven equally inadequate in the management of pain. Narcotics lead to addiction and all the problems thereof; synthetic pain relievers are ineffective; and tranquilizers cause more problems than they control. Drugs practically never actually control pain; they essentially never cure the cause of the pain; and they lead to depression, habituation, and mental confusion.

Beginnings of the Research

With this background fully in mind, in 1963 I began research on alternative techniques for relief of pain. After I had spent two years on basic research in pain physiology, Melzack and Wall's gate control theory of pain provided me the mental stimulus to hypothesize that electrical stimulation of the dorsal columns of the spinal cord might relieve pain. Eighteen months of further research led to the first use of this technique in 1967. The theory was excellent; the practice, mediocre.

We know that the largest sensory nerve fibers, Beta, do not report pain, but that activation of Beta fibers inhibits incoming information from the "C" fibers, which are largely responsible for chronic-suffering pain. Electrical stimulation of the Beta fibers, concentrated in the dorsal columns, should relieve pain below that level. Indeed, it can and often does. Mechanically, however, the equipment needed to do the stimulation safely and chronically is still not perfected. Thus, there are risks of paralysis (far less than with cordotomy), infections, leakage of spinal fluid, and other bad outcomes; but also there are frequent late (six months to three years) equipment failures necessitating removal and/or replacement.

Furthermore, the simplistic attitude that pain can be removed without reference to the patient's mental status is no more true with electrical stimulation than with destructive surgery. From the beginning of my work with stimulation, I recognized the tremendous importance of the lifestyle, personality, and attitude of the patient. Thus, between 1967 and 1971, I did about thirty dorsal column stimulator implantations—but I turned down sixteen patients for every one implanted! With the growing realization that dorsal column stimulation left no answer for at least ninety-four percent of chronic pain patients, I began looking at comprehensive or wholistic systems for managing pain.

My first major consideration was chiropractic. I realized that many patients reported pain relief after manipulation. Although useful in acute back pain, however, manipulation is of little benefit to the patient after surgery. Acupuncture is similarly limited in its application, with greatest success in acute pain. Various forms of psychotherapy, including the body therapies (Reichian, Rolfing, etc.), have been of little help for the invalid pain patient.

Then I learned of Fordyce's approach to chronic pain—behavioral modification or operant conditioning. From 1966 to 1971, he had treated 100 patients in an eight-week program where their complaints of pain were ignored, drugs were gradually withdrawn, and patients were assigned simple physical tasks like walking and sitting for increasing time periods. Results were remarkably good, especially considering the simplicity of the program. Sixty percent of the patients improved. But only about thirty percent maintained the improvement once they went home. Nevertheless, such improvement in patients who had not been helped by medical, pharmaceutical, or surgical therapy is impressive.

Developing the Program

Armed with this information, I returned to La Crosse to set up a comprehensive program designed to include all the modalities that seemed applicable to pain:

> acupuncture
> electrical stimulation
> physical exercise
> behavioral modification
> heat
> ice
> massage
> psychotherapy
> drug withdrawal
> nerve blocks and denervations (rarely and in highly
>   selected situations).

The first year, we treated 400 patients in a hospital program that averaged thirty-two days. Psychiatric consultation and group sessions three mornings a week were discontinued after one year in favor of Biogenics® (Autogenic Training and Biofeedback). Gradually over the next year and a half it became obvious that the most important modalities were physical exercise, Biogenics, and external electrical stimulation. Massage, ice, heat, and acupuncture were quite secondary. Except for cancer pain and tic douloureux, nerve denervations were indicated only in selected back problems where the pain seemed to originate from spinal facet joints that partially overlapped from degenerative disc disease. Indeed, this latter pathology is apparently the cause of a majority of back and sciatic pain.

Drug withdrawal is accomplished fairly easily if pain relief and psychological insight develop during the treatment program.

During the past 4 ½ years, we have treated 1,300 patients. About 350 of these have had the benefit of the complete Biogenic program and all the indicated therapy.

Analysis of Problems Treated

In dealing with each patient, we must first rule out a *correctable* physical problem. The comprehensive overview has revealed only about one patient in a hundred for whom additional major diagnostic tests are indicated. Corrective surgery has been needed in about six patients. *Diagnoses have included:*

Postfusion lumbar disc syndrome	36%
Postsurgical lumbar disc syndrome	24%
Degenerative lumbar disc syndrome	10%
Degenerative cervical disc syndrome	10%
(with or without surgery)	
Miscellaneous, including	20%

    Migraine headaches
    Tension headaches
    Postherpetic pain
    Paraplegic pain syndrome
    Phantom limb pain
    Postsurgical pain
    Posttraumatic pain
    Pain due to cancer
    Rheumatoid arthritis
    Osteoarthritis
    Postcordotomy dysesthesia
    Thalamic pain syndrome
    and a variety of unusual pain states.

About forty percent of the patients have had Workmen's Compensation claims. The patients with previous back surgery have averaged four earlier operations. Patients have also had two to three other operations, usually for various dysfunctions of internal organs (cholecystectomy, appendectomy, gastrectomy, hysterectomy, hemorrhoidectomy, etc.).

Drug use is common, with almost all patients taking three to ten drugs—the most common being codeine, Percodan®, Valium®, Talwin®, Librium®, aspirin, Tylenol®, Elavil®—but the entire range of analgesics, mood drugs, and tranquilizers is seen.

Assessing the degree of pain at the time the patient comes in and for later follow-up, we have for the past 2 ½ years used the following pain profile:

1. How much of the time do you have pain? (0–100%)
2. How severe is your pain? (mild, discomforting, distressing, horrible)
3. How much does pain inhibit your physical activity? (0–100%)
4. What drugs and amounts are you taking?
5. How does the pain affect your personality?

The average patient scores 43,332, although the range goes from 12,122 to 44,444.

Examination reveals mainly stiffness, poor mobility of the back and neck, and the common surgical scars. Minor nerve damage is common in the operated patients—i.e., absence of ankle jerk or a slight decrease in response to pinprick and touch in the foot and calf.

Having decided (for almost all patients) that further diagnostic tests are not indicated and that the physical component of the pain is nerve injury—partial damage—or scar, we are ready to suggest therapy. In all patients with spinal pain, at some time within the first week, Marcaine™ blocks of the appropriate facet joint nerves are done under fluoroscopic monitoring. If the procedure is successful—that is, if pain is relieved for two to twenty-four hours—then permanent destruction of the affected facet nerves is indicated. Unfortunately, for most operated patients—especially those with fusion—facet nerve blocks and denervations give incomplete relief of pain. Almost all patients except those previously unoperated, then, require the full twelve-day program.

During the next twelve days, patients are tried on at least three types of external electrical stimulators: Stim-Tech™, or Neurex™, Elec-treat™, and the Liss Pain Suppressor™. Both the pulse characteristic and the pattern of use vary on these stimulators—from twenty-four hours per day to three minutes four times a day; from 10 cycles to 20,000 cycles per second; from minimal sensation to tolerance of intensity. With this variety of equipment, ten percent of patients achieve total pain relief; about twenty percent achieve sixty to eighty percent relief; and twenty percent have forty to fifty percent pain relief.

Acupuncture is considered for those who desire it. About ten per-cent of patients are benefited markedly by acupuncture, but ninety percent of these do equally well with external electrical stimulation. Massage, heat, and ice are offered to all patients to try for themselves purely for partial symptomatic relief.

Limbering physical exercise is begun the second day, with super-vised sessions once a day and procedures to do alone once a day. As they progress, all patients are encouraged to take up cardiovascular strengthening exercises, mainly one of the aerobics programs.

The most important part of the comprehensive program is Biogenic training. Patients receive five hours a day of guided mental exercises, which include relaxation, physiological balancing, mental focusing, special personal goal-oriented programming, psychological insight, and spiritual awareness. A systematic progressive program is taught. Additionally, patients have half an hour each day with either the physician or a registered nurse. They are encouraged to work at least three hours per day with biofeedback equipment and cassette tapes of the Biogenic mental exercises. They also continually evaluate electrical stimulation. Occasionally, private hypnotic ses-sions, including life regressions, are used to reinforce the insight exer-cises.

During the second week, private counseling is done on two consecu-tive days by a talented psychic minister. Patients often comment that they gained more from those two half hours than they had earlier in three years of psychotherapy.

Numerous lectures supplement the mental exercises; they include discussions of anatomy, physiology, psychology, stress, nutrition, drugs, moods, and spiritual goals. Patients are encouraged to request drug withdrawal programs, and these are written individually for each patient. In about ten percent of patients, Elavil is added, and a similar number of patients try Cobroxin™. Occasionally, Dilantin™ is added to the Elavil. For those patients on large dosages of narcotics, it is usually necessary to switch them to methadone for gradual withdrawal.

Some Problems and Conclusions

The greatest shortcoming of the Pain Rehabilitation Center approach—with its two-week program and most patients from out of town—is the lack of follow-up and reinforcement. It is most difficult to encourage patients who live hundreds of miles away, and it is equally difficult to cooperate with their home physicians, most of whom do not truly understand either the philosophy or the treatments underlying the program. Spouses rarely accompany their mates to the program so that we also miss the opportunity for more marital counseling. Until there are sufficient programs to allow patients easy access to refresher courses near their home, this problem seems insoluble.

An equally serious problem is the American system of payment for medical care. A majority of patients expect some third party to care for them—Medicare, medical-surgical insurance, welfare, etc. However, all those programs are notoriously ill-prepared to cover rehabilitation expenses; the third party system was set up primarily to cover such serious acute illnesses as accidents, surgery, infections, and heart attacks. Most third party coverage is anything but comprehensive! Indeed, even the major medical policies rarely pay for biofeedback, acupuncture, or even electrical stimulators. Despite the fact that medical costs are cut tremendously by outpatient treatment, most third party coverage insists upon hospitalization to even have payment considered. Such requirements are directly opposed to the recently introduced certification of need required for hospitalization. Until these inconsistencies are corrected, the comprehensive treatment of pain will undoubtedly remain a relatively infrequent event. Despite interest expressed by many of the over 400 physicians who have visited in La Crosse, very few have attempted to set up similar programs. Most are unwilling to give up their current practices to take up an entirely new and different approach to patient care. Undoubtedly, the real future of the wholistic approach lies with young physicians who are attuned to treatment of the whole patient.

Bibliography

Fordyce, W. E.; Fowler, R. S.; Lehmann, J. R.; and Delateur, B. J. "Some Implications of Learning in Problems of Chronic Pain." *Journal of Chronic Disorders* 21 (1968): 179–190.

Green, Elmer E.; Green, Alyce M.; and Walters, E. Dale. "Voluntary Control of Internal States: Psychological and Physiological." *Journal of Transpersonal Psychology* 2 (1970): 1–26.

Luthe, Wolfgang, and Schultz, Johannes. *Autogenic Therapy*. Vol. 1–6. New York: Grune and Strattion, 1969.

Melzack, R., and Wall, P. D. "Pain Mechanisms: A New Theory." *Science* 150 (1965): 971.

Mixter, W. J., and Barr, J. S. "Rupture of the Intervertebral Disc with Involvement of the Spinal Canal." *New England Journal of Medicine* 211 (1934): 210.

Shealy, C. Norman. "The Pain Patient." *American Family Physician* 9 (1974) 130–36.

Bibliography

Part IV

Non-Western
Approaches to
Wholistic Healing

27

Effie Poy Yew Chow

Chinese Medicine: Contributions to Wholistic Healing

The way that can be mapped is not the eternal Way.
The name that can be named is not the eternal Name.

DIFFERENTIATION between Western and Eastern thought may be, in part, quite clearly identified by these lines, recorded by one of China's most preeminent Taoists, Lao-Tzu, in the sixth century B.C. [1,2,3] These are the opening words of the *Tao Te Ching*, a work embracing a way of life, the Tao, that has been practiced for over two millennia and is still being practiced today. The *Tao* conveys the understanding that a concept that may be scientifically defined, proven, or particularized is, by the fact of its definitive nature, not a conceptualization of the totality or ultimate reality. This reflects an ideology not entirely unique to the East, yet distinctly at variance with the predominant mode of Western thought, knowledge, and science—specifically health science. The ability to conceive of universal forces that cannot be contained by the written word and that go beyond the limitations of scientific delineation is essential to the Chinese perspective of life and of health. Western health science, however, has relied exclusively on definitive scientific data for the determination of what is to be considered real, functional, or effective.

Wholistic health is a movement in both Western and Eastern thought that recognizes the existence of life forces that have as yet to be adequately "named" or "mapped" for incorporation into conventional Western health science. Yet these forces have been tapped as effective healing energies by traditional practices of other world cultures, the rituals of ancient civilizations, and the discoveries of current wholistic medical research.

The contribution of Chinese medicine to wholistic health will be discussed in this chapter from a number of approaches: firstly, from the inherent history, theory, and philosophy of the system; secondly, from the manner in which Chinese medicine is carried out in everyday practice and living; and thirdly, from the way in which the systems of both Chinese and Western medicine are cooperating successfully to provide both preventive and critical care for the massive population of the People's Republic of China. The practical wholism that characterizes all phases of Chinese medicine will become increasingly apparent as we move from theory to practice to national health care systems. Because of the limited space, however, it will be possible to introduce the reader to only the surface aspects of this tremendously complicated and fascinating system of philosophy and medicine. It is hoped that you as the reader will be intrigued enough to search further on your own into this essentially wholistic system—Chinese medicine.

1. Wholism in the History, Philosophy, and Theory of Chinese Medicine

The Chinese culture has, until the twentieth century, based its system of health care entirely on principles of universal life energies recognized as early as the second, or possibly third, millennium B.C. The accounts of Confucius (sixth century B.C., Chow dynasty) date China's early philosophical development as far back as the third millennium B.C. and the reign of, most notably, Tuang Ti or the Yellow Emperor.[4,5,6] Chinese dictionaries record the Yellow Emperor's reign as dating from 2697 to 2597 B.C.; however, many academicians consider the accounts of Confucius and other records referring to the existence of the Yellow Emperor as legendary.[7,8] Nonetheless, in Chinese culture, the authorship of the *Nei Ching Su Wen*, the classic treatise on Chinese healing arts, is attributed to the Yellow Emperor.[9,10,11,12] This classic work, although a philosophical edict on life, is considered to include much of the substance upon which Chinese medicine is based.

Although the first legible Chinese medical texts to be found are considered to date no earlier than 540 B.C., the medical symbology used in these texts is generally believed to have originated in the thirteenth and fourteenth centuries B.C.[13,14] Because Chinese writings were first produced as bone engravings (the "oracle bones"), which have deteriorated beyond legibility, it is impossible to attribute exact dates to the origins of the earliest recorded works.[15,16] The *Book of the I-Ching (Canon of Changes)*, attributed by Chinese culture to Fu Hsi, whose reign predated even that of the Yellow Emperor, is considered by other scholars to date no further back than the first half of the first millennium B.C.[17,18] Regardless of the precise degree of antiquity attributed to the Chinese classics, these works present the symbolic interpretation of vital life forces and universal principles that underlies the entire structure of Chinese medical theory and practice.

Perhaps the most fundamental symbology of the Chinese philosophical system is represented by the terms *yin* and *yang*, which first appear in the *Book of the I-Ching*.[19,20] Yin and yang symbolize the two forces that sustain the universe. The interplay and resistance, union and separation, of the yin force and yang force, forever in motion in the paradoxical balance of opposing unity, form the power of the universe, and bestow power on all things within the universe. The yin force is associated with all that is dark, cool, negative, and feminine. The yang force is light, warm, positive, and masculine. The balance of these forces is harmony; the imbalance of these forces brings war, famine, disease, pestilence—chaos to the universe.

Just as the yin and yang forces dominate the universal flow of energy, so too the human creature, who is seen in Chinese culture as a microcosm of the macrocosmic whole, is dominated by the yin and yang. The *Nei Ching Su Wen* teaches that disease occurs when the balance of yin and yang within us is disturbed. The *Nei Ching* states:

> If Yin and Yang are not in harmony, it is as though there were no autumn opposite the spring, no winter opposite the summer. When Yin and Yang part from each other, the strength of life wilts and the breath of life is extinguished. If such a body is exposed to the dew and the wind, then colds and fever will set in. . . . If Yang is predominant, then the body will grow hot; the pores close and the patient begins to breathe heavily and gasp for breath. Fever will arise; the palate will become dry; the person becomes tense and irritable. . . .[21,22]

The concept of dual inseparable forces is not unfamiliar to Western science. In fact, the "negative" and "positive" polarities recognized as necessary to the balance of Nature may be considered to represent the same basic principle as the Chinese yin/yang forces. The Western theory of the immunological competence or incompetence of the body to ward off infection or disease may also be compared, in principle, to the Chinese theory of the balance of yin and yang polarities and its relationship to health and well-being. However, although these comparisons may be drawn, the concept of balance, as the essential characterization of all entities, is most distinctly the fundamental precept of Chinese medicine.

The Chinese doctor can perceive an imbalance in yin and yang, and which of these is the dominating or subsiding force, by studied and experienced knowledge and a finely tuned sensitivity to the characteristics exhibited by predominant yin or predominant yang. Specific human body parts—indeed all physical entities—are considered to be more yin or more yang by nature, according to the appearance, function, and character of the particular entity, as empirically observed, and its similarities to the essential qualities of either the yin or the yang force. No entity, however, is solely yin or yang, but merely is characterized by one force to a greater degree than the other. Even the yin and yang forces themselves are not totally without the essence of the other. As the *Nei Ching* states—

> There is also yin within yin, and yang within yang. Thus from early morn to the middle of the day the yang of Heaven is effective; this is the "yang within yang". From midday until dusk, the yang of Heaven is again effective, but now it is the "yin within yang". From the first dark of night until the cock's first crow, the yin of Heaven is effective; this is the "yin within yin". From the cock's first crowing until the early morning hours, the yin of Heaven is again effective, but now it is the "yang within yin".[23,24]

The Chinese perceive no entity as entirely one way exclusive of another; rather all entities are seen as microcosms of the macrocosmic whole, exhibiting not a lack or an antagonism, but only proportionately greater and lesser degrees of all that is.

Doctrine of the Five Elements

The totality and interrelation of all entities is more elaborately symbolized by the Doctrine of the Five Elements, believed to have been introduced to Chinese philosophy by Tsou Yen in the third century B.C.[25,26] This doctrine may have been adapted from Indian philosophy[27,28] and the theory of three elements. Various philosophies of the ancient civilizations believed in birth/death or consumption/ regeneration cycles of matter as manifested by three, four, or five basic elements. The Pythagorean school of Greece (fifth century B.C.) based its philosophy on the cycles of four elements—water, air, earth, and fire.[29] The early Thai philosophy also accepted four basic elements.

The Chinese doctrine of five elements—fire, earth, metal, water, and wood—is the central concept of a network of associated senses, forces, phases, anatomies, and states of being that correspond to one another on the basis of the elemental functions. The interrelation of the five elements is a simultaneous sequence of regeneration and consumption, which may be stated as follows:

Wood gives way to fire.	Wood consumes earth.
Fire gives way to earth.	Earth consumes water.
Earth gives way to metal.	Water consumes fire.
Metal gives way to water.	Fire consumes metal.
Water gives way to wood.	Metal consumes wood.

This conceptualization of the consumption and regeneration of material substance may be recognized as a more concrete symbology of the eternal dynamic sustained by the abstract forces of yin and yang. The correspondences of each of the five elements were empirically evolved in much the same way that particular entities became associated with either the yin or the yang force—that is, by a subtle and complex association of characteristics. That the odor termed *scorched* is associated with fire may be more evident to the Western mind than the association of metal and *rotten*, or water and *putrid*; yet with some consideration it is possible to sense, if not define, the nature of each association. The five elements and their correspondences are shown in Table 27.1.[30]

The doctrine of the five elements is a symbology structure as essential to the Chinese healing arts as the conceptualization of yin and yang, and it serves to guide the physician in identifying the body/mind energies and their representations in the harmony of universal forces.

The Flow of Chi

The most intricate of the Chinese symbology systems is the conceptualization of the flow of body/mind energies, the Chi, its paths through the body along the energy meridians, and its points of concentration, or acupoints. The meridians and points are conceived in

TABLE 27.1
The five elements and their correspondences

In terms of the macrocosm:

Five elements	Five seasons	Five taste qualities	Five colors	Five atmospheric influences	Five stages of development
wood	spring	sour	blue	wind	birth
fire	summer	bitter	red	heat	growth
earth	late summer	sweet	yellow	humidity	change (puberty)
metal	autumn	sharp	white	drought	maturity
water	winter	salty	black	cold	storage

In terms of the microcosm:

Five elements	Five sense organs	Five structural elements	Five Fus	Five Tsangs	Five emotions
wood	eye	sinews	bile	liver	anger
fire	tongue	blood vessels	small intestine	heart	joy
earth	mouth	muscles	stomach	spleen	anxiety
metal	nose	hair	large intestine	lung	sadness
water	ears	bones	urinary bladder	kidneys	fear

relation to the greater and lesser degrees of yin or yang dominant in three body areas and associated body organs and functions. The predominant yin or yang force influences the path of Chi, its direction, points of concentration, and linkage with specific body areas, parts, and organs. The *Nei Ching* devotes its second part, the *Ling Shu*, to practical application of the symbology systems developed in the first part, the *Su Wen*. In the *Ling Shu*, the points and meridians are graphically represented and show little or no discrepancy from the various acupuncture charts in use today.[31,32]

The current recognition, in the West and the East, of the phenomenal utility of acupuncture is perhaps largely responsible for the growing respect for cultural symbology systems, conceptualization of life forces and energies, and their relationship to the sustenance of human well-being. The monitoring of body/mind energies toward a state of being attuned with the harmony of universal forces is practiced, not only by the Chinese people, but in other cultural and theoretical systems as well. Curanderismo, Indian shaminism and herbology, Philippine healing, and Black folk medicine are only a very few of the cultural healing systems that are based on principles of balance and harmony of vital life forces as related to a higher universal power. Even within the realm of Western science, particularly in advanced studies in nuclear physics, relationships between undefinable phenomena of universal energy systems and the life forces of human body/mind energy are being recognized.[33]

The wholistic health movement is reintroducing and developing energy concepts and cultural practices in recognition of the vital impact they may have on human well-being. *Wholism*, by the nature of the word itself, implies a conceptualization of the totality and interrelation of all entities and forces, knowledge of harmony and balance, and a respect for all systems and practices that tap the sustaining life forces—whether scientifically or symbologically oriented. An overriding result of the wholistic health movement is a new sense of the nature of health with a special emphasis on the maintenance of well-being and prevention of disease.

2. Wholism in the Practice of Chinese Medicine

Chinese medicine, by the nature of its philosophical foundation, is functionally preventive. Diagnosis, for the Chinese physician, is not a process of symptomatic analysis for the purpose of isolating a pathological disorder. It must be recognized that Western health science has developed this ability far beyond the capacity of any other health care system, and with tremendous results. The Chinese physician, however, in the process of diagnosis, is seeking to detect disturbance to the balance of yin/yang forces and its precise effect on the course of the Chi. The Chinese people do not seek the diagnostic services of a physician only when there are symptoms present to analyze, but rather on a regular basis to determine if all continues well within. An old story in Chinese culture tells of the patient who will pay his doctor as long as he stays well; if he becomes ill he will reject that doctor as incompetent and go to another. As Chang Chung-ching (frequently referred to as the Hippocrates of the East) wrote in the third century B.C., "Forestalling the ill and treating it before it is apparent is work of a superior order."[34]

Diagnostic Techniques

The tools of Chinese diagnosis involve no instruments or technological apparatus. They are the five senses, a finely acute sensitivity, and a studied and experienced intelligence of the Chinese medical classics and subsequent writings. Examination is a four-phased process: inspection, auditory perception, questioning, and sphygmology.

Inspection involves thorough examination of the body orifices, which correspond to internal body organs, and determination of their color, texture, resilience, temperature, pulsation, odor, and other significant characteristics that may indicate the presence of an external or internal imbalance. The soles of the feet, palms of the hand, nails, and hair are also inspected for the extent of perspiration or deterioration, color, texture, and other significant characteristics. Urine and feces are examined for significant color, odor, and volume as well as consistency, frequency, or retention.

Auditory perception involves analysis of the patient's voice, breath, and cough. Specific qualities of voice—e.g., laughing, weeping, groaning, singing—indicate imbalances as well. Similarly, the manner of breath inhalation and exhalation corresponds to particular organs and functions. Coughing is appraised for characteristics exhibiting internal or external imbalances.

Sphygmology, or reading of the pulses, is considered the most utile of the four diagnostic procedures. Its development is attributed to Pien Ts'io or Pien Ch'ueh as early as the fourth or fifth century B.C.[35,36] As with each of the other diagnostic procedures, the function is to detect the status of the yin/yang forces and the effect on the Chi; if an imbalance is present, the physician is able to determine the severity and probable course of the condition as well as its presence. (In this sense, the diagnostic procedures are prognostic as well.) Three individual pairs of pulses, each both superficial and deep, can be palpated at the radial artery on each wrist. Thus, by palpating both wrists, twelve pulses can be felt, each pulse relating to one of the twelve organ systems or physiologic areas. The relationships are shown in Table 27.2.[37,38,39]

Each pulse should produce a specific sensation if the related organ is in good health; for example, the "heart pulse should be like the ringing sound of a sickle"—rich at first, then trailing off; the spleen pulse should alternate in regular rhythm; and so on.[40] Imbalances are identified in such terms as groping, choking, tender, limping, wavering to and fro, tangled as weed, and numerous others providing a rich gradation of sensations, each indicative of the presence and degree of an imbalance in a specific physiologic area. There are twenty-eight such different qualities to each pulse position.

Although the purpose of sphygmology, and each of the other diagnostic procedures, is to identify an imbalance before a pathological

TABLE 27.2
Relationship between Pulses and Organs

Left Radial Artery	Superficial (piao)	Deep (li)
Inch (Ts'un) pulse	small intestine	heart
Bar (Kuan) pulse	gall bladder	liver
Cubit (Ch'ih) pulse	urinary bladder	kidney

Right Radial Artery	Superficial (piao)	Deep (li)
Inch (Ts'un) pulse	large intestine	lung
Bar (Kuan) pulse	stomach	spleen/pancreas
Cubit (Ch'ih) pulse	"triple warmer"	"controller of the heart" pericardium

disorder develops, the use of sphygmology to precisely determine the nature and course of an existing pathological disorder is also highly effective and is currently being recognized as such by Western physicians. Several European physicians who have studied sphygmology— for example, Van Nghi or Darras—report that they were able to make "startling diagnoses which were subsequently verified by clinical tests."[41] In studies conducted jointly by French and Chinese physicians, the French doctors' clinical diagnoses coincided with seventy-nine percent of the diagnoses specified by Chinese doctors based entirely on pulse readings.[42] Nonetheless, the principles of Chinese medicine, which are truly wholistic in nature, advocate the use of sphygmology for prevention—before crisis intervention is necessary— and equally advocate the use of all the diagnostic procedures together, no one being adequate of itself alone. The *Nei Ching Ling Shu* states that diagnosis by inspection and auditory perception is lucid (ming), by sphygmology is intelligent (shen), and by questioning is workmanlike (chung). To use only a single method, however, is chung, to use two is shen, but to use all is both shen and ming.[43]

The parallels between Chinese medicine and wholistic health become increasingly apparent as we move from the philosophical foundation based on awareness of sustaining life energies, the preventive function of diagnosis based on respect for the totality of an individual's internal and external life patterns, to the methods of treatment that are an outgrowth of the philosophical basis and function of diagnosis. The yin/yang forces and elemental cycles are perceived as the regulating dynamic of all entities and functions of the universe in Chinese philosophy, while human life patterns and relationships to the universe are perceived as the regulating influence on the balance of the universal dynamic in the body/mind microcosm. Methods of treatment rely on the monitoring of body/mind energy patterns and the modification of life habits and behaviors to maintain (or regain) the ultimate harmonious balance essential to well-being.

Although the scope of this chapter does not allow a detailed accounting of the complex methodologies involved in the various Chinese treatment methods or lifestyle practices used to maintain or regain good health, it is possible to describe certain of the treatments and practices on the basis of their underlying principles. The conceptualization of dual and inseparable sustaining forces as symbolized by the yin/yang, and of simultaneous and cyclic consumption and regeneration as symbolized by the five elements, represents a dynamic also perceived in relation to the regulatory influences of the treatments and practices. Tonification and sedation, or stimulation and preservation, are the dual unified functions inherent in the specific treatment methods as well as the life habits and practices adopted for the maintenance of good health.

Both the physician and the family in Chinese culture provide a supportive framework for developing moderation in daily living habits. Excessive stimulus or excessive sedation, or the total influence of one without the other, is strongly advised against. One must not sleep too much or too little; eat too much or too little—or an excess of yin foods or yang foods; work too much or too little; expose oneself to too much heat or too much cold; and so on. Only by maintaining a balance in one's relationship to the environment may one prevent an imbalance of the microcosmic relationship to the macrocosmic whole. Specific practices undertaken to maintain a harmonious relationship with the environment—such as medication, breathing exercise, massage, and the martial arts—assist the individual to develop skills in tonification and sedation that will not subject the Chi to an excess of either.

Because treatment and practical techniques are based on the principle of balance—between the dual regulatory influences and their relationship to the dual universal forces—they may be used to prevent excesses and therefore imbalance, or to produce excesses to allow the recovery of balance. The manipulative therapies (i.e., treatments or practices that directly manipulate the flow of Chi), such as acupuncture, moxibustion, acupressure, cupping, massage, external (physical) exercise, and internal (respiratory) exercise, may be used either to tonify or preserve the body/mind harmony, or to stimulate or sedate the Chi in the case of imbalance.

Acupuncture

Acupuncture treatment (and the related treatments acupressure and moxibustion) is perhaps the most direct and graphic of the manipulative therapies in that the pathways and points of concentration of the Chi are precisely outlined and clearly accessible. Acupuncture regulates the Chi by insertion of fine needles into the points of intensity. If there is an excess of concentration (congestion), the needle is manipulated to disperse the Chi or sedate the excessive concentration. If the point is blocked, preventing the intensity of Chi in the point, the needle is manipulated to stimulate the point, eliminate the blockage, and reactivate the intensity of Chi. Acupressure operates entirely on the same principles but differs in that finger pressure is the manipulative tool rather than needles. Moxibustion, which is believed by some scholars to have been developed in the Stone Age,[44,45] before the existence of metal tools or needles, involves the burning of *moxa* or mugwort (*Artemisia vulgaris*) on the points. Moxibustion may be used in conjunction with acupuncture or independently; however, certain acupoints are forbidden in the use of moxa, and the correct positioning of the patient's body is of greater significance.

Cupping, which is believed to have been developed in the third or fourth century B.C.,[46] refers to the use of heated cups applied to a body area to produce suction, which in turn disperses congestion. Cupping does not act on the points, but rather on larger body areas corresponding to the location of general congestion. For example, in the case of bronchial congestion, a burning substance together with medicinal herbs is placed in the cup and then removed when the desired degree of heat is attained. If there is specific lung congestion, the cup is then placed on the back or chest in the area nearest the center of congestion and, as the cup cools, a suction is created. Similar treatment applies to congestion of the Chi in other body areas. The Chinese perceive breath to be a manifestation of Chi, similar to the Greek concept of *pneuma*, and in this sense, bronchial congestion is no different from a congestion of Chi in any other area of the body.

Massage

The use of massage, like the treatments just described, acts on external body areas to stimulate or sedate the Chi and therefore affect internal body organs. A complex system of hand movements to be used on specific body areas produces particular effects on corresponding organs and organ functions. This system was developed numerologically and incorporates the energy meridians as well as the eight Kua, which are the primary hand motions and corresponding body areas.[47] As with all treatments, massage may be used to tonify and preserve, as well as to stimulate or sedate the Chi.

Exercises

Internal (respiratory) exercise is a direct manipulation of Chi in the sense of its manifestation as breath, or pneuma. The state of being to be assumed in the practice of respiration exercise cannot be objectively defined; it is a phenomenon of consciousness that must be subjectively recognized. The three basic principles of respiration exercise may yield an indication of how it is generally to be performed; they are relaxation and repose (Sung Ching Wei Chu); association of respiration with attention (I-ch'i Ho'i); and interaction of exercising and resting (Lien-yang Hsiang-chien).[48] Various breathing exercises are carried out in particular postures in accord with the three principles. Respiration exercise is perhaps the most highly conscious of the treatments and practices, requiring the individual to act in concentrated unity with the philosophical conceptualizations on which it is based. The effect is to enhance Chi or, in the case of illness, regenerate the failing Chi. External (physical) exercises are performed in conjunction with respiratory exercise as a balance of the inner (yin) and the outer (yang) activities.

Physical exercise is also significant in its own right. Although all of the martial arts involve the balance of yin and yang, Tai Chi is the most developed of these arts in terms of this concept. Tai Chi is a series of movements performed in a slow, regular, coordinated, and natural manner while breathing is regular, deep, and quiet. The number of movements involved depends on the school of Tai Chi; for example, the modified Chin School, as taught by Kuo Lien Lee, consists of 64 movements; the Yang Tai Chi has over 200 movements; a third school has only 38. In each of the Tai Chi schools, however, it is taught that the mind, sense organs, internal organs, and limbs must all be in harmony. Harmony must be developed such that the bones are not disordered in movement and will oscillate if the individual is pushed or jarred. Tai Chi, and other practices of Chinese physical culture, may be viewed as the art of maintaining internal and external balance while in movement.

It is not difficult to recognize the similarity of the Chinese manipulative therapies to those incorporated in the practice of contemporary wholistic health. Indeed, as consistent with the wholistic health movement, specific Chinese therapies such as meditation, Tai Chi, and acupressure are incorporated into wholistic practice. Other wholistic forms of manipulative therapy may not rely on the precise methodological or philosophical structures of the Chinese techniques, but nonetheless, they may be recognized as based essentially on the same principles. The terms Chi and bioenergy lend themselves to obvious comparison. Postural integration, Rolfing, Autogenic Training, polarity/balancing techniques. Feldenkrais method, certain Reichian techniques, various forms of massage and dance, reflexology, and other wholistic practices all go far beyond the theory of simple calisthenics to embrace the wholistic concept of internal/external and body/mind harmony.

The treatments and practices that manipulate or monitor the Chi are a major constituent of Chinese medicine; however, there are other forms of treatment as well. Most notably, the use of herbs and other natural substances (including foods) to influence the balance of yin and yang has existed in China since its earliest recorded history and, according to Chinese culture, as early as the reign of Shen-nung preceding the Yellow Emperor.[49,50] Chinese medicine is one of the richest sources of known herbal, mineral, and animal medicaments, incorporating the empirical knowledge of several millennia. Medicinal treatment, like all of the treatments and practices, is used preventively to tonify the Chi and preserve balance, or, in the case of illness, to restore balance by stimulating or sedating the Chi. Each medicament is identified for yin or yang properties empirically known to affect specific body parts, organs, functions, or conditions. Other treatments and practices in Chinese medicine include hydrotherapy, sun therapy, spiritual healing, dream counseling, and certain forms of orthopedics and surgery.

3. Wholism in Cooperative Systems: A New Approach to Health Care

Traditional Chinese medicine, and many other world cultural and theoretic medical practices, have much to offer modern-day health care systems, whether the bases of their information are philosophical/empirical or rational/scientific. The wholistic health movement, which incorporates all effective health care practices, is largely responsible for making this fact known and the knowledge and practices accessible, not only in the United States, but on an international level.

Wholistic health, though the term may be specifically American, must be recognized as an international movement. The World Health Organization in Geneva, Switzerland, has published a considerable amount of information concerning the efficacy of cultural and alternative healing practices in many countries of the world.[51,52] As just one example, the National Research and Development Board of Zaire has recently funded a major research project to investigate all aspects of the country's traditional healing practices to possibly "integrate them into the country's health services."[53]

The most intriguing example, in relation to the context of this chapter, of the efficacy of a truly wholistic perspective on national health care is the system currently existent in the People's Republic of China.

Contemporary Medicine in China

The Chinese culture had very little contact with Western medicine previous to the turn of the century. In the last decades of the nineteenth century, there were approximately one hundred European and American physicians living in China.[54] However, the influence of the West was to dramatically increase: several Western medical schools, hospitals, and clinics were established in the early twentieth century. By 1928, the advent of the regime of Chiang Kai-shek, Western medical facilities had become the sole source of people's health service, and the practice of traditional Chinese medicine was outlawed.[55]

In 1949, at the time of the establishment of the People's Republic of China, some forty thousand physicians trained in Western medicine were responsible for the health care of the entire population of China—800 million persons.[56] Great numbers of the population, especially in rural areas, were not receiving care or were continuing to seek the services of traditional practitioners despite the illegality of doing so. In 1949, the leaders of the new People's Republic urged all practitioners of traditional Chinese medicine, some five hundred thousand, to resume their practice, side by side with the Western-trained physicians.

Although initially a great emphasis was put on the value of traditional medicine, and Western doctors were exhorted to adopt various traditional practices and remedies, the two medical systems remained fairly separate. Traditional Chinese doctors continued to practice primarily in rural areas where Western health services were minimal or nonexistent, and Western medical practice was predominant in the urban areas. Certain isolated traditional practices, primarily herbology, were taught in the medical schools; however, the general scope of medical education remained Western in theory and in most practices.[57]

Trend toward Synthesis of East and West

The lack of integration between the two systems was considerably modified in 1965, when the national health service policy called for a greater exchange between urban and rural medical personnel. Rotating mobile teams of health professionals from urban centers spent periods of time with traditional practitioners in the rural areas. The effect was to familiarize traditional practitioners with Western methodology, while at the same time providing Western-trained medical personnel with an experiential knowledge of traditional practice. In 1966, a synthesis of the two systems was further advanced by the establishment of a corps of "barefoot doctors," i.e., local villagers who were trained by the visiting urban medical teams in the basics of Western health care and by local traditional practitioners in the fundamentals of Chinese medicine.[58] The barefoot doctors serve their native villages and the surrounding countryside by initiating preventive care programs, referring persons to more highly trained traditional and Western medical personnel as needed, and treating minor injuries and illnesses by both Western and traditional practices. Traditional practice is often more heavily relied on by the barefoot doctors, however, because it does not require expensive or elaborate equipment, the rural residents are generally more receptive to the medical theory of their own culture, and its function is more generally preventive.

Nonetheless, the cooperation and exchange between traditional practitioners and Western medical personnel led to a greatly heightened awareness of the tremendous potential of a blend of the two systems in urban clinical settings as well as rural areas. In the past decade, the national health care policy of China has been to combine the two systems at all levels. Medical college curricula have been fundamentally revised to incorporate both Western and Chinese medicine in a well-integrated and highly practical system adaptive to both urban clinical and rural settings. Dr. E. Grey Dimond, who has visited the People's Republic of China, describes the curriculum of a medical school he observed:

> . . . nine months: At the medical school, a coordinated course combining anatomy, physiology, biochemistry, Chinese traditional medicine, and political education. A second phase of this program coordinated pharmacology and microbiology in a lecture laboratory course identified as Prevention of Essential Diseases. The microbiology class . . . consists of studying throat cultures . . . working in the laboratory to identify the organism . . . maintaining laboratory notebook. One could describe the course content as traditional but with a clinical orientation. . . .
> . . . six months: Lecture in clinical demonstrations and internal medicine, surgery, obstetrics, and gynecology. . . .
> . . . nine months: Out to the countryside to do practical medical work with their teachers. The medical school faculty and the students of medicine and surgery. In the evenings, clinical and basic science lectures are given by the faculty using the classrooms of primary schools in the countryside. The students also receive formal instruction in the recognition, collection, [and] use of herbs, and learn to use acupuncture. This is also the period during which the role of public health and preventive medicine is learned by on-the-job training. Students and faculty also engage in manual labor together, tilling a shared plot or doing road work, etc.[59]

One-month vacations, and two-month periods of physical fitness, military training, and manual labor occur between terms. Acupuncture, herbology, and preventive care are especially emphasized in all medical college curricula; certain training programs— for example, barefoot doctor training—are particularly comprehensive of the traditional treatments and practices.

Recent Developments

By the early seventies, most hospitals in China had both Western and traditional medicine treatment areas, with combined treatments also taking place (usually within the Western treatment wing). Several

Chinese hospitals have large departments, fully staffed and equipped, that operate entirely by combined treatment procedures. One very brief example of how combined treatment is remarkably effective in critical care is taken from Shui Wan Wu's *China Medicine As We Saw It:*

> On April 1, 1971, Yao Ching-lu, an aged peasant of the Shuikaochuang production brigade in the western suburb of Tientsin, contracted acute appendicitis with diffuse peritonitis. When he was admitted to Nankai Hospital, he was found to have paralytic ileus and was in critical condition. He was treated immediately with acupuncture, herb medicines taken orally and applied locally in conjunction with decompression of the gastrointestinal tract and saline-glucose infusions. Soon his pain was lessened, and the next day his abdomen became softer. On the fourth day, he began to take food and was discharged well from the hospital on the tenth day.
> . . . Through a long period of clinical practice, it has been shown that the use of combined Chinese and Western medicine in the treatment of acute abdominal disease reduces the number of surgical procedures, expands the scope of non-operative management, improves the cure rate and lowers the incidence of complication. [60]

American physicians who have observed the national health care program in the People's Republic of China (including those who wrote *China Medicine As We Saw It* and many others) can testify to innumerable cases in which the combined methodologies of Western and Chinese medicine produce excellent results. It is of special interest that traditional Chinese treatments do not produce harmful and debilitating side effects as is frequently the case with Western pharmaceutic and/or surgical treatment. Using combined treatment methods such as those developed in the People's Republic, natural herbs may replace harmful synthetic drugs, and surgery can often be avoided.

As indicated by the national health policy of China and its very significant successes, world cultural tradition has a great deal to offer modern medical care. As Dr. E. Grey Dimond remarks in reference to Western attitudes and traditional medicine, "In spite of our tendency to think of *them* as isolated, we may find that there is much for *us* to learn." [61]

The wholistic health movement has done much to attain wider

recognition and acceptance of this fact. It has reintroduced world cultural traditions and concepts of internal and external balance, energy systems, preventive care, self-responsibility, and the theoretical validity of many non-Western, nontechnological healing systems. Chinese medicine, as the philosophy and practice of balance, harmony, and moderation, and as a current national health policy incorporating combined treatment procedures from both the East and the West, contributes, in turn, a great deal to the wholistic health movement.

Notes

1. Pierre Huard and Ming Wong, *Chinese Medicine*, trans. George Wiedenfeld and Nicolson Limited (New York and Toronto: McGraw-Hill World University Library, 1968).
2. Stephen Palos, *The Chinese Art of Healing* (New York: Bantam, 1972).
3. Heinrick Wallnoefer and Ann von Rottauscher, *Chinese Folk Medicine*, trans. Marion Palmeda (New York: Bell, 1965).
4. Huang Ti, *The Yellow Emperor's Classic of Internal Medicine*, trans. Ilza Veith (Berkeley, Los Angeles, and London: University of California Press, 1970).
5. Pierre Huard and Ming Wong, op. cit.
6. Heinrick Wallnoefer and Ann von Rottauscher, op. cit.
7. Huang Ti, op. cit.
8. Stephen Palos, op. cit.
9. Huang Ti, op. cit.
10. Pierre Huard and Ming Wong, op. cit.
11. Stephen Palos, op. cit.
12. Heinrick Wallnoefer and Ann von Rottauscher, op. cit.
13. Pierre Huard and Ming Wong, op. cit.
14. Stephen Palos, op. cit.
15. Pierre Huard and Ming Wong, op. cit.
16. Stephen Palos, op. cit.
17. Ibid.
18. Heinrick Wallnoefer and Ann von Rottauscher, op. cit.
19. Fu Hsi, *I-Ching, Book of Changes*, ed. Ch'u Chai and Winberg Chai, trans. James Legge (New York: University Books, 1964).
20. Heinrick Wallnoefer and Ann von Rottauscher, op. cit.

21. Huang Ti, op. cit.
22. Heinrick Wallnoefer and Ann von Rottauscher, op. cit.
23. Huang Ti, op. cit.
24. Heinrick Wallnoefer and Ann von Rottauscher, op. cit.
25. Stephen Palos, op. cit.
26. Heinrick Wallnoefer and Ann von Rottauscher, op. cit.
27. Stephen Palos, op. cit.
28. Heinrick Wallnoefer and Ann von Rottauscher, op. cit.
29. Hippocrates, *The Genuine Works of Hippocrates*, trans. Francis Addams, vol. 1 (London: Sydenham Society, 1849).
30. Stephen Palos, op. cit.
31. Effie Poy Yew Chow, *Acupuncture: Its History and Its Educational Significance to Western Health Practices in the U.S.A.* (Santa Barbara, Calif.: The Fielding Institute, 1975).
32. Marc Duke, *Acupuncture* (New York: Pyramid, 1973).
33. Evarts Loomis and J. Sig Paulson, *Healing for Everyone* (New York: Hawthorn, 1975).
34. Pierre Huard and Ming Wong, op. cit.
35. Ibid.
36. Stephen Palos, op. cit.
37. Effie Poy Yew Chow, op. cit.
38. Stephen Palos, op. cit.
39. Shui Wan Wu, *The Chinese Pulse Diagnosis*, trans. Poon Chak Keung (San Francisco: Writers Guild of America West, 1973).
40. Heinrick Wallnoefer and Ann von Rottauscher, op. cit.
41. Ibid.
42. Stephen Palos, op. cit.
43. Pierre Huard and Ming Wong, op. cit.
44. Ibid.
45. Stephen Palos, op. cit.
46. Ibid.
47. Ibid.
48. Ibid.
49. Ibid.
50. Heinrick Wallnoefer and Ann von Rottauscher, op. cit.
51. V. Djukanovic and E. P. Mach, *Alternative Approaches to Meeting Basic*

Health Needs in Developing Countries (Geneva: World Health Organization, 1975).

52. *Health by the People* (Geneva: World Health Organization, 1975).
53. Family Health Division Press Release No. 06/76, dated March 23, 1976 (Geneva: World Health Organization).
54. Pierre Huard and Ming Wong, op. cit.
55. Effie Poy Yew Chow, op. cit.
56. Ibid.
57. Joseph R. Quinn, ed., *Medicine and Public Health in the People's Republic of China* (Baltimore: U.S. Dept. of HEW, Geographic Health Studies, John E. Fogarty International Center for Advanced Study in the Health Sciences, DNIH No.NIH73-67, 1973).
58. Ibid.
59. Joseph R. Quinn ed., *China Medicine As We Saw It* (Baltimore: U.S. Dept. of HEW, Geographic Health Studies, John E. Fogarty International Center for Advanced Study in the Health Sciences, DNIH No.NIH75-684, 1974).
60. E. Grey Dimond, "Medical Education and Care in the People's Republic of China," *Journal of the American Medical Association* 218, no. 10: 1552–57.
61. Ibid.

Bibliography

Acupuncture Anesthesia (A translation of a Chinese publication of the same title). Geographic Health Studies Program, John E. Fogarty International Center for Advanced Study in the Health Services, 1975. (Baltimore: U.S. Dept. HEW, Public Health Services, NIH)

"AMA Group Finds Chinese Medicine Excels in Some Areas." *Journal of the American Medical Association* 22 (1974): 1703–04.

Beau, George. *Chinese Medicine* (New York: Avon, 1972).

Bergson, Anika, and Tuchack, Vladmir. *Zone Therapy*. New York: Pinnacle, 1974.

Cerney, J. V. *Acupuncture without Needles*. New York: Parker, 1974.

Chan, Pedro. *Wonders of Chinese Acupuncture*. Alhambra, Calif.: Borden, 1973.

Chinese System of Healing. "Wayside" Grayshott Hindhead, Surrey: Health Science Press, 1964.

Chuange, Dr. Yu-Min. *Chinese Acupuncture*. Hanover, N.H.: Oriental Society, 1972.

Dimond, E. Grey. *More Than Herbs and Acupuncture*. New York: W. W. Norton, 1975.

Finger Acupressure. Los Angeles: Price/Stern/Sloan, 1974.

Five Elements of Acupuncture and Chinese Massage. New York: Health Science Press, 1973.

Freedman, Maurice, ed. *Family and Kinship in Chinese Society*. Stanford, Calif.: Stanford University Press, 1970.

Greel, H. G. *Confucius and the Chinese Way*. New York and Evanston: Harper and Row, 1960.

Kiev, Ari. *Transcultural Psychiatry*. New York: Free Press, 1972.

Lavier, J. *Points of Chinese Acupuncture*. New York: British Book Centre, 1965.

Li, F. P. "Traditional Chinese Medicine in the United States." *Journal of the American Medical Association* 220 (1972): 1132–35.

Li Shih-chen, comp. *Chinese Medicinal Herbs*. Translated and researched by F. Porter Smith, M.D., and G. A. Stuart, M.D. San Francisco: Georgetown, 1973.

Mann, Felix. *Acupuncture: The Ancient Art of Chinese Healing*. London: William Heinemann Medical Books, 1972.

McGarey, William A., M.D., *Acupuncture and Body Energies*. Phoenix: Gabriel, 1974.

Namikoski, Tokiyiro. *Shiatsu*. Tokyo: Japan Publications, 1969.

Paul, Benjamin D., ed. *Health, Culture and Community*. New York: Russell Sage Foundation, 1955.

Ruben, W. S., and Griffith, Joseph. *Tai Chi*. New York: Lancer Books, 1970.

Shiang, E., and Li, F. P. "The Yin-Yang (cold-hot) Theory of Disease." *Journal of the American Medical Association* 217 (1971): 1108.

Smith, Arthur H. *Proverbs and Common Sayings from the Chinese*. New York: Dover, 1965.

Snow, Edgar. *Red China Today*. New York: Random House, 1970.

Stephens, William N. *The Family in Cross-Cultural Perspective*. New York: Holt, Rinehart and Winston, 1963.

The Dimensions of Healing. Los Altos, Calif.: The Academy of Parapsychology and Medicine, 1972.

The Meridians of Acupuncture. London: William Heineman Medical Books, 1970.

Tokei, Koichi. *What is Aikido?* Tokyo: Rikugei, 1962.

Tom, Po-Chin. *Acupuncture and Moxibustion*. San Francisco: Chinese World Press, 1965.

Yu-Lan, Fung. *A Short History of Chinese Philosophy*. Edited by Derk Bodde. New York: Macmillan, 1964.

28

Acupuncture:
Healing the Whole Person[*]

Richard J. Kroening, Michael P. Volen, and David Bresler

Introduction

FOR SEVERAL YEARS, occasional visitors from the West have returned from China with reports of the successful use of acupuncture in the treatment of various medical problems.[1] These reports remained largely curiosities in the United States until the recent improvement of relations between China and the West brought much new information and stimulated considerable interest in acupuncture.[2] Most spectacular were reports of the use of acupuncture as an anesthetic that permitted patients to remain awake and alert during surgery while experiencing no pain.[3,4]

Acupuncture anesthesia has now been investigated in the West, and its effects appear to be much more subtle than those of chemical anesthetics.[5] In order to be most successful, thorough rehearsal of the operative procedure with the patient is necessary, for the effectiveness of analgesia can be impaired if the patient becomes frightened or excited. Although preoperative rehearsal is utilized routinely in many Chinese hospitals, it is rarely employed in the West. As a result, acupuncture for surgical analgesia has not been enthusiastically advocated except perhaps for obstetric deliveries and oral surgical problems.[6,7]

However, acupuncture is much more than a technique for producing surgical analgesia. It is a complete system of medicine, based upon the philosophy and world view of the culture from which it arose. Its origins have been lost in antiquity, but it has been estimated that acupuncture has been practiced since the third century B.C. Thus, it may well be the world's oldest system of wholistic medicine. In addition, it should be noted that more individuals have been treated by acupuncture in the course of human history than by any other formalized system of medicine.

The Tao

The classical Chinese conceptions of the human organism and the cause and treatment of disease are intrinsically linked to the philosophical constructs of traditional Chinese thought. Man is a reflection of the universe, a microcosm in the macrocosm, and both are subject to the same universal and divine law, the law of the Tao. To live according to the Tao is to adapt to the Order of Nature and to live in accord with the Ultimate Principle.

If one does not live according to the Tao, the resulting disharmony may be manifested as physical and/or psychological disease. Therapy must be directed toward the reestablishment of balance and harmony if it is to have long-term effectiveness.

Yin and Yang

Yin and yang denote the twin polarities that regulate both man and the universe (see Table 28.1). Although Taoist philosophy describes yin as negative and female, and yang as positive and male, the terms negative and positive are used in the same sense that modern physics describes an electron as negative and a proton as positive. A proton, although positive, is not superior to an electron. In the same manner, yin and yang refer to the opposing polarities, forces, or tendencies that form all living entities.

TABLE 28.1
Polarities of Yin and Yang

Yin	Yang
Negative	Positive
Feminine	Masculine
Passive	Active
Earth	Sky
Moon	Sun
Plain	Splendorous
Soft	Hard
Right	Left
White	Black
Even	Odd
Dark	Light
Cold	Warm
Emptiness	Fullness

Yin and yang exist only in relation to each other, for, according to the writings of the ancient Chinese, within each Yang there exists Yin, and within each Yin must be Yang. Nothing is pure yin or pure yang. There is always some yin and some yang in every living object, as can be seen in the Taoist symbol shown in Fig. 28.1. Thus, for example, no one is completely male or female; rather, masculinity and femininity are both present in each individual in varying degrees.

Homeostasis

Yin and yang forces ebb and flow, and this undulatory process affects, not only individual health and character, but all events in the universe. Their pulsation is found in the contraction and dilation of the heart (systole and diastole), and in the inhalation and expiration of the lungs.

Yin and yang relationships exist in the interaction of the parasympathetic and sympathetic divisions of the autonomic nervous system. Overactivity of the sympathetic nervous system produces what the Chinese call "excess yang" ailments, whereas overactivity of the parasympathetic nervous system produces "excess yin" ailments. Yin and yang may also be reflected by the manner in which blood sugar is

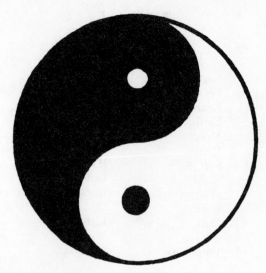

Fig. 28.1 Taoist yin/yang symbol

regulated by insulin and glucagon, and by the way in which central nervous system activation and sleep are regulated by norepinephrine and serotonin.

The goal of Chinese medicine is to maintain or restore balance between yang and yin, thus ensuring proper health. In Western medicine, the term *homeostasis* refers to a similar concept in which a balance of opposite forces is maintained to ensure proper functioning of physiological systems.

Meridians of Acupuncture

The ancient Chinese discovered that pressing, puncturing, or burning certain loci on the skin could alleviate pain, affect the course of certain ailments, and influence the functioning of internal organs. Of particular importance was the fact that widely separated loci affected the functioning of the same organ. These points were connected, and the resulting lines were given the name *Ching* or *meridian* (see Fig. 28.2).

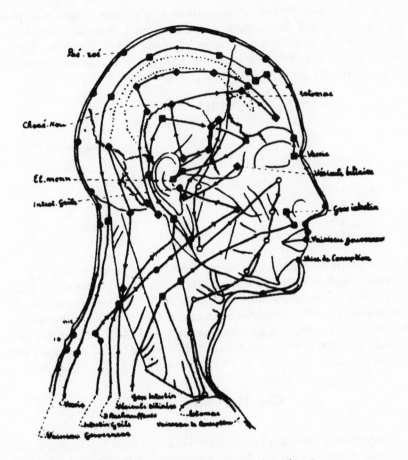

Fig. 28.2 Acupuncture meridians of the head

Originally, twelve double meridians were described, with each pair placed symmetrically on either side of the body. Each meridian corresponded to one of twelve internal organs conceptualized by traditional Chinese medicine. In addition to these twelve paired meridians, two important nonpaired control meridians were postulated: the Governing Vessel, which follows the spine and runs along the midline on the dorsal surface of the body, and the Conception Vessel, which runs along the midline on the ventral surface of the body. These two, plus six less-important lines, were called the eight "special" meridians. Later, "extra" meridians and "muscle" meridians were added, but in practice, the most commonly used acupuncture loci lie on the twelve main meridians and the two control meridians.

TABLE 28.2
The Acupuncture Meridians

Yin	Yang
Lung	Large Intestine
Spleen	Stomach
Heart	Small Intestine
Kidney	Bladder
Liver	Gall Bladder
Circulation-Sex	Tri-Heater

The Chinese divided the twelve meridians into six yin-yang pairs representing the twelve traditional internal bodily functions (see Table 28.2). Two of these meridians are obscure to Western medicine: the circulation-sex (also called the heart constrictor or pericardium) meridian probably relates to the endocrine system, while the tri-heater (also called the triple warmer) meridian relates to the "heat" of respiration, digestion, and reproduction.

Chi: The Energy of Life

Traditional Chinese philosophers believed that the universe was permeated with a vital life force or energy that they called Chi. This energy was thought to circulate continuously through the acupuncture meridians of all living organisms. This concept of an intangible life force is not unique to the Chinese, but exists under different names in many other religious and philosophical traditions.[8]

If the circulation of Chi is impeded or blocked in a given meridian as a result of external events (such as trauma, cold, dampness) or internal factors (such as fear, anger, sorrow), an abnormal surplus or deficit of Chi may result. The organ linked to the meridian then becomes unbalanced. This affects the entire organism, and is ultimately manifested by the presence of pain or disease.

Diagnostic Techniques

Before treating a patient, the traditional acupuncture practitioner first attempts to diagnose the nature of the imbalance of energy, utilizing a variety of diagnostic techniques. These include a careful inspection of the general appearance of the patient, skin coloration, texture of the hair, color of the tongue's coating, and a general examination of the mouth, nose, eyes, and teeth. The rate and clarity of breathing, the patient's tone of voice and manner of speaking, and the determination of any foul or characteristic odors also provide important diagnostic information.

The balance of the meridians is also assessed by careful examination of the radial pulses (see Fig. 28.3). By palpation of these pulses, the traditional practitioner is reportedly able to discern which of the meridians is malfunctioning, and whether this disturbance is due to increased or decreased Chi flow.

POSITIONS OF PULSE DIAGNOSIS

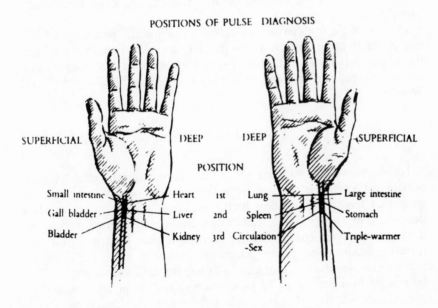

Fig. 28.3 Traditional Chinese pulse diagnosis

The link between philosophy and practice is demonstrated by the use of the yin-yang principle for arriving at a diagnosis: yin is associated with cold, internal, and reduced functioning, while yang is related to overheating, external, and hyperactive functioning.

Acupuncture Therapy

After a diagnosis has been made, the acupuncturist prescribes a course of acupuncture therapy. According to traditional Taoist philosophy, stimulation of appropriate acupuncture loci results in a restoration of balanced energy flow, which then permits the affected organ (and eventually, the entire organism) to return to its normal homeostatic state.

Acupuncture loci may be stimulated by insertion of fine, solid needles, by intense heat (moxibustion), or by massage (acupressure), depending upon the problem being treated. Modern technology has made available a variety of new techniques including electrical stimulation of the needles, ultrasound stimulation, and even laser beam stimulation.

The rationale underlying the selection of specific points and techniques for treating a given illness involves a variety of rather complex theoretical relationships that are beyond the scope of this chapter. The interested reader is referred to the books by Palos,[9] Mann,[10,11,12] and Beau.[13]

Tonification-Sedation

Tonification-sedation, one of the fundamental principles of acupuncture therapy, is derived from the concept of yin and yang. In simplified terms, tonification techniques are utilized to replenish a deficiency of energy, while sedation techniques are employed to reduce an excess of energy. Either technique may be appropriate for restoring balance, depending upon the nature of a specific illness.

For example, chronic fatigue in a thin, pale, asthenic individual may be related to a deficiency of yang energy, and tonification would be appropriate. On the other hand, sleep difficulties in a heavy, red-faced, plethoric individual may be related to an excess of yang energy, and sedation would be indicated.

This type of approach is representative of the wholistic nature of acupuncture therapy. Acupuncturists do not isolate and treat a specific medical symptom; they see a problem as a single manifestation of the general condition of the individual. Acupuncture therapy involves the whole person, and the skilled acupuncturist treats the patient, not the disease.

Acupuncture facilitates the organism's own tendency toward homeostasis and health, and results are accomplished through the body's natural mechanisms of recovery and regeneration. This differs from Western medicine, which generally relies upon the introduction of some external substance to modify events within the body. Consequently, acupuncture seems to be most effective in those situations where the body's own life support and regenerative capacities are not too severely compromised.

Mind and Body

Practitioners of Western medicine often attempt to distinguish diseases of the body from diseases of the mind, but it is becoming increasingly clear that this is a false duality. The state of the mind and body are inseparable, and both are involved to some degree in every illness.[14]

Traditional Chinese medicine does not distinguish between mind and body, but views psychological and physiological symptoms as manifestations of a unitary underlying energy imbalance. In this context, it is interesting to note that many acupuncture patients who achieve relief of physical symptoms also report feelings of relaxation, well-being, and occasionally even mild euphoria.

Relationship of Individual and Environment

In the Western world, it is generally accepted that one can practice medicine without an underlying philosophy or religion; even an atheist can be an accomplished surgeon. But in the medical world of traditional China, this is inconceivable. Without proper knowledge of cosmic relationships and intense study of the weather, seasons, stars, and planets, medical treatment is impossible. Anything that affects the planets, seasons, and climates is thought to also affect the organs, tissues, and emotions of man.

Western scientists are only now beginning to appreciate the powerful influence of climate on disease. For example, it is now known that cases of coronary occlusion occur more often on cold, cloudy days than on warm, sunny days. Chinese observers described this phenomenon nearly five thousand years ago.

Traditional Chinese health care practitioners considered diet to be one of the most important factors in health and disease. Foods were evaluated in terms of their relative yin and yang energy. Certain types of grains and meats were thought to be either harmful or beneficial, depending upon the energetic status of a given individual. The flavor and color of foods were also considered to be extremely important.

It is difficult to determine if these complex correspondences have therapeutic validity or are merely superstitious customs handed down across generations. Nevertheless, the underlying importance of these general principles remains valid. The individual cannot be isolated from the environment in which he lives and the food he eats.

Environmental factors may be even more important for contemporary man than for the Chinese who lived centuries ago. Modern man must face unprecedented environmental pollution, processed foods that lack critical nutrients, and the stresses of a noisy, crowded technological society. These and other environmental factors that affect health and disease must be carefully considered by contemporary practitioners, just as ancient acupuncturists considered the wind and the cold and the dampness.

Acupuncture as Preventive Medicine

It has been reported that acupuncture was utilized primarily as a form of preventive medicine in ancient China.[15] Villagers would consult their acupuncturist periodically in order to diagnose and correct an imbalance of energy before it had become sufficiently serious to produce any detectable physical symptoms. Should this prove to be accurate, it represents a highly sophisticated form of preventive medicine, compared to which our present methods of examination appear somewhat crude.

It is not inconceivable that there were once acupuncturists capable of recognizing extremely subtle manifestations of impending disease. It is well known that stimulation of certain acupuncture points acts as a general tonic for many individuals, even in the absence of illness. For example, needling Tsu-san-li, a major acupuncture point, is said to be associated with increased production of immunoglobulins,[16] and many acupuncturists believe that periodic stimulation of this point may prevent certain minor illnesses.

Western Theories of Acupuncture

A considerable amount of research has now been conducted to explore possible mechanisms of action of acupuncture. In particular, neurophysiological research on the nature of pain has produced several theories that attempt to explain how acupuncture can relieve pain.[17] A discussion of this research is well beyond the scope of this chapter, and no comprehensive explanation has yet been widely accepted. However, it seems likely that acupuncture involves a complex mobilization of the immune/inflammatory system, peripheral neural stimulation, and subtle psychological factors.[18]

Does this mean that the traditional theory of energy flow has no practical validity? The answer to this depends upon the perspective of the questioner. Modern physics has shown that matter and energy are not distinct, but represent two aspects of the same phenomenon. In some situations, it is easier to explain a given phenomenon in terms of matter; in others, in terms of energy. Likewise, all events in the organism, whether psychological or physiological, involve both matter and energy. Thus, it does not seem at all contradictory to think in terms both of energy flow and of physiological mechanisms in order to explain what is happening when acupuncture is performed.

Future of Acupuncture in the West

Traditional Chinese medicine approaches the concepts of health and disease from a different perspective than Western medicine, and its ideas and terminology often seem strange or unfamiliar to most Western physicians. In addition, Western medicine has become increasingly specialized, and it has not been clear where acupuncture, which approaches the treatment of the patient as a whole, should fit into this system of specialization. Thus, many physicians, while interested in the potential of applicability of acupuncture, are not sure how it could be included in their own medical practice, and few have access to formal training programs.

It is hoped that this situation will change as acupuncture is more thoroughly investigated in this country. Acupuncture research is now being conducted at many medical schools in the United States, and some have begun training programs in acupuncture for medical students and staff. Most physicians who have seriously investigated acupuncture agree that it is a safe and effective form of therapy, although there is still disagreement as to how it works.

It seems strange that acupuncture is less readily available in the United States, with its sophisticated health care system, than in most other countries of the world. We hope that new state laws will be enacted to license, regulate, and set standards for the practice of acupuncture. As medical schools become more actively involved in teaching acupuncture to medical students and physicians, patients will have greater access to well-trained acupuncture practitioners, and as more and more people are successfully treated by acupuncture, they may help provide the impetus to bring about these changes.

Notes

1. David E. Bresler and Patricia Wisen, *Acupuncture: A Selected Bibliography 1800-1972* (Los Angeles: National Acupuncture Association, 1973).
2. Arthur W. Galston, "Attitudes on Acupuncture," *Yale Review* 61 (1972): 312–17.
3. James Reston, "Now, About My Operation in Peking," in *New York Times Report from Red China* (New York: Avon, 1971).
4. E. Gray Dimond, "Acupuncture Anesthesia: Western Medicine and Chinese Traditional Medicine," *Journal of the American Medical Association* 218 (1971): 1558–63.
5. David E. Bresler, Richard J. Kroening, and Michael P. Volen, *Acupuncture for Control and Management of Pain* (Beverly Hills, Calif.: Center for Integral Medicine, 1971).

6. Charles Ledergerber, "Acupuncture and Electrotherapeutic Research," *International Journal of Acupuncture* 2 (1976): 105–18.
7. Richard J. Kroening and David E. Bresler, *Acupuncture for Facial and Dental Pain* (Beverly Hills, Calif.: Center for Integral Medicine, 1976).
8. Stanley Krippner and Daniel Rubin, *The Energies of Consciousness* (New York: Gordon & Breach, 1975).
9. Stephan Palos, *The Chinese Art of Healing* (New York: Herder and Herder, 1971.
10. Felix Mann, *The Treatment of Disease by Acupuncture* (London: Heinemann, 1963).
11. Felix Mann, *The Meridians of Acupuncture* (London: Heinemann, 1964).
12. Felix Mann, *Acupuncture: Cure of Many Diseases* (London: Heinemann, 1971).
13. Georges Beau, *Chinese Medicine* (New York: Avon, 1972).
14. A. T. W. Simeons, *Man's Presumptuous Brain* (New York: E. P. Dutton, 1962).
15. Stanley Krippner and Daniel Rubin, op. cit.
16. Peking Acupuncture Anaesthesia Co-Ordinating Group, "Preliminary Study on the Mechanism of Acupuncture Anaesthesia," *Scientia Sinica* 16, no. 3 (1973): 447–56.
17. David E. Bresler, Richard J. Kroening, and Michael P. Volen, op. cit.
18. David E. Bresler and Richard J. Kroening, "Three Essential Factors in Effective Acupuncture Therapy," *American Journal of Chinese Medicine* 4, no. 2 (1976): 81–86.

29
Ronald D. Grisell

Kundalini Yoga as Healing Agent

KUNDALINI YOGA, on a physical level, is primarily an integrated lifestyle for vitality, happy mentality, and longevity. From such a base, man can begin his ascent. There is a spiritual level, but that will not be discussed here. As practiced from day to day, this yoga is physical-psychological preventive medicine, but there exists an array of techniques to readjust imbalances and to help the mind-body heal *itself*. Space limitations prevent detailed description of more than a few specific techniques, but an attempt will be made to present a general framework in which to understand the workings of Yoga. The author takes no responsibility, however, for anyone who attempts any of the techniques mentioned briefly in this paper without thorough instruction from a qualified practitioner. Like the finest precision space vehicle, these powerful methods are designed to carry a precious passenger straight to the highest attainment; minor mistakes in application can be dangerous.

Basic Yogic Theory

Particularly emphasized in Kundalini Yoga are high states of consciousness and awareness, attained through a careful combination of three basic parts of Yoga: Laya Yoga (sound current and mantra), Karma Yoga (practice), and Gyan Yoga (philosophy). Yet no domain of existence is ignored, in line with the philosophy or theory of Yoga,

441

which will now be outlined in part. The ultimate objectives of perfection and union cannot be achieved unless all parts work in total harmony, including psychological and psychic as well as physiological mechanisms. ". . . you must have energy so that your dead computer may live and pass on the signal to you and may compute all that you want to do in this society. We call this energy, in the olden science, the Kundalini."[1] *Kundal* means the "curl of the hair of the beloved," an image that must have expressed profound romantic contentment to the ancients. The spiritual nerve, *kundalini*, is in 3½ coils like a snake, and can be awakened by the mixing of the two primal forces— *prana* (life force of the atom; positive) and *apana* (eliminating force; negative)—near the base of the spine. The kundalini then rises through the central nerve until it reaches the higher centers and activates man's psychic powers. This is imagery, and not intended to correspond directly with something physical. It is a model, useful in fixing the concentration. Physically, the pineal gland is thought to be caused to secrete something by the rising kundalini "heat." There may also be a pulsation or "radiation" at 3½ to 4 cycles per second, possibly of waves of neural excitation, which produces a superalert state, in addition to mustering vast latent mental capacities. It is believed that the pineal-pituitary glandular system can open transmental capabilities. Normally, the process is blocked; but with a balanced life and by means of an exquisitely timed combination of chanting, breathing, application of locks (isometric contraction of muscles and constriction of sphincters), mudras (roughly, postures, positions, applied pressures), exercises, and meditations, the kundalini can be raised. Laya Yoga is partly the process of reversing the gravitating tendency of the kundalini. In general, the kundalini approach to physical problems can be more rapid, in its effective synthesis, than any one type of Yoga.

Mantras and Sound

On the surface, Laya Yoga includes sound—the chanting of mantras, or the imagining of the sound on the breath. However, it is undeniable that the spoken word has powerful effects both externally, on others, and internally. Large areas of the brain are active in speech and hearing. Electrical repercussions appear to extend far into many other areas, including those for association and for sight.[2] Alerting excitations and the inhibitions working together with them pass up and down between cortex and an activating system (reticular activating system) deep in the base of the brain near the spinal cord, which extensively regulates both conscious and subconscious mental processes as well as modulating incoming and outgoing signals of the spinal cord and other large nerve trunks to the head. Therefore it is not surprising that massive psychophysiological reactions should result from the hearing or the pronouncing of a word. It might be expected also that rhythmic repetition of actual or imagined utterances would set up complex but more or less periodic waves of electrical and chemical activity in the brain, reducing extraneous thoughts and distractions as one possible result. Pavlov has shown long ago that a surprisingly wide variety of repetitive stimuli induce sleep. Especially effective, of course, are various verbal rituals (for example, counting sheep, monotonous lectures). Words spoken derogatorily in a group about one of its members, particularly about that person's greatest fears and insecurities, can have an amazing effect on adrenal and sweat glands, hair, body temperature, heart rate, and other organs or functions. On the positive side, it therefore stands to reason that specific patterns of brain waves can orchestrate grand symphonies of neurohumoral and glandular secretions, eliciting the finest emotions—as can a real symphony in an appreciative listener. More crudely, chanting *rah, rah,* . . . at a football game can excite both team and spectators to a feverish pitch. In an interesting corollary, chanting *ma, ma,* . . . was once demonstrated to the author and several other persons in his presence to have a reproducible weakening effect in the lifting strength of arms and legs without prior knowledge or suspicion that this would prove to be the case; whereas chanting *ra, ra,* . . . seemed to increase the chanter's lifting capacity. Careful experiments remain to be done. It so happens that a coordinated combination of the sounds *ra* (representing "sun energy" or positive, generating force) and *ma* (representing "moon energy" or negative, receptive force) comprises the Rama mantra, deceptively simple and difficult to chant properly.[3] In this mantra, *ra-a, ma-a* is chanted at approximately one repetition per four seconds. (Tempo as well as rhythm may well be important for respiratory reasons, as will be amplified below.)

Mantras, as a class, display an economy of phonemes—a surprisingly small number of certain "primal" sounds. *Ra* and *ma* recur in many. The sounds *sa* (infinite), *ta* (life), *na* (death), and *ma* (rebirth, light) are especially important and occur in combinations, e.g., *sat* (true infinite), *nam* (name, or manifested existence), *ram* (ancient, primal sound current), but *never out of sequence*. Mantras are chanted in what is called a complete *pranayam*, a rhythmic cycle of breath motions. Many mantras acutely force one to take a measured inspiration in order to complete the pranayma, which is elegantly designed to prevent inhalation during execution. Note that sounds accompanying the breath can involve emotional inspiration, as well.

The Fundamental Rhythm in Kundalini Yoga

In addition to rhythm, tempo, and sequence, the *number* of repetitions has significance perhaps beyond its obvious importance in any physical exercise set. The numbers 2, 4, 8, 16, 32, . . . had a profound permeation through ancient technology, and they had an extensive symbology associated with them that seems largely lost today. For example, there is a very fundamental rhythm in Kundalini Yoga called the *ashtang*: sixteen beats in two cycles of eight, four strokes up and four strokes down, alternating in each cycle. Another example is the ancient Sixteen Finger Breath, which is well illustrated by part of the Ungali pranayam:

inhale:
sa-sa-sa-sa-sa-sa-sa-sa-sa-sa-sa-sa-sa-sa-sa (fifteen separate or "broken" strokes);
exhale:
ta-ta-ta-ta-ta-ta-ta-ta-ta-ta-ta-ta-ta-ta-ta;
inhale:
na-na-na-na-na-na-na-na-na-na-na-na-na-na-na;
exhale:
ma-ma-ma-ma-ma-ma-ma-ma-ma-ma-ma-ma-ma-ma-ma.[4]

The four parts constitute the *panj shabad*, or *five* basic sounds—five, including *sa-ta-na-ma*, which means roughly "I am Truth,"—and *sixteen* fingers, including the whole parts in addition to their fifteen component strokes. Yet here is more than a wholistic number theory.

Ronald Grisell

It is not understood in entirety, but to catch a glimpse of some of the subtlety of ancient thought, consider the famous Fibonacci sequence 1, 1, 2, 3, 5, 8, 13, 22, ... Notice the property, possibly relating to biology, that differences between adjacent numbers reproduce the whole sequence. Similarly, sums of adjacent pairs reproduce. Among an astounding variety of additional properties, the Fibonacci sequence is related to the Greeks' Golden Section. A modern-day mystical mathematical society has been founded around this sequence, and it even publishes a journal (*Fibonacci Quarterly*); but it would be wrong to impute to this group the fanatic fervor of the ancient Pythagoreans. The sequence does occur in various phyllotactic structures, with more or less accuracy, throughout nature. The ancients utilized prime factors of these numbers, such as 11 ($2 \times 11 = 22$), which is the "number of infinity in the world of material," and 22, which is the "infinite number of longing and mastery." Now, the unifying observation is that, in analogy with the Fibonacci series, the accumulating sums (sum of the first n terms) are always 1 less than the next ($n + 1$ term); e.g., $1 + 2 + 4 + 8 = 15 = 16 - 1$. Thus, 16 is the sum of its factors plus itself as the whole. (A pairwise sum of adjacent terms is analogous to an accumulated sum in that the former is the truncation of the latter to the last two terms. Incidentally, there are interesting sequences "in between" the powers of 2 and the Fibonacci, where sums of the preceding three terms determine the next, or sums of four, etc.) The number 11 occurring in many kundalini exercises also arises as one of the accumulated sums of the Fibonacci sequence, excluding the first, redundant 1 which is there mainly to get things going. So does 32 (= 1 + 2 + 3 + 5 + 8 + 13). Mysticism in this case may precede (or follow!) understanding. One can perhaps understand the awe inspired in both ancient and modern numerologists considering many revelations of modern mathematics: e.g., that crystal structures, atoms, and fundamental particles can be classified according to a higher number theory (groups)—at least partially in the case of particles. Biology has yet to find a deeper order, but one of the inventors of the computer, Alan Turing, has suggested that symmetrically and periodically fluctuating chemical reactions may have much to do with complex living forms, cell division, and growth. It would be too much of a digression to mention the many more-recent and better-known developments in morphogenesis, nonequilibrium thermodynamics, etc.

Breath Control

The above aspects of Mantra Yoga are embedded as areas in a more encompassing science of breath control, *pranayama*. Wholistic symbology is ostensibly involved; but much more profoundly, periodicity of breath is thought in Yogic philosophy to influence strongly all other life rhythms, and thereby the regularity and organization so important to life. Physiologically, it is not so far-fetched that there may be a degree of coupling or entrainment between lungs, stomach, heart, intestines, etc. All these, by the way, are innervated parasympathetically through the vagus or X-th nerve, and modulated sympathetically through the reticular activating system (R.A.S.) mentioned earlier, as well as in regions between this and the spine (medulla and pons). There may also exist mechanical coupling simply due to rhythmic volume changes, but these remain speculative. Young, athletic people often show a heartbeat arrhythmia (literally "lack of rhythm") when breathing quietly and deeply at rest; their hearts slow down slightly near the end of each breath. Apparently this is normal. People are sometimes alarmed, if not frightened into seeing a doctor, when their hearts miss a beat. This also happens primarily during periods of deep rest, particularly in bed while dropping off to sleep or waking up. The possibility is suggested that the regulated breathing in many types of Yoga might have specific therapeutic effects on abnormal heart arrhythmias, spastic colon, or other disorders in line with its general relaxing and vitalizing effect on these organs. In Raja Yoga, for example, breath is frequently used to massage and to "pump." There is an interesting possibility that deep breaths may have a pumping action on the spinal cord and on the dural sac containing it and the cerebrospinal fluid. Moreover, there is evidence that the fascinating cerebrospinal fluid pump is due to a coupling with blood pulsation in the abdomen.[5] On the whole, it is noteworthy that such an important area as biological rhythmicity (physiological and circadian) is virtually uncharted by modern science.

Before leaving the subject of mantras, it should be emphasized that breath control is merely the base of a pyramid. To indicate the upward progression of this pyramid, the "Mahan jap" or "linked jap" will be mentioned, particularly as it may be of interest in psychiatry and counseling.[6] After careful meditative preparation, perfect concentration is achieved by each member in a group. Then, the panj shabad, *sa-ta-na-ma*, is started by one person at random and taken up immediately by another as the first person ends; thereafter, it is taken up one person at a time around the group, but in no predetermined order—something like a Quaker prayer session. It is believed that there is some kind of "group energy" that shifts from person to person, not necessarily guided by individual will or desire. A sublime sensitivity may develop in proportion to the number of participants plus twice that number squared. Thus the number of awarenesses that must be taken into account in a jap with ten people is 410—about four hundred times the sensitivity of a single person; one hundred persons have a combined sensitivity about a hundred times the sensitivity of ten. Again, the whole must be counted with the parts. In ways similar, a married couple can improve their ability to listen to one another; to be silent and act as a unit. As Yogi Bhajan puts it, "after arguing and yelling at each other until they can yell no more," it is well, to prevent this negativity from affecting other areas of their relationship, to sit down opposite each other and alternatingly exhale a forceful and high-pitched *wha guru*! (For more details, such as stimulation of the "life nerve" by pressing thumbs together, see S.S.S.H. Singh's article on meditation.[7]) In other group chants, just as individuals contribute to the current of sound, so could a group consciousness acting as a unit. If this group concept is expanded to include the entire universe in the large and in the small (there is thought to be life force even in the most elementary of particles) then some grasp is gained of the so-called sound current.

"Breath is life" perhaps in the sense that oxygen and nitrogen molecules have some interactive, organizing influence, but this almost alchemical topic of Yoga will not be discussed, as not much is known about prana, scientifically. The end result of breathing, oxidation, is evidently necessary for what are normally termed "living" organisms; the earth itself or a gigantic, learning computer hooked up to motors and sensors being excluded, for example; but some form of electron exchange appears to be necessary in anaerobic organisms, such as some bacteria, and it is doubtful that even the viruses that are parasites on these bacteria can get by without some form of oxidation-reduction. In humans, the process of respiration involves infusion of oxygen into the hemoglobin of the blood via the lungs, then circulation to the capillaries, diffusion or transport of oxygen into the cells, and finally an awe-inspiring factory of chemical reactions. Unlike many respiratory therapists, the Yogis seem to have taken all of these stages into account in their integrative approach. Each stage of respiration is regulated in a ladder of reflexlike networks of nerve cells extending to and up the spine in ever more complicated loops or rungs far up into the brain; every loop controls and modulates lower rungs and in turn is regulated by higher; the highest are concerned with volitional control. Contraction of the diaphragm muscles and expansion of the chest will continue weakly and erratically if only the lowest of the brain loops is intact (in the medulla). A higher region (in the lower pons) imparts rhythmicity but itself alone produces a peculiar gasplike breathing unless moderated by a still higher region (in the upper pons) just below the R.A.S. The proximity of the latter two systems may have something to do with the close relationship between the alpha-rhythm of relaxed and meditative states on the one hand, and slow, deep breathing on the other. It is a property of loop systems that a disturbance or a rhythm in one tends to cause a similar effect in the others, usually in a reversible manner.[8] With these considerations, the complicated causes and effects to be described may be more understandable.

Combined Exercise Meditations

Breath rhythm is the key to many Kundalini Yoga *kriyas* (combined mental-mantra-breath-lock-exercise-meditations). One kriya to balance the aura (nearly visible emissions including possibly gases, light, ions, and electrons) and to generally strengthen the nervous system entails a twenty-two-count breath: inhale in four equal parts to the mantra *sa-ta-na-ma*; hold for sixteen counts, and exhale in two counts with a silent *wahe guru* (expresses ecstasy in enlightenment). In many kriyas, the breath should be as even and periodic as possible. It is interesting in this regard that the R.A.S., which is largely responsible for synchronization and coordination of the brain, is affected by incoming sensory signals from the ears and from the massive system of sense receptors in and around the lungs and chest cavity.[9]

Together with the stretching motion and sounds, mental concentration on the breath is important in achieving desirable effects. This, among other factors, is illustrated by part of the antidepression and brain synchrony meditation:

Sit in easy pose (lotus, or cross-legged position) with an erect spine. The hands are in gyan mudra (pinching-like hand position) with first finger on top of the thumb. Raise the upper arms parallel to the ground and bring the mudras in front of the eyes so the thumbs and forefingers touch. Open the eyes wide and stare beyond the hands to the horizon. Then inhale deep and separate the hands 36 to 45 inches (to the side, so the elbows are about at right angle, 90°) while keeping the eyes fixed. Then inhale back to the original position. The elbows will move a little, but keep them relaxed. Start with a slow movement, one cycle of the breath taking about 4 seconds. As the hands go outward, mentally vibrate "SA." As they return, vibrate "TA." Then for the second repetition "NA" on the inhale, and "MA" on the exhale. Meditate on the life energy of the breath. The mental feeling of stretching the breath from a single point (between the eyes) to the width of the arm spread is essential.[10]

Many essential directions have been left out here due to space restrictions. Others will be mentioned later in relation to therapy for marijuana usage. A careful practice of this meditation can alleviate confusion, scatteredness, lack of motivation, and feelings of alienation due to separation and discord between the hemispheres. Perhaps the bilaterally symmetric movement of the arms is coupled with the (also bilateral) movement of the lungs for an augmented effect. As to how this and other kriyas for balance and coordination of mind might work, EEG studies have indicated that they result in much lower bilateral interhemispheric correlations at rest and higher correlations when alert than in certain types of mental disturbance, such as schizophrenia and obsessive neurosis.[11]

In the second part of another kriya, the right index finger is alternately pressed against the right and left nostrils so as to close them in synchrony with (1) inhalation through the left, (2) holding forty-five seconds, (3) exhalation in four equal parts through the right nostril. After a few minutes, a change is made to eight equal parts. This follows a first part of the kriya which prepares one by ridding of self-doubt and by balancing energies that lead to increased radiance and personal beauty. While in lotus position with a straight spine, the second part continues by focusing the attention at a point between the brows. This directs the mind to adjust its waves to relate to the world.[12] Such are seemingly very complicated effects brought about by relatively simple means: since the sensory nerves to each nostril are paired with opposite hemispheres, the old Yogic theory that sun energy (dominant) and moon energy (submissive, receptive, magnifying) can be balanced by the breath would seem to apply. However, with our present lack of understanding of the role hemispheric interaction plays in consciousness, it may be a bit premature to posit. All that can be said is, these techniques work, somehow. Incidentally, preliminary results indicate that there is a reverse effect: nostrils appear to alternately open and close with an average but highly variable period of about ninety minutes (unpublished studies of several laboratories, including our own and the Kundalini Research Institute), under quiet conditions in individuals free of congestion, colds or other respiratory problems.

In other areas, such as improved concentration or distraction from pain, supportive evidence for the efficacy of breath techniques can be found. For example, the Lamaze-Pavlov method for painless childbirth has gained much popularity, if this is evidence of success. Hypnosis can make effective use of breath in relaxation. In most instances, however, it is difficult to judge just how much is due to will power and how much due to subconscious effects of breathing. Hypnosis could be nothing more than a skill at self-manipulation of mental states, in which external cues from the hypnotist and internal behavior are merely symbolic, or patterns of pretense.

"Breath of fire" might conjure images of fakirs and fakers, but there is no connection. This breath is strong but shallow and rapid (two or three per second), with no pause. Exhalation consists of pulling the navel forcefully inward; chest muscles remain as relaxed as possible. Inhalation occurs naturally by the slight volume expansion of the abdominal muscles. It is normally done in a cross-legged sitting position, with a certain positioning of hands, teeth, and tongue, as described in M. S. S. G. S. Fowlis's article on Breath of Fire.[13] Effects were found to be:

1. Cleansing of the blood, for blood related disorders
2. Higher voltages generated by the nerve cells
3. Increased global alpha rhythm
4. Mental constancy, i.e., concentration, will power
5. Extra endurance
6. Expansion of lung capacity
7. Ability to hold the breath (in swimming, diving, etc.)
8. Increased peripheral circulation

9. Detoxification (removal of toxins and deposits from drugs, smoking, and bad nutrition from the lungs, mucous lining of airways).

Some understanding of the physiology of this important exercise has been gained through a study of heart rate, blood pressure (systolic and diastolic, and time of recovery), and tidal volume.[14] (*Systolic* is, roughly, maximum pressure; *diastolic*, minimum; time of recovery refers to return to normal or base rate; tidal volume is volume of air inspired with normal breath—about ½ liter in the young adult male.) It was found that systolic pressure increased about as much as in moderate running in place. Time of recovery was much less for breath of fire than for this moderate exercise. Tidal volume increased after eight minutes with breath of fire as much as the maximum increase with heavy running in place. Heart rate increased very little with breath of fire. Consistent with this, but contrary to what one might expect, no relations were found between breath of fire and hyperventilation.[15] The exercise can be done for twenty minutes or more.

Complementary to the dynamics of breath are several static factors in kundalini kriyas: position of hands and fingers, pressures on fingertips, orientation and focal length of eyes, concentration of mind, isometric contraction of certain muscles and constriction of sphincters, and a whole kinesiology of posture. "The whole body has been made to adjust to all the complications of postures and positions that can activate the brain's thoughts, extension, and performance, so that man can experience what he wants to know, and that is the unknown of himself."[16] Space prevents mention of all but a few glandular effects of these static factors.

There is no gland or organ that some kriya does not stimulate, and this is the aim of a complete regimen. Proper combinations of posture; pressure on fingertips, palms, and heels (stimulating nerves and meridians); muscular contraction; and flexions of the spine can drain lymph glands from groin and thigh areas. Thyroid and parathyroid are stimulated by letting the head fall back, rolling it from side to side at prescribed intervals, on occasion with a mantra. The pineal is stimulated, rather oddly, by directing and focusing the eyes on the midpoint between the eyebrows; but also by the most basic techniques of "raising the kundalini" mentioned earlier. The pituitary gland, together with the pineal, is central to many kriyas concerned with higher consciousness, and interestingly, the old Yogic theory of a two-way connection between the pineal-pituitary complex and the sex organs is being borne out by recent studies of certain hormones and enzymes (e.g. estradiol, testosterone[17]). Hence, the health of the sex organs may be improved by unlikely meditations—such as that described by S. S. S. H. Singh in *Creative Happiness*,[18] in which wrists are twisted approximately at right angles with a precise and complicated grasp between the hands, thumbs pressed together; eyes are closed and focused at the brow point; and several other conditions are concurrently met. One result of the more physically rigorous exercises is to release toxins from bad diet. Moving the waist from side to side will stimulate, and certain muscular contractions will rejuvenate, the liver. In a kind of synergy, the state of the sex organs is thought in Yogic science to have a reverse effect on the state and quality of consciousness: a substance called *ojas* is believed to be released into the bloodstream, as a kind of "distillate," possibly related to the sex hormones. Ojas is considered to be the product of a many-stage refinement process, beginning with food and air. As the last stage, it is a very precious and a very potent substance which "lubricates" nerves and stimulates the pineal and pituitary glands. In concluding this list, which is far short of completeness, the importance of sexual organs, hormones, and enzymes should be taken into account in the maintenance of mental and physical health, if not in actually repairing dysfunction. In addition, the brain-gland relationships should not be disregarded.

In Kundalini Yoga theory, concentration on an organ with an image or visualization of that organ in a state of health will improve or correct a malfunction. A partially consistent Russian view on this is well expressed by Asratyan and Simonov.[19] Perhaps this can explain the power of variously directed concentration, mentioned above, in many of the kriyas. In Western physiology, the power of the brain in regard to physical therapy appears to be largely overlooked—or belittled at best. One exception is the excellent discussion of cortex and sexual energy and several other topics of a more wholistic, integrated neurology-physiology, to be found in Peat's *Mind and Tissue*.[20]

Kundalini Approaches to Therapy

In summary, the general principles of kundalini approaches to therapy are as follows:

1. Cleansing of bowels, lungs, blood, lymph, etc. by eliminative kriyas, fasting, and washing of nasal passages (neti), thereby cutting off supply routes to invasive diseases
2. Improving nerve and muscle strength by breathing exercises, limbering flexions, and appropriate pressures
3. Maintaining proper function of endocrine glands by means of mudras
4. Keeping the body *flexible*, *active* and *balanced* by postures
5. Balanced, vegetarian diet (to be discussed below)
6. Avoidance of excessive *direct* sunlight on large areas of skin (indirect is necessary)
7. Hair should be clean and covered to prevent static and accumulation of dust and to retain oils (special combs of wood are recommended)
8. Maintenance of constancy and equilibrium by kriyas, diet, proper clothes, and colors (white is recommended, both for temperature regulation and for psychic health)
9. Generally, rules of physical and biological system science are followed:
   a. In therapy, perturb the mind and body only so far as to correct (see f below)
   b. Take cycles and rhythms of the body system into account
   c. Allow treatments to thoroughly permeate and come to completion
   d. Take the law of karma, or conservation of energy, into account
   e. Allow for the fact that momentum is also conserved: do not try to correct a condition or dysfunction too quickly
   f. For every action, there is an equal and opposite reaction—this holds for complex people as well as in simple physics

Nutritional Considerations

Important to a final discussion of some specific therapeutic applications are certain dietary principles of Kundalini Yoga, with which the generalities will now be concluded. The reader is referred to Hawkins's article on Food and Health for a much more comprehensive treatment. In general, humans are omnivorous—not wholly noncarnivorous. Concerning meat versus vegetables and fruit:

An ideal diet yields maximum energy from a small input and produces little waste. Of the three major foodstuffs, carbohydrates alone most closely meet these criteria. . . . Yet, despite "house-cleaning" problems, a balance of all three major foodstuffs is essential. . . . Our bodies too need prefabricated building blocks rather than individual atoms of carbon, oxygen or nitrogen. . . . Before being absorbed, they [fats and proteins] are enzymatically cleaved into their respective subunits. . . . Although the percentage distribution of their subunits varies from substance to substance, they are common to all foods—plant and animal alike. This means that the more complex fat and protein moieties in meat and eggs offer no nutritional advantage over their counterparts in dairy and vegetable products.[21]

Yogis recommend only about a third to a fourth the daily protein that Western nutrition experts do, but Yogi-recommended protein (milk, yogurt, nuts and certain legumes) is of higher biologic value. The residues of metabolism of these forms of proteins are more efficiently and reliably eliminated by the liver, kidney, and digestive system. Additionally, meat is also frequently contaminated by hormones and toxins administered to or resulting from the processes of breeding, fattening, and slaughtering.

Another main principle of diet is the maintenance of proper blood pH (a measure of acidity or alkalinity, optimally at 7.40). Meat, fish, and eggs produce acidic blood, and provide a burst of energy—as practiced by some athletes who eat steak before contests—but the energizing effect is short lasting and inefficient, and may also create stress and tension as an aftermath. On the other hand, some blood acidifying foods are necessary, but the blood pH can be adjusted properly by eating a diet consisting of about two-thirds alkaline-producing foods, such as sweet and sour fruit, green vegetables, pulses, legumes and even lemons (which one may imagine as being acidic in effect as well as taste). Yogic therapy teaches that slightly alkaline blood is the purest form, and essential for good health and a calm demeanor.

A third principle is that "concentrated" foods are to be minimized, in that they overly tax the digestive system, disrupt the balance of other organs, and increase blood acidity. For example, in addition to being highly concentrated, sugar has definite correlations with various heart and circulatory conditions and possibly with breast cancer.[22,23] "Concentrated" does not necessarily mean dehydrated or low-fiber foods, but refers more to the perturbing effect on the digestive system. Fats like butter, oil, and margarine are approximately neutral as far as blood pH is concerned, but they are difficult to digest and may cause excessive acidity in the upper gastrointestinal tract.

A related consideration is the rawness of foods. Fresh green vegetables and fruits, for example, retain maximum content of vitamins and minerals, but they must be balanced with cooked foods, which lubricate—i.e., prevent too much roughage from clogging the digestive tract at narrowed points and valves. Of course, cooking degrades starches so that they can be more readily digested, as well as warming them and thereby accelerating the process of absorption, but it also tends to extract the oily vitamins. The Yogis have developed cooking methods that make food more assimilable and provide richly saturated oil bases to lubricate and energize the body. Incidentally, it is not at all clear that the maximizing of polyunsaturated fats, as often recently recommended by various Western dietary authorities, is beneficial or even safe. A great portion of the body, including cell membranes, is composed of saturated fatty acid side groups in lipids, and according to the first principle here, our bodies would most efficiently utilize nutrients that are structurally similar to human tissue.

Yogic diet may be considered by some to be "faddist," but when one considers the incredible, and often contradictory, proclamations of such authorities as the Food and Drug Administration and the American Medical Association, some caution is perhaps justified. As a case in point, the National Academy of Sciences recommends a thirty per cent excess over their already admittedly "generous" daily allowance of protein to allow for incomplete absorption. In India, such overloading is thought to contribute to a special form of autointoxication. Whether this is in fact true or not, unnecessary taxation and inefficiency go against kundalini dietary principles—and against common sense.

Therapeutic Application

Using and illustrating the above principles, the remainder of this chapter will be devoted to particular therapeutic applications—which, however, are not necessarily the most exemplary applications of Kundalini Yoga, nor are they intended to supplant psychiatric or medical methods, particularly in regard to proper diagnosis, emergency or surgical procedures, or other forms of treatment.

Drug Rehabilitation

As one application of Yogic diet, long-time or heavy users of marijuana can benefit especially from the antidepression and brain synchrony meditation mentioned above, combined with appropriate beet and banana fasts.[24] More important than any specific physical therapy, in some cases, is the loving guidance and inspiration by another person; such attention can be critical in this and other types of drug damage, where alienation from parents and society is often a factor. Medical and physical techniques can have only a limited effect by themselves on certain severe types of depression, for example. Again, the Yoga is not intended to replace other professional treatment. The range and scope of what nonprofessionals might do to assist doctors and psychiatrists and to help relieve overload on clinics and other community resources, in the framework of Kundalini Yoga, has been well outlined recently.[25]

Migraine and Other Severe Headaches

Yoga may be used to ameliorate a variety of tension- or pressure-related nonmigrainous head pain. Many of the commonly practiced kriyas to release eye and muscle tension involve slowly rolling the head and bending it far forward, chin into chest.[26] Headache caused by muscle spasms in the scalp above the eyes can be relieved by a kriya which, among other aspects, involves pressing the base of the palm against the bridge of the nose (supratrochlear and supraorbital nerves). Alternatively, pressure on the infraorbital nerves just under the protrusion of the cheek bone relieves spasms in lower muscles near the eyes and nose. Important and concurrent reductions of tension in other areas (back, abdomen, shoulders, and intestine) is achieved in a continuing series of exercises focusing the mind, increasing circulation to the face and head, improving balance, and working on the sexual force.[27] Simple headache can be due to constipation. Circulation and eliminative kriyas are effective in removing toxins and in readjusting blood flow.[28]

Neck bending to relieve migraines is illustrated by the following general procedure for the prodromal stage (nausea, loss of vision or appearance of spreading, jagged patterns in the visual field, weakness, drowsiness, depression, salivation), found effective in several cases by the author. Lie down comfortably with a thick, soft pillow under the back of the head so as to bend the neck as far forward as bearable. (It is not yet clear precisely what the bending does physiologically, but it could be affecting the cerebrospinal fluid pressure.) The room should be absolutely dark (as anyone experiencing this kind of migraine will testify!). In addition, various mantras may be chanted or mentally vibrated; they have an arousing effect on the sympathetic nervous system. Sympathomimetic chemicals (such as desert tea or ephedra) might have an antimigraine effect, but this has not yet been thoroughly tested.[29] Nothing, so far, requires any particular Yogic skill, but in a second stage, symptomatic relief can be had in a significant percentage of cases by means of Yogic techniques for increase of temperature in the extremities or in one extremity (brain temperature goes down, by a kind of negative feedback). This has been well proven also in recent years by workers in the field of biofeedback.[30] However, a third phase of psychotherapy to find and eliminate any deep-seated stresses may well prove more permanently beneficial by curing the causes.[31] Here, Kundalini Yoga offers a variety of self-aids: brain balancing and thought-eliminative kriyas (e.g., two described by S. S. S. H. Singh that work on the "conflict personality area"[32,33]). Finally, hypertensive headaches are treated in the long term by diet and by kriyas designed to decrease blood pressure. More will be said on diet below, where the cause of headache is discussed.

Hypertension and Arteriosclerotic, Ischemic and Degenerative Heart Disease

Evidence exists both for and against practically every theory as to the cause of essential hypertension, which, together with other heart and circulatory conditions related to it in complex ways, is the *number one killer of Americans* and many other peoples. It is possible that there are many types of hypertension. Neurogenic and endocrine aspects are under investigation at this laboratory, and evidence continues to accumulate that essential hypertension may have frequent elements of dysfunction of neural control, among other possibly concurrent causes (kidney disease; hormonal abnormalities; psychogenic factors such as continual emotional disturbance; obscure metabolic disorders; ischemic lesions of the brain and other tissues, particularly kidney; eliminative dysfunction for blood-pressure-regulating agents). Sensors in major arteries (carotid sinus, aortic arch) send signals to the brain (medulla), which then controls arteriolar constriction, cardiac output, and other parameters of the cardiovascular system and may modulate a wide range of glandular systems. It is unfortunate in this regard that long-term studies of the effects of kriyas on efficiency and precision of neural control, circulation (which is under extensive and complex regulation by the central nervous system), and as yet ill-defined factors of balance of the nervous system (stability, equilibrium or "set" points, homeostasis) have not been made scientifically by the medical profession. Undue skepticism and lack of funds for support of this kind of research are certainly major impediments.

There could well be a dietary factor: arteriosclerotic and degenerative heart disease in general appears to be more directly correlated with high sugar in the diet than with dietary cholesterol (or even with serum triglyceride levels, which include cholesterol produced endogenously by the liver). (Ahrens presents a good review of this complicated situation.[34]) Another so-called concentrated food, salt, tends to keep arterial pressure high, and a reduction of this element in the diet can often successfully treat essential hypertension. Moreover, there is much individual variation in reaction to sugar, which tends to implicate heredity as an important factor; however, exercise seems to counteract a potential diabetogenic effect of sucrose.[35] Kundalini Yoga is not alone, of course, in espousing daily morning exercise, but it is almost unique in the amount and type: two to three hours of special exercises in the very early morning and again in the early evening, or at other times of the day. Incidentally, in several studies on senescent conditions, particularly atherosclerosis, it has been found that elderly people can adapt to moderate exercise, even if they have not been getting sufficient exercise for some time.

In closing this section, one of the related and major diseases of old age, atherosclerosis will be discussed, particularly as one of the culminations, apparently, of a lifetime of imbalance of some kind—the avoidance of which is much emphasized by most Yogas. Lipid deposits called *atheromatous plaques*, containing a large amount of cholesterol, form in the subintimal layer of large arteries. In later stages, fibroblasts interpenetrate the plaque-degenerated areas, causing progressive *sclerosis*. Arteriosclerosis occurs when calcium precipitates in the lipids to form calcified plaques, hardening the arteries. In spite of the furor about dietary cholesterol, it is far from clear that this is even a minor cause, as discussed briefly above. As the Yogis have claimed, however, the cause may very well be dietary in the main, with elements of lack of exercise. Although not much is known definitely about its cause, recent developments in dietary therapy are not receiving the attention they deserve. It has been found that vitamin E promotes oxidation in many ways and opposes many effects of excess estrogen, such as the development of "age pigment."[36] Vitamin E can protect the liver against damage by toxins, one of the points considered most important in Kundalini Yoga. Yet, it inhibits destructive oxidation as involved in aging and cancer and possibly in the damage of membranes in such critical areas as heart and capillaries. It accelerates clot removal and inhibits clot formation in blood vessels, but E also promotes normal clotting in wounds. Taken together with vitamin C, in megadosage, it appears to remove many of the causes of high blood pressure. Other vitamins that can improve circulation by opening small vessels are folic acid and niacin. Perhaps one reason why vitamin E has not been considered highly by the medical profession is that, as a colleague expressed it, "It doesn't work like a drug—a big dose doesn't immediately force the blood pressure down. Sometimes, in fact, the first effect is to strengthen a damaged heart, raising the blood pressure for a few days."[37]

In view of the exciting possibilities of vitamin E, it is not irrelevant in this regard that a major portion of the kundalini diet involves vegetable oils, fresh greens, and many other vegetables rich in this fat-soluble vitamin, and also that Yogis do tend to live a long, and full, life.

Notes

1. Stated by Siri Singh Sahib Harbhajan Singh Khalsa Yogiji during lecture series on Kundalini Yoga—the Yoga of awareness, University of California at Los Angeles, Extension Division, 1972.

2. V. S. Rusinov, ed., *Electrophysiology of the Central Nervous System* (New York: Plenum, 1970).

3. S. S. S. H. Singh, "Meditation on Rama," *Journal of Science and Consciousness*, 10 (1975): 49 (Kundalini Research Institute, 8191 Monte Vista, Claremont, CA).

4. S. S. S. H. Singh, "Ungali Pranayam," *Journal of Science and Consciousness* 10 (1975): 5.

5. G. Du Boulay et al., "Further Investigations on Pulsatile Movements in

the Cerebrospinal Fluid Pathways," *Acta Radiologica Diagnosis* 13 (1972): 496–522.

6. S. S. S. H. Singh, "Mahan or Linked Jap," *Journal of Science and Consciousness* 10 (1975): 48.

7. S. S. S. H. Singh, "Meditation," *Journal of Science and Consciousness* 6 (1974): 20.

8. R. Grisell, *Methods of Modelling Neural Networks*, vol. 1 (Pomona, Calif.: Multidisciplinary Publications, 1976): 138–40.

9. G. Moruzzi, "Synchronizing Influences of the Brain Stem and the Inhibitory Mechanisms Underlying the Production of Sleep by Sensory Stimulation," in *The Moscow Colloquium, Electroencephalography of Higher Nervous Activity*, ed. H. H. Jasper and G. D. Smirnov, Supplement no. 13, The International Journal of Electroencephalography and Clinical Neurophysiology (Montreal: The EEG Journal, 1960): 231–56.

10. S. S. S. H. Singh, "Anti-depression and Brain Synchrony Meditation," *Journal of Science and Consciousness* 10 (1975): 54.

11. A. S. Aslanov, "Correlation between Cortical Potentials in Patients with Obsessive Neuroses." Also: O. M. Grindel, and V. S. Rusinov, "Correlation Analysis in Central EEG Rhythms of the Healthy Human Cortex." Both in *Electrophysiology of the Central Nervous System* (New York: Plenum, 1970).

12. S. S. S. H. Singh, "Two Pranayams To Balance Mental Energy," *Journal of Science and Consciousness* 10 (1975): 55.

13. M. S. S. G. S. Fowlis, "Breath of Fire," *Journal of Science and Consciousness* 10 (1975): 24–26.

14. J. N. S. Glassman, P. Shotler, and M. Daniels, unpublished study, June, 1975. (Documented in the research records of the Kundalini Research Institute, Claremont, Calif.)

15. M. S. S. G. S. Fowlis, unpublished study, July, 1974. (Documented in the research records of the Kundalini Research Institute, Claremont, Calif.)

16. Stated by Siri Singh Sahib Harbhajan Singh Khalsa Yogiji during lecture series on Kundalini Yoga—the Yoga of Awareness, University of California at Los Angeles, Extension Division, 1972.

17. C. H. Sawyer, "Activation and Blockade of the Release of Pituitary Gonadotropin as Influenced by the Reticular Formation of the Brain," in *Reticular Formation of the Brain*, edited by H. H. Jasper; L. D. Proctor; R. S. Knighton; W. C. Noshay; and R. T. Costello (Boston: Little, Brown, 1958). E. Steinberger and M. Chowdhury, "Control of Pituitary EHS in Male Rats," *Acta Endocrinologia* 76 (1975): 235–41. E. Steinberger, "Hormonal Control of Mammalian Spermatogenesis," *Physiological Review* 51 (1976): 9–45.

18. S. S. S. H. Singh, " 'Creative Happiness' Public Talk at Unitarian Church," *Journal of Science and Consciousness* 6 (1974): 10–13.

19. E. Asratyan and R. Simonov, *How Reliable Is the Brain?* trans. B. Belitsky (Moscow: Peace Publishers, n.d.).

20. R. Peat, *Mind and Tissue: Russian Research Perspectives on the Human Brain* (Pomona, Calif: Multidisciplinary Publications [575 N. Hamilton St., 91768], 1976).

21. J. W. S. Hawkins, "Food and Health, Part 1," *Journal of Science and Consciousness* 6 (1974): 8–14.

22. R. S. Ahrens, "Sucrose, Hypertension and Heart Disease: An Historical Perspective," *The American Journal of Clinical Nutrition* 27 (1974): 403–22.

23. G. Hems and A. Stuart, "Breast Cancer Rates in Populations of Single Women," *British Journal of Cancer* 31 (1975): 118–23.

24. S. S. S. H. Singh, "Anti-depression and Brain Synchrony Meditation."

25. M. S. S. G. S. Fowlis, "Help for the Drug Damaged Drop-ins," unpublished paper available from Kundalini Research Institute Publications, Pomona, Calif.

26. S. S. S. H. Singh, "Exercises for Tension and Periodic Headache," *Journal of Science and Consciousness* 7 (1974): 30–31.

27. S. S. S. H. Singh, "The Navel Center and Elimination," *Journal of Science and Consciousness* 10 (1975): 5–22.

28. S. S. S. H. Singh, "Elimination and Circulation Kriya," *Journal of Science and Consciousness* 7 (1974): 15–17.

29. R. Peat, personal communication, April, 1976.

30. Y-J. La Vallée and Y. Lamontagne, "Les Applications Thérapeutiques de la Rétroaction Biologique," *L'Union Médicale du Canada* 103 (1974): 264–71.

31. C. N. Legalos, "Biofeedback and Psychotherapy," in *Biofeedback: Behavioral Medicine*, ed. L. Birk (New York: Grune and Stratton, 1973).

32. S. S. S. H. Singh, "Beggar's Meditation," *Journal of Science and Consciousness* 10 (1975): 28.

33. S. S. S. H. Singh, "Eliminating Thoughts You Dislike," *Journal of Science and Consciousness* 10 (1975): 29.

34. R. S. Ahrens, loc. cit.

35. L. H. Opie, "Dietary Sucrose in Relation to the Development of Ischemic Heart Disease," *The American Heart Journal* 89 (1975): 674–75.

36. R. Peat, *Nutrition for Women* (Eugene, Ore.: Blake College, 1975).

37. Ibid.

30

H. Leonard Jones

The Tibetan Art
of Healing

Health is related to *life*—how we are created, grow, live, and die. It is how we are and how we feel, as well as how we relate to those around us.... It is related to the environment within which we live in all its forms.... As with many living organisms, the whole can be healthy while a piece is sick or dying, and yet we know the sick piece cannot but affect the whole. The converse is not true, for if the whole is sick and dying all the parts die also.... The ancients knew this well, for the shaman faced with illness dealt both with the ill person and with the community. As the shaman removed the ill part, the whole community was engaged in coming together, joining their energies in a variety of activities which regenerated the whole at the same time as dealing with the part. [1]

SHAMANISM—the belief in an unseen world of gods, demons, and ancestral spirits, responsive only to the shaman's trance and magic—applies primarily to the religious systems and phenomena of the north Asian, Ural-Altaic people. [2] It has its counterpart in Tibet in the pre-Buddhist religion of Bon. This was dominated by concerns of healing (either in the physiologic sense of curing disease or in the extended sense of overcoming transgression) and with restoring the world to its presumptive proper state. Bon would thus be defined as a healing cult, and it is presumed to remain in small and remote areas of the country today.

Buddhism was introduced into Tibet from India in the seventh century A.D. It has had a profound influence on the people and their way of life ever since. About half the males have been monks. The fourteen successive Dalai Lamas have been both the spiritual and political leaders. The laity has been devout. Religious mantras— Sanskrit invocations to a deity—prayer wheels and flags, stone heaps and monuments to saints, many of whom were great physicians, have abounded everywhere.

The Northern or Mahayana School of Buddhism—with its ritualistic aspect, the Tantra; the great stress on compassion; and the use of prayers while giving or taking medicine—is espoused by Tibet. This contrasts with the Hinayana Buddhism in India, where the practice of medicine by members of the Order of Monks is discouraged. Thus the history of medicine in Tibet is closely intertwined with its history of Buddhism.

The most recent (1973) and major reference on Tibetan medicine is an English translation by Rechung Rimpoche Jampal Kunzang.[3] It includes thirty-one chapters from the second book of the most important treatise, the *rGyud-Bzhi*, and two chapters from the fourth book thereof. The latter are entitled "Examination of the Pulse and Veins" and "Examination of the Urine." The second book includes chapters on embryology, anatomy, physiology, indications of approaching death, causes of disease, symptoms, classification of diseases, everyday conduct, conduct during the seasons, food and drink, dietary rules, taste and digestive qualities of medicines, action of medicines, pharmacology, surgical instruments, health rules, diagnosis of diseases, general rules for treating diseases, humoral pathology, and required qualities and duties of a doctor and nurse. There is also a biography of the great physician-saint gYu-Thog, anatomical and other plates, as well as a bibliography of European works on Tibetan medicine.

Rechung's *Tibetan Medicine* is the first really comprehensive work on the subject to appear in English. Like most, if not all, translations from Tibetan medical writings, it encountered enormous difficulties, too numerous and complex to amplify here. Not the least of these is the difficult language itself, which was created about eleven hundred years ago from an ancient Indian syllabic. Incidentally, the quantity of medical literature translated into Tibetan is much greater than the number of medical volumes and manuscripts written in the land itself over the years.[4] The literature embodies many ancient Indian medical works as well as traditional Chinese ones. Here it must be noted that Lamaist medicine, owing to its overemphasis on the "demon-conditioned" aspect of certain diseases such as infection, has fallen far behind Chinese medicine in this particular field.[5] The integration of traditional Chinese medical tenets into their own philosophy of healing could not always have been easy for Lamaist doctors. The Chinese concepts of the yin and yang polarity and all its ramifications, their "occult anatomy" and pathology—to name just three examples—differed considerably from the comparable Tibetan ones.[6,7]

It seems appropriate here to comment that it takes a long and arduous time to become a Tibetan doctor. Usually thirteen years of foundation studies are required before years of theoretical and practical bedside training and many examinations. It has been necessary for the genuine healer to take precautions against unscrupulous moneymakers. The cardinal rule of occult science is ever stressed: "When you attempt to take one step towards knowing hidden truths, you have to take three steps simultaneously towards knowing your own weaknesses and towards the perfection of your character!"[8] Moreover, the elite physician generally requested no fee, although it was customary for the patient to pay according to his means and then in the form of natural produce and presents. In sum, then, it appears that Tibet is the only country in the world whose art of healing has remained essentially unchanged for centuries—at least until comparatively recently.[9] In spite of this—or perhaps because of it—Tibetan medicine is highly respected throughout central Asia, for it has a remarkable record of success in healing.[10]

Against this very brief background, the scope of the remaining discussion must be limited to the most pertinent and selected aspects of the Tibetan art of healing: the causes and mechanisms of diseases; symptoms, signs and diagnosis; modes of treatment; and the most dominant concepts and practice of that healing which can be reasonably adopted now (and later after more research) by those engaged in the assessment and therapy of the whole person in the wholistic spheres of body, mind, and spirit.

According to Buddhist philosophy, the long-term cause of disease is ignorance, which in turn gives rise to anger, greed, and apathy. Any one or more of these three "poisons of the mind" can lead to an imbalance of the three humors or fluids. In Tibetan humoral pathology, based on the Indian theory, these substances are known as "air", "bile" and "phlegm", which are not known to us by those names, but by their "subtle equivalents," which symbolize respectively "mind," "energy," and "inert matter," as nearly as can be rendered in translation of the Sanskrit. They permeate the whole body, but govern, above all, the brain, abdomen, and bowels. An excess of bile (energy) results in so-called hot diseases, predominant in the summer; too much phlegm (inert matter) evokes "cold diseases," mostly in the winter. An excess of air (mind) aggravates either hot or cold diseases, usually in the spring or fall.

The accessory or immediate causes of disease include poor diet, bad habits and behavior, accidents, weather changes, and wrong medicines or amounts thereof, any of which can upset the balance of the three humors. This can also pave the way for "demonic influences" leading to psychosis. Usually these or other serious disorders are believed to be the consequence of errors in thought, word, and deed committed during previous lives on earth—the cause-and-effect concept of the karmic life force in reincarnation.

Even though bodily cleanliness is briefly mentioned as one of many good habits in the prevention of disease,[11] it is well known that none but the most prosperous Tibetans seem to pay much attention to it. The foremost reason given is that "pure thoughts are incomparably more important...."[12] Another reason is that water is thought to collect vital energy. Still another is the extremely dry alpine climate, which is unfavorable to colonization of bacteria. Moreover, psychogenic factors are well recognized by Tibetan doctors as etiologic in some skin diseases, just as they are by Western dermatologists and other physicians. Less accepted by the latter are the putative favorable influences of wearing such objects as an otter skin against goiter or turquoise jewelry for liver complaints.

Cancer occurs far less frequently in Tibet than in the West. This has been attributed to the absence of such contributory factors as poor diet, improper food preparation and processing, toxic contamination of water supply, excessive venery, smoking, and community air pollution. The root causes, however, are believed to reside in psychological and emotional areas, which are diminished among Tibetans by their generally more selfless attitudes toward others, their equanimity through self-regulation and spiritual conduct.

It would serve little useful purpose here—even if there were enough space—to recount the many other different diseases imputed partly or wholly to various combinations of disharmony of the three humors. Nor would it be worthwhile to give their classification into "hot" and "cold" diseases, as well as their associated symptoms and signs. Suffice it to mention that 404 common diseases are recognized, of which 101 are ascribed to unbalanced humors.[13]

Just as today's well-trained internist or diagnostician places prime importance on a good, comprehensive history, so also does the Lamaist physician stress the significance of symptoms in arriving at an accurate diagnosis. Thus, disease descriptions include various combinations of the following symptoms: easy fatigability; weakness; restlessness; insomnia; hypersomnia; hunger; thirst; shivering; cough; sputum; shortness of breath; palpitation; difficulty in swallowing; vomiting; hiccup; indigestion; diarrhea; stiffness, aches, and pains in joints; sneezing; urinary frequency; and "suppression of natural function."

Physical examination is not as comprehensive, but includes inspection of the body for such conditions as signs of malnutrition, abnormalities of the skin, eyes, ears, nose, and tongue (for example, pallor, jaundice, or dryness), abdominal swelling, and tenderness to palpation of any part of the body. Meticulous attention is paid by the Tibetan doctor to examination of the pulse, with three fingers or each of his hands over both radial arteries of the patient. Minute descriptions of many different kinds of pulses indicate that they often give clues to the diagnosis. The general rule is that the normal basal pulse rate is about five times the respiratory rate.

The urine is inspected with great care as to its color, clarity, foaming characteristics, and sediment. The sputum, vomitus, and feces are also inspected.

It is highly pertinent here to refer to Blofeld's book *The Tantric Mysticism of Tibet*, which is recommended as a practical guide for those interested in this subject and the practice of tantric meditation.[14] The author, an English "devoted" Buddhist for forty years, points out the dangers of unguided or improperly guided tantric meditation: "Wrongly applied they [tantric methods] could lead to madness and worse than madness." The following is quoted from an interpretive summary of Blofeld's book by a brilliant Los Angeles attorney:

The basic principles of Tantric Buddhism...[contrast] with Christian theology emphasizing piety and scholarship. "Tantric" means "to weave" indicating activity.

The quest to transmute ego and selfishness into desirelessness, bliss and service is sacred. It is attained in the stillness of the heart. The quest requires great effort and is long; all sentient beings must be liberated according to Mahayana Buddhism, but Vajrayana is the Short Path and all help must be used. Heaven is taken by storm.

Secrecy is important and one must recognize everything as Nirvana. One must hear all sounds as mantras and all beings as Buddha. Christians would say we should see all things as good—holy; pray without ceasing and recognize Christ in everything.

Mantras are sacred invocations recited in a special tone of voice.... When repeated [they] produce both minor and startling changes in consciousness. Maximum effects are achieved by harmonious coordination of body, speech and mind in mudra, mantra and dyana.

Tantric adepts see all good above the duality of good and evil. Compassion and self control are essential. Harm and harassment are evil.

Visualization and centering on a point controlling thoughts are essential in integrating body, speech and mind.... Psychic and material symbols play an important role, e.g. the yinyang and mandala as indicative of relatedness and wholeness and the universe beyond outside the borders of the circle.

To keep count and for the recitation of the mantras, rosaries of 108 "beads" (of carved bone) of varying size and color are used. Christian rosaries of 33 or 66 beads used in Novenas with "Hail Mary" and "Our Father" furnish Christian analogs.

Mantra is clung to for the proper state of mind when one passes from the physical body into the bardo prior to reincarnation. [There were] similar practices in Christianity until the Middle Ages when "the art and craft of dying" was lost.

Carl Jung found substantiation for his theories of the unconscious in "The Tibetan Book of the Dead," but suggested that persons born into the West and Christianity are not by accident and should master their own religion before attempting others. That insight by the one who Arnold Toynbee said had done more than anyone in history to elevate the human soul is valid and should not be taken lightly.

The advanced souls in the West who may have sojourned in the East in previous lives will find Tantric Buddhism valuable in their sacred quest to know what we call "God" by a thousand different names. [15]

There are general rules for the treatment of diseases: adoption of good health habits; mild decoctions to prevent the spread of contagious disease; gentle laxatives as indicated, especially during convalescence; importance of taking medication as prescribed and of not suppressing "natural" functions such as vomiting and bowel movements; as well as aggressive attempts to cure certain diseases before they become entrenched and thence more difficult or impossible to cure.

When a diagnosis is in doubt, the Lamaist physician makes use of the diagnostic or therapeutic trial. This consists of the prescription of one of several mild decoctions or soups for different suspected disorders. This principle is consistent with the time-honored dictum of *primum non nocere*—"above all, do no harm"—so often lost sight of and the cause of so many adverse reactions in the current Western practice of disease-oriented crisis medicine, with its "half-way technology."[16]

Most medicinal herbs are (or used to be) gathered on a mountain to the north of Lhasa, the capital of Tibet, near the monastery of Sera.[17] Great care is taken in the choice of plants, which could be beneficial or harmful, more or less effective, depending on the season and on location on sunlit or northern slopes. Rechung, in his chapter on pharmacology, classifies forms of medicine into: decoctions, powders, pills, syrups, oily medicine, ash-like medicine, concentrated medicine and medicinal wine.[18] Numerous mixtures from the flowers, fruit, leaves, sap and/or roots of plants are listed under each category for various conditions. Sometimes one or more metals—especially gold, silver, zinc, iron, and mercury—or stones, are added to a prescription, as is the custom in India. Other remedies are based on the belief in strange analogues between certain substances and parts of the body, reminiscent of folk medicine in other countries. For example, ox gall is used to treat eye weaknesses, the spleen for abscesses, a dog's tongue for healing wounds, and its liver as a remedy for leprosy.[19]

Surgery is used as a last resort and then only for wounds and abscesses; rarely for other conditions, depending on established causes, and thus not for exploratory purposes.

Cauterization is used for sickness due to air imbalances (nervous diseases). Cold compresses and bloodletting are employed in bile disorders (energy imbalances); hot compresses and cauterization for "cold diseases" of phlegm (inert matter).

According to Rechung's chapter "Notes on Practices Continued in Tibetan Medicine up to the Present Time," cupping and bloodletting (for hypertension and certain other circulatory problems) should be done at the proper time, and provided there are no contraindications such as pregnancy or "air" disease. Moxa or moxabustion should be performed with a golden needle placed over the appropriate vein and through tinder which is lit at the upper end. The needle is removed the instant the fire touches the body. It should be used only on the crown of the head for air (nervous) diseases. It can be performed on other parts of the body for digestive diseases, convulsions, dropsy—diseases caused by air and phlegm—but not those due to bile (e.g., not for febrile diseases or jaundice). Curiously enough, acupuncture, though deemed by the Chinese to go hand in hand with moxa, is barely mentioned by Rechung.[20] Burang, however, states that it is generally practiced with care and reserve and even then by highly qualified specialists.[21] They should be familiar with not only the nearly 900 different points of needle insertion, but also the postulated currents of life forces of energy, invisible and eluding anatomical and material qualifications.

A list of eight mixtures is presented as being used at the present time. Only two of these are quoted as representative:

> Srog-hdzin-bchu-dug, which has 16 ingredients: cloves, black aloewood, nutmeg, a mineral drug called sho-sha, costus speciosus, saffron, frankincense, sandalwood, lime, rush, yellow pigment, shandril, sha-chhen, salt, ginger, piper longum. It is used against nervous diseases and melancholia. To be taken in beer, or about one teaspoonful of hot water…which has three ingredients: soma plant, syrup, camphor. These three mixed together, should be taken with beer. Used for vomiting, against bone fractures, tuberculosis and leukorrhea.[22]

It seems reasonable to assume that most if not all of the foregoing modalities are still being used in Tibet even after the Chinese occupation seventeen years ago. Although all Western drugs are available in China, or at least those parts visited recently by a scientific delegation,[23] traditional remedies are still widely prescribed. Chairman Mao's exhortations to combine Western and traditional medicine are enthusiastically espoused, since classical China's rich materia medica is "the product of 2,000 years of the people's struggle against disease."[24]

How much of the ancient Tibetan art of healing can be a reasonably valid contribution to modern wholistic healing or health? Several such aspects have already been suggested. Certainly the responsibility of the person for his health, with certain exceptions, is a major and recurring theme in both. So are the maintenance of good health, mental and spiritual growth, as well as prevention of disease through good habits and self-regulation. The importance of a natural, well-balanced diet and conservatism with respect to hazardous diagnostic and therapeutic modalities are other examples in common.

The emphasis on harmony and balance in both is striking: the Tibetan symbolism of phlegm, air, and bile—which mean, respectively, inert matter, mind, and energy—requires a balance of these for health. In some respects, but apparently not all,[25] this concept is comparable to one definition of wholistic health,[26] which is "the balanced integration of the individual in all aspects and levels of being— body, mind and spirit, including interpersonal relationships and our relationship to the whole of nature and our physical environment."[27] Evarts Loomis devotes a whole chapter to harmony and balance in his *Healing for Everyone—Medicine of the Whole Person.*[28] It does not seem irrelevant here to mention the growing recognition of the importance of functional differences between the right (intuitive) and left (analytical) sides of the brain, the neglect of the former, and the need to bring them into better balance.[29]

Roy Menninger recently wrote a significant editorial in the *Annals of Internal Medicine* entitled "Psychiatry 1976: Time for a Holistic Medicine." He deplores the mind-body dualism—the polarizing dichotomy between the "objective" physicochemical concepts of physiology and pathology on the one hand, and the more abstract religiopsychiatric conceptions of the psyche on the other. He states further that the possibility that some of the self-improvement techniques and experiences may have profound effects on pathologic conditions resistant to traditional treatment is too important for medicine to ignore. He concludes that "breaking the grip of these dualities will permit medicine to recapture the whole person as the focus of attention and reduce those dehumanizing preoccupations with the disease alone, the psyche alone, the liver or pancreas alone, the psychosis alone. This *is* holistic medicine for a society that needs to learn from the medical profession how to be an effectively caring society."[30]

Epilogue

My personal interest in Tibet was heightened during a year (1969– 70) of volunteer service on the staff of the United Mission Medical

Center in Kathmandu, Nepal. At the request of the late Dr. Bethel Fleming, the founder of that hospital (also called Shanta Bhawan),[31] I saw the highest local spiritual leader, the Rimpoche, several times in consultation at the two-thousand-year-old Buddhist temple at Swayambutinath. Always gracious and charming, he invited my wife and me to his private quarters on each occasion.

In 1973, while serving with CARE/MEDICO in Kabul, Afghanistan, my wife and I traveled to Dharamsala, the hill station in northern India, for a holiday. This was climaxed by our private audience with His Honor the Dalai Lama, which lasted almost an hour. We were greatly impressed with his fluency in English, knowledge of world affairs, spirituality, and dedication to the future of Tibet and Tibetans everywhere.

The office of the Dalai Lama arranged for us to meet his personal physician, Yeshi Dhonden. He examined my wife for a chronic neck disorder; this included a history through an interpreter and a meticulous palpation of her cervical and radial pulses. He exerted pressure over her cervical spine, resulting in a loud, cracking sound. Her symptoms immediately disappeared and have remained absent to this day. Unfortunately, my own cervical osteoarthritis (worse than hers, by clinical and X ray documentation) did not respond to either manipulation or herbal pills! This court physician was writing a book on Tibetan medicine which on completion I hope to obtain and have translated into English.

About two years after we saw Yeshi Dhonden, he was invited to make rounds at a teaching hospital of Yale University Medical School.[32] He examined a female patient selected by a member of the staff. The diagnosis was unknown to him and the staff. After long inspection of her body and palpation of her pulse, he personally examined a specimen of her urine, vigorously stirring and smelling it. Through an interpreter, his diagnosis was delivered in a "soft bilingual fugue" of flowery circumlocution: a metaphor of an unwanted open gate and eddying currents of an eroding and flooding river, which actually described a congenital heart defect and its ensuing cardiorespiratory impairment. His diagnosis was then confirmed in more prosaic terms by the only professor there who knew it as established through more "sophisticated" prior studies: "congenital heart disease—interventricular septal defect, with resultant heart failure."

Notes

1. Leonard J. Duhl, "The Health Planner: Planning and Dreaming for Health and Wellness," *American Journal of Health Planning* (October 1976): 7–14.

2. *Encyclopaedia Britannica*, Macropaedia, 15th ed., s.v. "Shamanism."

3. J. K. Rechung, *Tibetan Medicine* (Berkeley and Los Angeles: University of California Press, 1973).

4. Theodore Burang, *The Tibetan Art of Healing* (London: Watkins, 1974).

5. Ibid.

6. Ibid.

7. John Blofeld, *The Tantric Mysticism of Tibet* (New York: Causeway Books, 1974).

8. Theodore Burang, op cit.

9. John Ervin, personal communication, September 1976.

10. Theodore Burang, op. cit.

11. J. K. Rechung, op. cit.

12. Theodore Burang, op. cit.

13. J. K. Rechung, op. cit.

14. John Blofeld, op. cit.

15. John Ervin, personal communication.

16. Ilza Veith, *Medizin in Tibet* (Leverkusen: Bayer, 1961).

17. Huang Ti, *The Yellow Emperor's Classic of Internal Medicine*, trans. Ilza Veith (Berkeley, Los Angeles and London: University of California Press, 1970).

18. J. K. Rechung, op. cit.

19. Huang Ti, op. cit.

20. J. K. Rechung, op. cit.

21. Theodore Burang, op. cit.

22. J. K. Rechung, op. cit.

23. E. E. Windhager, "Medical Trade School or Academic Institution?" *Alumni Quarterly* (Ithaca, N.Y.: Cornell University Medical College Alumni Association, Fall, 1975): 11–12.

24. Louis Lasagna, "Herbal Pharmacology and Medical Therapy in the People's Republic of China," *Annals of Internal Medicine* 83 (1975): 887–93.

25. Theodore Burang, op. cit.

26. Giuseppe Tucci, *Tibet: Land of Snows* (New York: Stein and Day, 1967): 154–70.

27. *By-Laws* of Association for Holistic Health, Inc. (San Diego: April, 1976).

28. Evarts G. Loomis and J. Sig Paulson, *Healing for Everyone: Medicine of the Whole Person* (New York: Hawthorn, 1975).

29. Robert E. Ornstein, *The Psychology of Consciousness* (New York: Penguin, 1972): 65–88, 161–97.

30. Roy W. Menninger, "Psychiatry 1976: Time for a Holistic Medicine," *Annals of Internal Medicine* 84 (1976): 603–4.

31. Grace N. Fletcher, *The Fabulous Flemings of Kathmandu* (New York: E. P. Dutton, 1967).

32. Richard Selzer, "The Art of Surgery," *Harper's Magazine* (January 1976): 75–78.

31

Chandrasekhar G. Thakkur

Ayurvedic Medicine: Past, Present, and Future

THE AIM OF Oriental medicine was not medication of the human being in parts; the sole purpose was very positive—to understand the human being as a whole. The first axiom that our ancestors, centuries ago, gave us was that knowledge of the part cannot yield knowledge of the whole. Believers in truth and searchers after peace of mankind considered *vidhya* ("knowledge"), *vitarka* ("logic"), *vigyana* ("science"), *smriti* ("remembrance"), *tatparata* ("adaptability"), and *kriya* ("practical knowledge") as the six pillars of success, and that for one who attains them there is nothing impossible in this world.

Centuries ago, the healing of a person was wholistic, but science then did not enjoy the prominence it now does and was "covered" by religion.

Let me put before readers in simple, plain, lucid language the basic concepts of Ayurvedic science. The five basic factors, or the protoelements, are earth, water, fire, air, and ether. These create the universe; they also create the body; and they form the diet; a relationship is thus established between macrocosm and microcosm. In other words, whatever is in the body (*pinda*) is in the universe (*Brahmanda*), and this analogy of the physio-universal interrelationship, or what is called "Pinda and Brahmanda Nyaya" is the most basic or original. It gives a message from the deep insight of the ancestors that the plants and various animal kingdoms also have life, and we in the human kingdom are associated with the universe, and all are part and parcel of one machinery.

Today's medical approach of understanding each and every patient is stereotyped and routine; instruments play a more important role than the eye. The examination of the patient is mechanical, whereas in the Ayurvedic system of medicine the person as a whole is examined according to the physical constitution of the self. It is believed that, when the sperm (*bija*) of father and ovum (*bija*) of mother unite for fertilization in the uterine cavity of the fallopian tube, around them is an excess of one of three protoelements—air, fire, and water—or of two or even all three of them. As a result, the developing person has an air constitution, a fire constitution, a water constitution, an air-fire constitution, a fire-water constitution, an air-water constitution, or a three-fold constitution. Therefore each individual patient, i.e., the person as a whole, differs from others. Logically, then, the practice of experimenting on rats, rabbits, guinea pigs, or dogs and then introducing a chemical substance into the human body with the hope of producing a like effect is not acceptable to Ayurvedic medicine.

Of the sciences of India in the form of Vedas, Upanishads, Vedantas, and Puranas, Ayurveda is one. The word *Ayur* means "life," and *Veda* means "science," and, in the words of Sushruta, one of the compilers of Ayurveda, "This science of life is everlasting and bestows merit, prestige, happiness, longevity, livelihood, and heaven." Charaka, another compiler of Ayurveda, says: "Hence those alone that act after due investigation are considered wise," and he adds, "A full conception of the science will never be achieved by the knowledge of only a part of it." And as far as scientific attitude is concerned, he was very clear that "all suffering which afflicts the mind or body has ignorance for its cause and all happiness has its basis in clear scientific knowledge." The exponents of this art and science of medicine were open minded and large hearted and openly proclaimed, "The whole world is the teacher for the wise and for the fool the whole universe is full of enemies."

Our ancestors, when they presented the therapy, first dealt with health. They dealt with the anatomy, physiology, daily regimen (both for the day and night), various seasons, diet, and all the aspects of personal and social hygiene. Here also the idea of treating the person as a whole appears very important. Diet is one point where Ayurveda scores over, and leaves aside, all other systems of medicine. Any ingreient, in Ayurveda, is not valued in terms of carbohydrate, fat, starch, protein, minerals, vitamins, or the calories it yields; instead, six types of tastes—sweet, sour, salt, bitter, pungent, and astringent—are taken into consideration. The action that produces heat or cold in the body is taken into account, and so are three local digestive actions (one in the mouth and upper portion called sweet postdigestive action; one occurring in the lower part of the stomach or duodenum called sour postdigestive action; and one in the lower part of the intestines called pungent postdigestive action). Further, each item in itself, having its own sweet, sour, or pungent digestive action, is taken into account. It therefore becomes easily understandable how what is poison to one can be nectar to another. Ayurveda prescribes a dietetic regimen, not only for a sick person, but also for a healthy man, according to age, season, country, digestive capacity, etc., of the individual human being concerned.

The idea of ectomorphic, endomorphic, and mesomorphic personalities advanced by Kresmer and Shelly was quite familiar to the ancient authorities on Ayurveda, if only in greater detail and with a wider connotation. Mention must also be made of Dr. William A. R. Thomson, who in his treatise *The Searching Mind in Medicine* attempts to describe the thin, lean personality on one side, the obese personality on the other, and the medium personality in between. Ayurveda, in comparison, deals with the air and water personalities on two sides and the fire personality in between. The description of the air, fire, and water personalities is given in such vast detail that the walking, talking, diet, sleep, and nature of each personality type are all spelled out. These details, of course, cannot be completely incorporated in the small compass of this essay. But just to give a glimpse, the air element is quick, water is slow and steady, fire is hot and radiant. By correctly diagnosing one's personality, what medicines, remedial measures, diet, etc., would agree with one was determined.

So a physician of Ayurvedic medicine is not merely a man of medicine. He has an insight into the society, and his foremost duty becomes how to keep a person fit and fine, free from illness. He knows his patient as a whole—there is no question of a heart, liver, or kidney alone walking into his office. He knows his patient from top to bottom, and he is aware of the effect of a particular dietetic item on his body, as also of change in environment.

Ayurveda was the first and foremost Oriental medicine that thought of body and mind separately and jointly. The three protoelements— air, fire, and water—in equilibrium maintain the health of the body, and any disturbance in the equilibrium creates disorder of the physique. Our ancestors were quite aware of the qualities of Sattva, Rajas, and Tamas—*Sattva* meaning "divine or noble," *Rajas* meaning "human," and *Tamas* meaning "animal or passionate." Of these three states of mind, Sattva has been considered as the quality, Rajas and Tamas being vitiations. When these three are in normal equilibrium according to one's own individual temperament, they maintain the mental health; any upset creates mental disorders. So you also find mental disorders described in the Ayurvedic system of medicine. Our ancestors were firm believers that mental agonies affect the physique, and, conversely, physical disorders have an effect on the mind. An authority like Osler in *Modern Medicine* has said in the chapter on nervous diarrhoea, it is an old and trustworthy theory and observation—one does not know why and how but it is true—that mental states profoundly affect the intestinal canal. When you measure with a thermometer the temperature of a person who complains of feverishness, mental upset and agony, and a burning syndrome in the body, the reading may be 98.4°F. or lower, and there would be no fever according to modern medicine. But Ayurvedic medicine recognizes the disorder as a mental fever or feverishness of the mind and would treat it with the help of *dhe* ("intellect"), *dhairya* ("endurance"), *atma* ("soul"), *vighyana* ("the science of it"), and with herbs like jatamansi, shankhapushpi, and brahmi, which help the mind. These herbs do not act as tranquilizers or mood elevators, but their strengthening of the nerves aids the body. Conversely, herbs like ashwagandha (*Withania somnifetra*) and shatavari, which act on the human physique, nourishing and improving nutrition, also have an effect on the mind.

On the one hand, Sir William Jones, English Orientalist, avers that "there is no evidence that in any language of Asia there was one original treatise on medicine, considered as science"—an obvious travesty of truth, in my opinion. But on the other hand, that we are not bolstering up bogus or even exaggerated claims on behalf of Ayurveda is sufficiently proved by what Will Durant has to say on the subject, in his famous work *Our Oriental Heritage*:

> In the latest system of Hindu medicine the illness is attributed to disorder in the body humours and treatment is recommended with herbs. *Many of its diagnoses and cures are still used in India, with a success that is sometimes the envy of western physicians* [Emphasis added.]

Surgery was well developed in ancient times. In the realm of plastic surgery, skin grafting was done and artificial noses or organs were prepared. Our ancestors were also conversant with the idea of infection. Sushruta refers to the spreading of such contagious diseases as smallpox, measles, conjunctivitis, and tubercular infection. But the sole responsibility was not thrown on any bacteria or viruses. It was the immunity of the human person as a whole that was of the utmost importance to the physician; he tried to understand the imbalance of air, water, and fire element in the body of the individual and worked to treat the conditions that fostered the attack of the bacteria or viruses. Treatments included body cleansing by various processes—in certain cases even mental processes, including meditation, prayers, and Gem therapy—and various cures like fasting.

Diagnosis is of great importance even today in Indian Oriental medicine. The physician tries various methods, pulse examination being one of the most important. Here the teachings of Lord Buddha are remembered: "There are the petals, the pollen, the corolla, and the stalk, but there is no lotus flower. There is this or that passing idea, this or that transitory emotion, this or that image but no organised whole behind them which can be called the ego or the self." Therefore it is stressed that an intelligent physician should endeavour to investigate correctly each disease by the use of three methods, i.e., authoritative instruction, direct observation and examination, and inference. It was very clearly said that the physician should first diagnose the disease and then decide the line of treatment and proceed with the treatment in the light of his observations. If the physician begins the treatment without diagnosing the disease properly, even though he may be the best therapeutist, his success depends purely on chance. But he who knows the differential diagnosis of disease, who is skilled in all kinds of therapeutics, and who is well versed in the knowledge of clime, season and dosage, achieves success with certainty. Therefore the intelligent physician, having investigated correctly the following ten factors, proceeds with the treatment. In doing this the understanding of each individual as a whole is the sole goal for a scientific-minded physician. So the physician is not merely a consulting medical authority pocketing his normal fees, but he becomes the friend, philosopher, and guide of the patient. The idea of wholistic healing and its basic principles and concepts are described in great detail in *Charak Samhita*.

Ten Factors to be Investigated by the Physician

1. Physical constitution.
2. Makeup. The makeup of a person is divided into eight types with a view to finding out the individual differences relating to strength and vitality. These eight types refer to skin, blood, flesh, fat, bone, marrow, semen, and the mind.
3. Compactness. A compact body has bones that are symmetrical and well knit, joints that are also well knit, and well-placed flesh and blood. Those with a well-compacted body are strong; those with an ill-compacted body are weak; and those with a moderately compacted body are moderately strong.
4. Bodily proportions. Length of life, strength, vitality, happiness, authority, wealth, and other desirable qualities are dependent on the proper proportions of the body. The contrary conditions are found in the case of the body that falls short of or exceeds the right proportions.
5. Homologation. Those to whom ghee, milk, oil, meat juice, and all the six tastes are homologous are strong, tolerant of hardships, and long lived. Those to whom dry things and only one of the tastes are homologous are of low vitality, unable to endure hardships, short lived, and admit of mild medication. Those of mixed homologation are of moderate strength.
6. Psychic makeup. The mind is termed the psychic element. It is of three kinds, and therefore human beings fall into three psychic groups.
7. Gastric capacity. The digestive capacity is to be judged in terms of capacity of ingestion and digestion—whether high, moderate or low.
8. Capacity for exercises. This is to be judged in terms of capacity for putting forth effort.
9. Age. Age denotes the state of the body as a result of the passage of time and is divided into three main parts—early, middle, and old age.
10. Disease condition in general.

Kenneth Walker in his work *A Doctor Digresses* says, "It is useless for me to search the shelves of my library because there is no medical text-book which defines health." However, the best definition of health is given by Ayurveda: When the three body protoelements—air, fire, and water—are in equilibrium; the gastric appetite is neither voracious nor weak nor irregular but is normal; the body nutrients—the food juice, the blood, the flesh, the fat, the bone, bone marrow, and the vital essence—are in equilibrium; the body excretions—sweat, urine, and evacuations—are properly made; and a person is bestowed with a pleasant and peaceful mind and soul; then the person is really a *swastha* (*swa*, "own," *stha*, "standing"); he is called a healthy one. This, again, gives us an idea of wholistic healing.

Herbology and Its Uses in Wholistic Health

Herbs have been used in the alleviation of the human body and mind, not only for centuries, but for several thousands of years. References to herbs are plentiful in Vedas and pre-Vedic times, going back from seven to ten thousand years ago. The American Indians perhaps possessed knowledge of the effect of herbs on the human system—a particular herb acting in a particular ailment—but, in the Ayurvedic system of medicine, each herb is explained according to the effect of taste, action, and digestive action in the human body, with the specific action on various elements, and how and why it works. Unfortunately, this knowledge is scattered; in my travels around the world I found that in one country Glycerriz is used for throat problems; in another for leucorrhoea in women; in another country for increasing breast milk; and in yet another country as a rejuvenator and revitalizer. So there is need for a comprehensive materia medica, which is a more vital necessity than research.

Principles of Ayurvedic Medicine

The first chapter and stanza in the most ancient text of Ayurvedic medicine starts with the words *deergha* ("very long") and *jeeviteeya* ("span of life"), illustrating that the main concern of Ayurveda was the issue of health, not the problem of disease and disorders. After dealing with health in detail, the ancestors dealt with the diagnosis and treatment of disorders. A remedy is called pure, effective, efficacious, and complete and the only real remedy if it subsides and cures one disease from the root cause and permanently, while one that subsides the disorders temporarily and gives rise to other disorders is called an impure and incorrect remedy. The physician, the nurse, the patient, and the medicine—these four are the pillars of the treatment. Each one of them has to possess four qualities, and only if all four are complete in the qualities can the treatment be successful. It was emphasized that the physician must be well versed in theory and practice; one who knew theory by heart but did not know practice at all was not considered praiseworthy, and it was enjoined that such a one should be taken to the king for prosecution and strict imposition of penalty, hanging not excluded.

The treatment is also divided into various types. For those whose body is full of vitiation, purification of the body is advised. Sweating, anointing the body with various oils, massages, vomiting with various emetics, mild laxatives, strong purgatives, various medicated enemas, nasal inhalations, and various body-cleansing programs were carried out, and are still carried out in Kerala in South India. This process is called Panchakarma. Experts in naturopathy who visited these centers were amazed at the results. For conditions like bronchial asthma, allergic cold, and various other types of disorders, body cleansing was carried out. The basic idea was that, just as a dirty cloth cannot catch fast color, so you can never cure a disease permanently if the body is full of vitiation. Here it should be clarified that the original Sanskrit words *Vata* ("air"), *Pitta* ("fire") and *Kapha* ("water predominant") have been very sincerely but misleadingly translated to signify body humors like wind, bile, and phlegm representing air, fire, and water in their gross sense, as excretions, but not in the real sense that they are the basic factors that maintain the body, and when vitiated by external or internal causes create disorders. Here again, the person as a whole was treated for his vitiation—not only the disease, but the patient as a whole, was taken into consideration. It is continually emphasized that each individual is a different entity, and the same mode of treatment is never prescribed for one and all. Three to four thousand years ago, treatment with herbs used only a single herb; later on, combinations and various compounds gradually came into use. Until the fifteenth century, there was "mercurial treatment," which used metals and minerals. The object of this hectic and drastic treatment was to cure the disease quickly and get the patient better fast, irrespective of diagnosis—like antibiotics that temporarily subside infection. However, people of their own choice in India today prefer the ancient medical treatment, which strikes at the root of the disease and takes into account the patient as a whole. The body cleansing program mentioned above is carried out only in those cases where the individual is strong and sturdy enough to go through the various processes. For pregnant women, infants and young children, and old, debilitated, and crippled persons, no body cleansing program is carried out; only soothing, cooling, subsiding, and allaying treatment with herbs and mild measures is employed.

We are often reminded of the fantastic modern medical achievements in the field of emergencies, where detailed diagnosis and analysis is carried out to determine the pathological and physiological changes occuring in the body by which the condition is brought on. But as far as cure is concerned, we often come across sentences in the modern medical textbooks like "Yet an ideal ingredient is to be found out to solve the situation." For most of the diseases, only control is available, and therefore the cure of a disease is not complete and ideal. The ancient Ayurvedic system of medicine, however, has shown its effect even in emergencies and in cases that have been labelled incurable and the patient has been left to his fate. Even though immediate miraculous cure is not obtained and more time is taken, the herbs and treatment of the patient as a whole have helped achieve success. It is not possible within the compass of this essay to quote all the legion of examples; so just two case histories follow.

1. A patient suffering from swelling all over the body, particularly on the leg and under the eyes (dropsy/ascites) had a medical report finding "albumin +4; pus cells plenty; red blood cells present number, plus infection; diagnosis: subacute nephritis, going into degenerative process." The patient was put on corticosteroids and other treatment, which failed. Ayurvedic treatment put the patient on a diet consisting only of skim milk, with no salt, and the juice of the pure herb punarnava (spreading hogweed), and slowly and gradually the patient recovered.
2. A millionaire from Ceylon was suffering from diabetes and had consulted all the leading physicians in the world. He was told that his condition could only be treated by insulin or the oral blood sugar–reducing agent. He had been undergoing this treatment for

many years and at times his condition deteriorated. He was put on the simple Ayurvedic line of treatment consisting of drugs like shilajit, the bitter drugs such as neem, karela, giloy etc., with brihat vasanta kusumakar. The patient reported from Colombo that his urine and blood have been tested and the urine shows no sugar while the blood sugar curve is normal. The treatment increased his strength and gave him normal health, which he had considered a dream of next-birth.

I am not trying to impress upon the readers the supremacy of the ancient medicines over the modern ones. *The idea is to bring out the basic difference of treating the patient as a whole and the disease separately.*

Ayurveda has branches like anatomy, physiology, personal hygiene, hygiene of seasons, materia medica, pharmacology, diagnosis, treatment, dietetics, nutrition, and various other branches, including treating ailments of children and women, and operative and postoperative treatment. In fact, an entire branch of surgery developed from this system of medicine and still exists today. It includes piercing the ear lobes and nasal septum.

Unfortunately, as India passed through a period of slavery, the science became stagnant for a time; but now that India has obtained independence and is on the path of development, it is expected that the message of Ayurveda will reach all the corners and nooks of the world. In India, universities are now accepting Ayurveda, and state governments are giving their patronage. Former prime minister Indira Gandhi evinced keen interest in reviving the ancient glory of India, and with a scientific and progressive outlook, research work has already started.

Sex forms an important part of life and must be considered when dealing with wholistic healing. During my visits to the United Kingdom, the Continent, and the United States, I found that the Kinsey reports and the efforts of Masters and Johnson amazed the new generation. The Indian philosophy of the Yogis, who preached and taught Yoga, was one of abstinence and celibacy. While *Charak Samhita* gives us an idea of how the masters believed in celibacy and abstinence, on the one hand, for a particular *sadhana* or attainment of worship, it also shows how sexual efficiency could be arrived at by a householder in his married life. Knowledge about sex is spread in Vatsyayana Kama

Sutra, which is in full praise of the woman. Here Ayurveda does not disagree. It says: "Willpower is the best rejuvenator and virilific, and woman is the best aphrodisiac, in whom are confided the five sense organs—hearing, touch, sight, taste and smell. The best means of stimulating one's manhood (the best agent of virilification) is an exhilarating sexual partner in the wife. When the desired sense objects yield great pleasure even if singly experienced by the senses, then what need be said of the person of the woman in whom the delectable objects of all the senses are found established together?"

Dealing with psychosomatic illnesses, impotence, rejuvenation, and revitalization, the masters gave the idea that, just as the wheels of a bullock cart require normal oiling and greasing, so the human body every year in the season of winter requires revitalizing and overhauling, and for that, a dietetic regimen, body cleansing, and treatment of the person as a whole is prescribed. In this scientific era, one thinks of such aphrodisiacs as yohimbine, an extract of the bark of an African tree, for quick erection and sexual stimulation. Contrary to this, Ayurveda deals with the body buildup, psychic makeup and overhauling of the whole testicular system, without recourse to any hormone but simply by herbs—and the theory behind all this is really amazing.

Astrology

The ancestors believed that the planets in various signs of the zodiac affect the environment, and their cosmic rays affect our physique and mind—in other words, medicine and astrology are interrelated. Thus the method of diagnosing and understanding the person as a whole by the use of astrology, as well as by palmistry, in the field of medicine forms a part of wholistic healing. The underlying principles are that Aries, Cancer, Libra, and Capricorn are quick signs; Taurus, Leo, Scorpio, and Aquarius are steady signs; and Gemini, Virgo, Sagittarius, and Pisces are dual signs (quick as well as steady). The temperament of a patient can be judged from the rising sign (which may be fixed, movable or dual). The sun and Mars stand for fire; Mercury and Saturn for air; and Jupiter, Venus, and the moon for water. In palmistry, the line of life, popularly so called, is considered as the line of the digestive system or of vitality; the line of the head is considered to be the line of the nervous system, ruled by the moon; and the line of the heart is the line of the soul or the sun. Even today, this integration of astrology and palmistry in detail is practised with such amazing success that when a patient comes, his birth horoscope or chart made in Hindu division is thoroughly scrutinized, including the planetary configurations at the time of birth, the transits of the passing planets, and major periods and subperiods. Here it may be explained that the first house in a horoscope rules over the head; the second over the face; the third over the extremities; the fourth over the chest; the fifth over the heart, abdomen and back; the sixth over the intestines; the seventh over the urinary system and kidney; the eighth over the genitoreproductory and excretory systems; the ninth over the thighs; the tenth over the knees; the eleventh over the ankles; and the twelfth over the feet. In the same fashion, each of the twelve signs ruling over twelve parts of the body, and the planetary configurations occurring, give the type of disorders—i.e., the first over health, the sixth over disease, the eighth over longevity—not to tell how long a man will live, but to understand the type of body and mind one is going to have, already has, or will have in the future.

Dr. Michio Kushi of the East-West Foundation, Boston, and Dr. Shen of Boston use physiognomy for purposes of diagnosis. There may be various Oriental methods—Chinese, Japanese, Indian, Korean, Egyptian—to treat the person as a whole. To understand the patient as a whole is the first and foremost task, but how and in what terms? Not merely as a victim of certain adventitious factors like germs, etc., but as a complex of certain basic factors that are liable to derangement and disorder through various causes such as age, diet, climate, season, and the rest; and having considered this, to go on to prescribe matching modes of treatment to restore him, not only to a state where his particular complaint has disappeared, but to a condition of happiness wherein the body and mind are equally involved. Ayurveda is a modern must because its appreciation and practice can materially contribute not only to mitigation of disease but more positively to the regeneration and revitalization of the individual as well as of society.

Bibliography

Charak Samhita, vols. 1–6. Original Sanskrit text and English as well as other vernacular translations combined. Vol. 1 deals in detail with the person as a whole. Sind Ayurvedic Pharmacy, 375, Kalbadevi, Bombay 2, India.

Chawkham, Moharashi Sushruta. *Sushruta Samhita*. Banaras, India: Sanskrit
    Series.
Thakkur, Chandrasekhar G. *Herbal Cures*. Sind Ayurvedic Pharmacy, 375,
    Kalbadevi, Bombay 2, India.
————. *Medical Astrology*. Kanya Books, 101 West 125th Street, New York,
    NY 10027, or Samuel Weiser, 734 Broadway, New York, NY

Directory of Organizations

THE FOLLOWING is a list of wholistic resources: organizations, centers, and groups. Some of these are established, well-recognized organizations. Others, by virtue of their newness and focus, remain quite unknown to the general public. The list is by no means comprehensive, nor do the editors mean to imply an endorsement of any of these resources by listing them here. The editors' purpose is to present sources that may be approached for further information.

Many groups are not in a position to answer questions from the public on a large scale. However, the majority appear to be involved in the wholistic healing movement and are usually willing to share information, exchange ideas, and advance purpose of the movement.

Wholistic Healing Centers

Alliance for Health and Wholeness
135 Madison Avenue, N.E.
Albuquerque, NM 87123
(505) 265-0221

A.R.E. Clinic
4018 North 40th Street
Phoenix, AZ 85018
(602) 955-0551
William A. McGarey, M.D.
Gladys T. McGarey, M.D.

Boston Center of Healing Arts
One Park Place
Boston, MA 02130

Center for the Healing Arts
11081 Missouri Avenue
Los Angeles, CA 90025
(213) 477-3981
Harold Stone, Ph.D., Executive Director
Jacquelyn McCandless, M.D., Medical Director

Center for Holistic Arts
2616 Front Street
San Diego, CA 92103
(714) 235-6388
Fred Weaver III, M.D., Consulting Director

Center for Wholistic Healing
212 San Jose Street, Suite 203
Salinas, CA 93901
(408) 422-YOGA
James W. Knight, M.D., Director

Hawaii Health Net
2534 South King Street
Honolulu, HI 96814
(808) 955-1555
Walter S. Strode, M.D., founder

Hering Family Health Clinic
2340 Ward Street, Suite 107
Berkeley, CA 94705
(415) 458-1992
Corey Weinstein, M.D.

Holistic Health Center
8907 Wilshire Blvd., Suite 200
Beverly Hills, CA 90211
(213) 652-5084
Patricia Phillips, M.S.W., Admn.
Coord.
Barry Vishny, M.D.

Meadowlark
26126 Fairview Avenue
Hemet, CA 92343
(714) 927-1113
Evarts G. Loomis, M.D., founder

P.S.I. Center
Endicott Building, Suite M
Greenhills Shopping Center
Cincinnati, OH 45218
(513) 742-2266
Robert Rothan, D.D.S., Director

San Andreas Health Council
531 Cowper Street
Palo Alto, CA 94301
(415) 324-9350

Leonard Duhl, M.D., Advisor

Wellness Resource Center
42 Miller Avenue
Mill Valley, CA 94941
(415) 383-3806
John Travis, M.D., Medical Director

Wholistic Health and Nutrition
Institute
150 Shoreline Highway, Suite 31
Mill Valley, CA 94941
(415) 332-2933, 332-2992
Richard L. Kozlenko, D.P.M.,
M.P.H., founder

National Organizations

Academy of Psychosomatic Medicine
Box 1053
Mountainside, NY 07092

American Academy of Physical
Rehabilitation
30 N. Michigan Avenue, Suite 922
Chicago, IL 60602

American Academy of Stress
Disorders
8 S. Michigan Avenue
Chicago, IL 60603
R. Grayson, M.D., President

American Art Therapy Association
Art Therapy Department
Hahnemann Medical College
Philadelphia, PA 19102

American Association For Health,
Physical Education & Recreation
1201 16th Street, NW
Washington, DC 20036

The American Association for the
Study of Headache
621 South New Ballas Road
St. Louis, MO 63141

American Chinese Medical Society
303 E. 71st Street
New York, NY 10021
E.C.K. Tong, M.D., President

American Chiropractic Association
2200 Grand Avenue
Des Moines, IA 50312

American College of Nutrition
146 Central Park West
New York, NY 10023
(212) 874-4650
Seymour L. Halpern, M.D.

American College of Preventive
Medicine
801 Old Lancaster Road
Bryn Mawr, PA 19010

American Congress of Rehabilitation
Medicine
30 N. Michigan Avenue, Suite 922
Chicago, IL 60602

American Dance Therapy
Association
2000 Century Plaza, Suite 230
Columbia, MD 21044

American Foundation for
Homeopathy
910 17th Street NW, Suite 428-31
Washington, DC 20006
H. L. Trexler, M.D., President

American Geriatrics Society, Inc.
10 Columbus Circle
New York, NY 10019
(212) 582-1333

American Group Psychotherapy
Association, Inc.
1865 Broadway
New York, NY 10023

American Health Foundation
2200 Grand Avenue
Des Moines, IA 50312

American Holistic Medical Association
Route #2 Welsh Coulee Road
La Crosse, WI 54601

The American Institute of Nutrition
9650 Rockville Pike
Bethesda, MD 20014

American Medical Association
535 North Dearborn Street
Chicago, IL 60610

American Nurses' Association
2420 Pershing Road
Kansas City, MO 64108

American Occupational Therapy
Association
6000 Executive Blvd., Suite 200
Rockville, MD 20852

American Physical Therapy
Association
1156 15th Street NW
Washington, DC 20005

American Physiological Society
9650 Rockville Pike
Bethesda, MD 20014
E. E. Selkurt, Ph.D., President

American Psychoanalytic Association
One East 57th Street
New York, NY 10022

American Psychological Association
1200 17th Street NW
Washington, DC 20036

American Psychological Association
Division of Humanistic Psychology
10088 Ascan Avenue
Forest Hills, NY 11373
(212) 268-3384

American Psychological Association
Division of Philosophic Psychology
Psychology Department
St. Catherine College
2004 Randolph Road
St. Paul, MN 55105
(612) 698-5571

American Psychosomatic Society
265 Nassau Road
Roosevelt, NY 11575

American Public Health Association
1015 18th Street NW
Washington, DC 20036
C. A. Miller, M.D., President

American Society of Contemporary
Medicine and Surgery
6 N. Michigan Avenue
Chicago, IL 60602
M. E. DeBakey, M.D., President

American Society for Psychical
Research
5 West 73rd Street
New York, NY 10023

American Society for
Psychoprophylaxis in Obstetrics
(Lamaze)
36 West 96th Street
New York, NY 10025

Association of Academic Physiatrists
30 N. Michigan Avenue
Chicago, IL 60602
J. F. Lehmann, M.D., President

Association for Holistic Health
Box 33603
San Diego, CA 92123
(714) 298-5965
David Harris, founder
Richard Svihus, M.D., board
member

Association for Humanistic
Psychology
325 Ninth Street
San Francisco, CA 94103
(415) 626-2375

Association for Transpersonal
Psychology
Box 3049
Stanford, CA 94305
James Fadiman, Ph.D., President

Biofeedback Research Society
University of Colorado Medical
Center
Box C268, 4200 East Ninth Avenue
Denver, CO 80220
Francine Butler, Executive Secretary

California Council for Therapy and
Rehabilitation through Horticulture
1021 South Fifth Street
Alhambra, CA 91803

EWAHA/ Council of Nurse-Healers
33 Ora Way
San Francisco, CA 94131

Federation of American Society for
Experimental Biology
9650 Wisconsin Avenue
Washington, DC 20014

Gray Panthers
3700 Chestnut Street
Philadelphia, PA 19104
(215) 387-0918

Holistic Health Association
Box 61426
Houston, TX 77208
(713) 795-4263
Elliott Goldwag, Ph.D., founder

International Academy of
Orthomolecular and Preventive
Medicine
624 Shartle
Houston, TX 77002
(713) 468-3570

International Association for
Psychotronic Research
Box 107
Cotati, CA 94928

International Childbirth Education
Association
Box 20852
Milwaukee, WI 53220

International Chiropractors
Association
741 Brady Street
Davenport, IA 52808

International College of Applied
Nutrition
Box 386
La Habra, CA 90631

The International College of
Psychosomatic Medicine
c/o Adam J. Krakowski, M.D.
210 Cornelia Street, Suite 103
Plattsburgh, NY 12901

International Cooperation Council
8570 Wilshire Boulevard
Beverly Hills, CA 90211
(213) 652-4190

International Kirlian Research
Association
144 East 90th Street
New York, NY 10028
(212) 854-5196

International New Thought Alliance
6922 Hollywood Boulevard, No. 811
Hollywood, CA 90028
(213) 464-8361

International Society for General
Semantics
509 Sansome Street
San Francisco, CA 94126
(415) 391-9187

International Transactional Analysis
Association
1772 Vallejo Street
San Francisco, CA 94123

La Leche League International
9619 Minneapolis Avenue
Franklin Park, IL 60131

National Acupuncture Research
Society
505 Park Avenue, Suite 1508
New York, NY 10022

National Association for Music
Therapy
Box 610
Lawrence, KS 66044
(913) 842-1909

National Association for Veterinary
Acupuncture
Box 5181
Fullerton, CA 92635

The National Health Federation
212 West Foothill Boulevard
Monrovia, CA 91016
(213) 358-1155

Parapsychological Association
c/o G. J. Pratt, M.D.
Box 152, University of Virginia
Hospital
Charlottesville, VA 22901

Religious Research Association, Inc.
2511 North Main
North Newton, KS 67117

Society of Biological Psychiatry
2010 Wilshire Boulevard
Los Angeles, CA 90057

Society for Psychophysiological
Research
Experimental Psychology Laboratory
Syracuse University
Syracuse, NY 13210

Society for the Scientific Study of
Religion
Box U68A
University of Connecticut
Storrs, CN 06268

Society for Wholistic Medicine
137 S. Garfield
Hinsdale, IL 60521

United Society of Physiotherapists
c/o Patrick Trotta, Ph.T.
40-24 Taylor Road
Fairlawn, NJ 07410

Training-Oriented Centers

Western Region

Academy of Divine Healing
Dynamics, Inc.
9915 Eddy Road
Carmel Valley, CA 93924
(408) 625-1397
Wayne Cook, Founder

Aletheia Psycho-Physical Foundation
515 N.E. 8th
Grants Pass, OR 97526
Jack Schwarz, N.D., President
(503) 479-4855

The American Center for the
Alexander Technique
812 17th Street
Santa Monica, CA 90403
(213) 451-3641

Autogenic Health Center
6401 Broadway Terrace
Oakland, CA 94618
(415) 658-5913
Vera Fryling, M.D., founder

Berkeley Psychic Institute
2545 Regent Street
Berkeley, CA 94704
(415) 548-8020
The Rev. Lewis Bostwick, Director

Biofeedback Institute of San
Francisco
3428 Sacramento Street
San Francisco, CA 94118
(415) 921-5456
George D. Fuller, Ph.D., Clinical
Director

Biofeedback Research Institute
6325 Wilshire Blvd.
Los Angeles, CA 90048
(213) 933-9451

California Institute of Asian Studies
3494 21st Street
San Francisco, CA 94110
(415) 648-1489, 648-2644
Frederic Spiegelberg, Ph.D.,
President

California Yoga Teachers Association
1736 Ninth Avenue
San Francisco, CA 94122
(415) 566-4100

Center for Chinese Medicine
Box 32072
Los Angeles, CA 90032
(213) 282-2141

The Center for Designed Change
215 Cleveland Court
Mill Valley, CA 94941
(415) 388-8872, 388-1163
Dick Vittitow, Codirector

Center for Energetic Studies
1645 Virginia Street
Berkeley, CA 94703
(415) 647-4011
Stanley Keleman, Director

College of Health Sciences
Bernadean University
3519 Thom Boulevard
Las Vegas, NV 89106
(702) 645-1825
Dr. Joseph M. Kadans, President

Center for Integral Medicine
465 North Roxbury Drive, Suite 811
Beverly Hills, CA 90210
Richard Kroening, M.D.
David Bresler, Ph.D.
(213) 459-3373

College of Natural Therapeutics
1434 Fremont Avenue
Los Altos, CA 94022
Roy B. Oliver, N.D., U.S.
Representative

College of Oriental Studies
939 South New Hampshire Avenue
Los Angeles, CA 90006
(213) 487-1235, 384-0850
Ven. Dr. Thich Thien-An, President

East West Academy of Healing Arts
33 Ora Way
San Francisco, CA 94131
(415) 285-9400
Effie Poy Yew Chow, Ph.D.,
President

Effectiveness Training Associates
(P.E.T.)
110 South Euclid
Pasadena, CA 91101
(213) 796-5107
Dr. Thomas Gordon

Esalen Institute
Big Sur, CA 93920
(408) 667-2335

Explorations Institute
1711A Grove Street
Berkeley, CA 94709
(415) 548-1004
James Elliott, founder

GENESA
4702 San Jacinto Terrace
Fallbrook, CA 92028
(714) 728-2822
Derald G. Langham, Ph.D., founder

High Point Foundation
2916 East Dakota
Fresno, CA 93726
(209) 222-2034
Viola Davis, Ph.D., Director

High Point Foundation and
Psychosynthesis Training Center
647 North Madison Avenue
Pasadena, CA 91101
(213) 681-1033, 797-8355
Edith Stauffer, Ph.D., Executive
Director

High Point Northwest Foundation
828 Casper
Edmonds, WA 98020
(206) 775-1090

Holistic Health Organizing
Committee
1030 Merced
Berkeley, CA 94701

Humanistic Psychology Institute
325 Ninth Street
San Francisco, CA 94103
(415) 626-4494

Institute for the Advancement of
Human Behavior
Box 2288
Stanford, CA 94305
(415) 321-1895

Institute of Holistic Health Education
3150 Mission Drive
Santa Cruz, CA 95065
(408) 475-8296

Institute of Postural Integration
1057 Steiner Street
San Francisco, CA 94115
(415) 929-0119
Jack W. Painter, Ph.D., Director

Institute for the Study of
Consciousness
2924 Benvenue Avenue
Berkeley, CA 94705
(415) 849-4784
Arthur M. Young, President
Kenneth R. Pelletier, Ph.D., Director

Institute for the Study of Human
Knowledge
Box 2045
Stanford, CA 94305
Robert E. Ornstein, Ph.D., President

Charles T. Tart, Ph.D., Director of
Research

Institute for the Study of Humanistic
Medicine
3847 21st Street
San Francisco, CA 94114
(415) 285-2854
Allen B. Barbour, M.D.

Kundalini Research Institute
778 William
Pomona, CA 91768
(714) 623-1738
M.S.S. Gurucharan Singh Khalsa,
Director of Research
Yogi Bhajan, Spiritual Director

The Massage Guild
3119 Clement Street
San Francisco, CA 94121

National Center for the Exploration
of the Human Potential
976 Chalcedony Street
San Diego, CA 92109
(714) 272-7330
Herbert A. Otto, Ph.D., Director

National College of Naturopathic
Medicine
415 Postal Building
Portland, OR 97204

The National Sex Forum
540 Powell Street
San Francisco, CA 94108
(415) 421-5035

Novato Institute for Somatic
Research and Training
1516 Grant Avenue
Novato, CA 94947
(415) 897-0336
Eleanor Criswell, Ph.D., Director

Nurse Consultants and Health
Counselors
1931 Union Street
San Francisco, CA 94123
(415) 346-1526
Jocelyne M. Nielsen, R.N., Director

The Polarity Health Institute
Shasta Forest Lodge
Fall River Mills, CA 96028
(916) 336-5141

Polarity Therapy Workshops
401 North Glassell Street
Orange, CA 92666
(714) 532-1633
Pierre Pannetier, N.D., Director

Psychosynthesis Institute
3352 Sacramento Street
San Francisco, CA 94118
(415) 922-9182

The Radix Institute
Box 3218, 225 Santa Monica
Boulevard
Santa Monica, CA 90403
(213) 395-1555, (805) 646-8555
Charles R. Kelley, Ph.D., Director

Reflexology Institute of California
275 Summit Avenue
Mill Valley, CA 94941

Selective Awareness Seminars
1230 University Drive
Menlo Park, CA 94025
(415) 328-7171
Emmett E. Miller, M.D., Director

Sematodontics of Phoenix
Box 15668, 3718 E. Indian School
Road
Phoenix, AZ 85060
(602) 955-5662

Tibetan Nyingma Meditation Center
2425 Hillside Avenue
Berkeley, CA 94704
(415) 843-6812
Tarthang Tulku, Rimpoche, founder
and Head Lama

Touch for Health/Kinesiology
1192 North Lake Avenue
Pasadena, CA 91104
(213) 791-1201
John F. Thie, D.C.

University of the Trees
Box 644
Boulder Creek, CA 95006
(408) 338-3855
Christopher Hills, founder and
Director

Well-Springs
11667 Alba Road
Ben Lomond, CA 95005
(408) 336-8177
Kay Ortmans, founder

Central Region

Chicago Center for the Alexander
Technique
116 S. Michigan Avenue, Suite 1300
Chicago, IL 60603
Goddard Binkley, Director

Christos School of Natural Healing
Box 1503
Taos, NM 87571
William LeSassier, N.D., Founder

Himalayan International Institute of
Yoga Science and Philosophy
1505 Greenwood Road
Glenview, IL 60025
(312) 724-0300
Swami Rama, Director
Rudolph M. Ballentine, M.D.,
Director

National College of Naturopathic
Medicine
3100 McCormick Avenue
Wichita, KS 67213
H. Gordon Hurlburt, N.D.,
Administrator

Oasis Center for Human Potential
12 East Grand Avenue
Chicago, IL 60611
(312) 266-0033

Rolf Institute of Structural
Integration
Box 1868
Boulder, CO 80302
(303) 449-5903
Ida Rolf, Founder

Eastern Region

American Center for the Alexander
Technique, Inc.
142 West End Avenue
New York, NY 10023
(212) 799-0468

Center for Human Life Styling
Box 6585
St. Petersburg Beach, FL 33736
(813) 247-2131
John C. McCamy, M.D., founder

Creative Education Foundation, Inc.
State University College at Buffalo
1300 Elmwood Avenue
Buffalo, NY 14222
(716) 862-6221
Dr. Sidney J. Parnes, President

Creative Growth Workshops
510 LaGuardia Place
New York, NY 10012

Dialogue House Associates, Inc.
45 West 10th Street
New York, NY 10011
(212) 228-9180
Ira Progoff, Ph.D., founder

East West Foundation
359 Boylston Street
Boston, MA 02116
(617) 734-3853
Michio Kushi, founder

Encounters
5225 Connecticut Ave., N.W.
Washington, DC 20015
(202) 530-4485, 363-3033
L. Tirnauer, Ph.D., Director

Healing Seminars
c/o Dr. Joyce Goodrich
315 East 68th Street
New York, NY 10021
Dr. Lawrence LeShan, Director

The Human Dimensions Institute
4620 West Lake Road
Canandiagua, NY 14424
(716) 394-8173
Jeanne and Fred Rindge

Humanistic Psychology Center
285 Central Park West
New York, NY 10024
(212) 873-3668
Carmi Harari, Ed.D., Executive
Director

The Institute for Bioenergetic
Analysis
144 East 36th Street
New York, NY 10016
(212) 532-7742

Institute for the New Age of Man
340 East 57th Street
New York, NY 10022
(212) 753-5457
John C. Pierrakos, M.D., Director

The Institute for PsychoEnergetics
126 Harvard Street
Brookline, MA 02146
(617) 738-4502
Buryl Payne, Ph.D., Director

National Humanistic Education
Center
Springfield Road
Upper Jay, NY 12987

National Institute for the
Psychotherapies, Inc.
330 West 58th Street, Suite 200
New York, NY 10019
(212) 582-1566

National Institute of Reflexology
Box 948
Rochester, NY 14603

New England School of Acupuncture
1330 Beacon Street, Suite 315
Brookline, MA 02146
(617) 738-1398
James Tin Yau So, N.D.
David Gold, M.D.

The Psychomotor Institute
25 Huntingdon Avenue, Suite 415
Boston, MA 02116
(617) 261-2622
Albert and Diane Pesso, Codirectors

Psychosynthesis Research Foundation
40 East 49th Street, Room 1902
New York, NY 10017
(212) 759-1480

Shiatsu Education Center
52 West 55th Street
New York, NY 10019
(212) 582-3432

The Tai Chi Association
211 Canal Street
New York, NY 10001

Canada

Canadian Institute of
Psychosynthesis, Inc.
3496 Marlowe Avenue
Montreal, Quebec, Canada
Martha Crampton, Ph.D., Director

Evering Consultants Ltd.
43 Eglington Avenue East, Suite 803
Toronto, Ontario, Canada M4P 1A2
Dr. Terry Burrows

New Horizons Research Foundation
Box 427, Station F
Toronto, Ontario, Canada M4Y 2L8

Yasodhara Ashram
Box 9
Kootenay Bay, B.C., Canada VOB
1XO
(604) 227-9220
Swami Sivananda-Radha, President

Miscellaneous Resource Organizations

Anthroposophic Press, Inc.
258 Hungry Hollow Road
Spring Valley, NY 10977
(books of Rudolf Steiner and other authors)

Cancer Control Society
2043 N. Berendo
Los Angeles, CA 90027
(213) 663-7801

The Council for Homeopathic
Research and Education, Inc.
36 West 44th Street, Rm. 812
New York, NY 10036
Claude H. Schmidt, Ph.D., President

Euthanasia Education Council
250 West 57th Street
New York, NY 10019

Foundation for Research on the
Nature of Man
402 Buchanan
Durham, NC 27708

Health Maintenance Center
1370 Avenue of the Americas
New York, NY 10019

Health Research Publishers
Box 70
Mokelumne Hill, CA 95245

Hidden Valley Health Ranch
Route 6, Box 881
Escondido, CA 92025
(714) 745-2742
Dr. Bernard Jensen, Director

Institute of Nutritional Research
Box 3413
Los Angeles, CA 90028

Inter-Health, Inc.
2970 Fifth Avenue
San Diego, CA 92103

Life Extension Institute
Stevens Tower
1185 Avenue of the Americas
New York, NY 10036
(212) 572-8300

Lucis Trust
866 United Nations Plaza, Suite 566-7
New York, NY 10017
(212) 421-1577
Alice Bailey, founder

New Dimensions Foundation
267 States
San Francisco, CA 94114
(415) 621-1126

Oncology Associates
1413 8th Avenue
Fort Worth, TX 76104
(817) 926-7821
O. Carl Simonton, M.D.

Pacific Research Systems/Nutrition,
Health & Activity Profile
2222 Corinth Avenue
Los Angeles, CA 90064
(213) 478-1718

Parapsychology Foundation
29 West 57th Street
New York, NY 10019
Eileen Garrett, founder

Psychical Research Foundation
Duke Station
Durham, NC 27706

SIECUS: Sex Information and
Education Council of the United
States
122 East 42nd Street, Suite 922
New York, NY 10017
(212) 611-7010

World Institute Council
777 United Nations Plaza
New York, NY 10017

Yes Educational Society
1035 31st Street NW
Washington, DC 20007
(202) 338-7874

Growth-Oriented Organizations

Western Region

Aikido of San Francisco
678 Turk Street
San Francisco, CA
(415) 441-6087
Robert C. Nadeau, Director

Ananta Foundation
214 Gridley Rd.
Ojai, CA 93023
Marcia Moore, founder

Anderson Research Foundation, Inc.
3960 Ingraham Street
Los Angeles, CA 90005
(213) 387-9164
Dr. Laurence Anderson, Director

Anthos Growth Center
24 East 22 Street, 8th Floor
New York, NY 10010
(212) 260-8148

Astara
792 West Arrow Highway
Upland, CA 91786

Asunaro Eastern Studies Institute
134 Acres
Sonoma, CA
(707) 996-9659
Noboru Muramoto, founder

Biocentric Institute
9255 Sunset Boulevard, Suite 716
Los Angeles, CA 90069
Nathaniel Branden

Bio-Energetics Northwest
3938 First NE
Seattle, WA 98105
(206) 639-9210
Alan M. Clarke, M.D.

Center for Being and Becoming
789 West End Avenue
New York, NY 10025
(212) 663-4372

The Center for Developing
Conscious Vision
4902 California Street
San Francisco, CA 94104
(415) 668-4528

Center for Human Communication
120 Oak Meadow Drive
Los Gatos, CA 95030
(408) 354-6466

The Center for Studies of the Person
1125 Torry Pines Road
La Jolla, CA 92037

Creative Bodywork Center
4338 California Street
San Francisco, CA
(415) 221-2683

Crossroads Communications, Inc.
325 9th Street
San Francisco, CA 94103

Devta
122 Ward Street
Larkspur, CA 94939
(415) 924-0406

East West Center of Macrobiotic
Studies
7511 Franklin Avenue
Hollywood, CA 90046
(213) 876-9153

East-West Cultural Center
2865 West 9th Street
Los Angeles, CA 90006
(213) 480-8325
Dr. Judith M. Tyberg, founder

Eckankar
Box 3100
Menlo Park, CA 94025

Eductivism
1777 Union Street
San Francisco, CA 94123
(415) 673-5200
Jack Horner, founder

EST: Erhard Seminars Training
1750 Union Street
San Francisco, CA 94123
(415) 441-0100
Werner Erhard, founder

Garden of Sanjivani
2083 Ocean Street Extension
Santa Cruz, CA 95060
(408) 425-0597

George Ohsawa Macrobiotic
Foundation
1471 10th Avenue
San Francisco, CA 94122

Getting in Touch
Box 1225
Los Gatos, CA 95030
(408) 353-3770
Rita and Lorne Bay, Directors

Guild for Growth
861 University Avenue
Palo Alto, CA 94301
(415) 326-3707

The Healing Light Center
138 N. Maryland Ave.
Glendale, CA 91206
(213) 244-8607
The Rev. Rosalyn Bruyere, Director

Health Concerns
2223 L Street
Sacramento, CA 95816
(916) 444-2134
James R. Walt, President

Hoffman Quadrinity Center
Fischer-Hoffman Process
1005 Sansome Street
San Francisco, CA 94111
(415) 397-0466
Bob Hoffman, founder

Holistic Childbirth Institute
1627 Tenth Avenue
San Francisco, CA 94122
(415) 664-1119

Inner Light Foundation
Box 761
Novato, CA 94947
(415) 897-5581
The Rev. Betty Bethards, founder

The Institute for Bioenergetics and
Gestalt
1307 University Avenue
Berkeley, CA 94702
(415) 849-0101
Michael B. Conant, Ph.D., Director

Institute for Conscious Birth
223 South Alexandria Street
Los Angeles, CA 90004
(213) 383-6713

Institute of Reality Awareness
8217 Beverly Boulevard, Suite 7
Los Angeles, CA 90048
(213) 658-8600
Leslie J. Kent, D.D., Director
Renee Stampler, D.C., Associate
Director

Internal School
1251 9th Street
Arcata, CA 95521
(707) 822-2908

Krishnamurti Foundation of America
Box 216
Ojai, CA 93023
(805) 646-2726

Lifespring
2237 Union Street
San Francisco, CA 94123
(415) 921-5433

Lomi School
2250 Bush Street
San Francisco, CA 94115
(415) 931-5924

The Love Project
Box 7601
San Diego, CA 92107
(714) 225-0133
Diane K. Pike, founder

Making Ways
40 Power Lane
Fairfax, CA 94930
(415) 652-4400

Mann Ranch Seminars
Box 570
Ukiah, CA 95482
(707) 462-3514

Meditation Group for the New Age
Box 566
Ojai, CA 93023

Metamorphosis Institute
550 Waldo Point
Sausalito, CA 94965
(415) 332-0569

Mountain Grove
Barton Road
Glendale, OR 97442
(503) 832-2211

National Family Communication
Skills Center
350 Sharon Park Drive, Suite A-23
Menlo Park, CA 94025
Win Colton, Director

Niscience, Inc.
336 West Colorado Street
Glendale, CA 91204
(213) 244-0113
Ann Ree Colton, founder

Odysseus
409B Alberto Way
Los Gatos, CA 95030

Open Door Clinic
1000 H Street
Eureka, CA 95501
(707) 822-2957
Gena Pennington, M.D., Director

Passage-Ways
818 Cherry Street
Santa Rosa, CA 95405
(707) 526-8800

Phenomenon of Man
Philosophy of Teilhard de Chardin
8932 Reseda Boulevard, Suite 204
Northridge, CA 91324
(213) 886-5260

The Philosophical Research Society,
Inc.
3910 Los Feliz Boulevard
Los Angeles, CA 90027
(213) 663-2167
Manly P. Hall, President

The Phoenix Institute
976 Chalcedony Street
San Diego, CA 92109
(714) 488-0626
Dr. Kathryn Breese-Whiting,
President

Polestar Foundation
20688 4th Street
Saratoga, CA 95070
(408) 867-1100

Prana Yoga Ashram
488 Spruce Street
Berkeley, CA 94708
(415) 527-8648
Swami Sivalingam, founder and
Director

Precision Psychodrama Institute
3960 Ingraham Street
Los Angeles, CA 90005
(213) 387-9164

Prometheus
401 Florence Avenue
Palo Alto, CA 94301
(415) 328-6137

PSI: Psycho-Spiritual Integration
One Northwood Drive, Suite 5
Orinda, CA 94563
(415) 254-1450
Ernest F. Pecci, M.D., Director

SAGE Seminars
1190 Park Avenue
San Jose, CA 95126
(408) 294-6606

SAGE: Senior Actualization and
Growth Exploration
2455 Hilgard Avenue
Berkeley, CA 94709
(415) 841-9858
Gay Gaer Luce, Ph.D., founder

Sandstone
21400 Saddle Peak Road
Topanga, CA 90290
(213) 455-9055
Paul Paige, Ph.D., Director

Self-Realization Fellowship
3880 San Rafael Avenue
Los Angeles, CA 90065
(213) 225-2471
Founded by Paramahansa
Yogananda

Shanom
1527 Shoreline Drive
Santa Barbara, California
(805) 299-1842

Shanti Nilaya
Box 2396
Escondido, CA 92025
Elisabeth Kubler-Ross, M.D.,
founder

SIMS: Students International
Meditation Society
1015 Gayley Avenue
Los Angeles, CA 90024
(213) 478-1569
Maharishi Yogi, founder

Soma Institute for Body Therapy
4676 Admiralty Way
Marina del Rey, CA 90291
(213) 823-7009

Structural Patterning Institute
300 Valley Street
Sausalito, CA 94965
(415) 332-3771
Judith Aston, founder

Subud, USA
Box 116
San Rafael, CA 94902

Sunrise Center
1554 - 46th Avenue
San Francisco, CA 94122
(415) 681-8133

Synergy Seminars
P.O. Box 855
Sausalito, CA 94965

Tahoe Institute
Box DD
South Lake Tahoe, CA 95729

Tatagata's Forest
Box 216
Ben Lomond, CA 95005
(408) 336-2336

The National Center for the
Exploration of Human Potential
222 Westbourne St.
La Jolla, CA 92037
(714) 459-2785
Herbert A. Otto, Ph.D., Chairman

The Topanga Center for Human
Development
2247 West Topanga Canyon Blvd.
Topanga, CA 90290

Unfolding Path
1578 Willowmont Avenue
San Jose, CA 95118
(408) 266-7051

United Church of Religious Science
3251 West Sixth Street
Los Angeles, CA 90020
(213) 388-2181
Ernest Holmes, founder

The Village Oz
P.O. Box 86
Point Arena, CA 95468

Vortex Institute
Box 73152
Fairbanks, AK 99707
(907) 452-5954

Whole Life Center
3437 Alma Street
Palo Alto, CA 94306
(415) 493-0561
Carl Ebnother, M.D.

Yogi Academy Foundation
3209 Burton Avenue, SE
Albuquerque, NM 87107

Zen Mission Society
Shasta Abbey
Mount Shasta, CA 96067
Rev. Juyu Kennett, Roshi, Abbess

Central Region

American Medical-Psychic Research
Assn.
135 Madison Avenue NE
Albuquerque, NM 87108
(505) 265-0221

Association for the Understanding of
Man
Box 5310
Austin, TX 78763

Boulder Center for the Healing Arts
855 Arapahoe
Boulder, CO 80302

Boulder School of Massage Therapy
2855 Walnut Street
Boulder, CO 80302
(303) 443-5131

Cambridge House
1900 North Cambridge Avenue
Milwaukee, WI 53202

Center for Creative Communication
666 Manhattan, No. 1
Boulder, CO 80303
(303) 499-5366

Center of Spiritual Awareness
Box 7
Lakemont, GA 30552
Roy Eugene Davis

Concept-Therapy Institute
Route 8, Box 250
San Antonio, TX 78228

Dream Counsellors Inc.
139 Madison Avenue, NE
Albuquerque, NM 87108
(505) 265-0221
Ralph Yaney, M.D.

ESP Research Associates Foundation
Suite 1630, Union National Plaza
Little Rock, AR 72201
(501) 375-5377
Harold Sherman, founder
Olga Worrall, member, board of
directors

Feathered Pipe Ranch
Colorado Gulch
Helena, MT 59601
(406) 442-8196

Fransisters and Brothers
2168 Lafayette Street
Denver, CO 80210

The Houston Center for Potential
Growth
1214 Miramar
Houston, TX 77006

Institute of Human Engineering
3680 E. Fall Creek Parkway
Indianapolis, IN 46205
(317) 923-6626

Institute for Living, Inc.
2309 Delancey Place
Philadelphia, PA 19103
(215) 546-7344

Le Centre du Silence (Mime)
701 Arapahoe Ave., Suite 206
Boulder, CO 80302
Avital, Director

Midwestern Institute of
Parapsycholology
Box 282
Mason City, IA 50401

Naropa Institute
1111 Pearl Street
Boulder, CO 80302
(303) 444-0202
Chogyam Trungpa, Rinpoche,
founder

Ontological Society
Sunrise Ranch, Box 328
Loveland, CO 80537
(303) 667-0599

Phoenix Institute
1400 Foothill Boulevard
Salt Lake City, UT 84108

Psyche Research Institute
10701 Lomas N.E., Suite 210
Albuquerque, NM 87112
(505) 292-0370

Psychic Research Foundation
203 North Wabash Avenue, Suite
1820
Chicago, IL 60601
Rev. Henry Rucker, Director

School of the Natural Order
Box 578
Baker, NV 89311
Founded by Vitvan

School of Yoga
517 Lovett Boulevard
Houston, TX 77006
(713) 522-8938

Spiritual Advisory Council
93 Spring Creek Road, Rt. 5
Lockport, IL 60441
Ethel Lombardi, founder

Spiritual Frontiers Fellowship, Inc.
800 Custer Avenue
Evanston, IL 60202

THEOS: They Help Each Other
Spiritually
11609 Frankstown Road
Pittsburgh, PA 15235
Bea Decker, Director

Unity School of Christianity
Unity Village, MO 64065
(816) 524-3550

Eastern Region

Arica Institute, Inc.
24 West 57th Street
New York, NY 10019
(212) 489-7430

Association for Research and
Enlightenment
Edgar Cayce Library and
Documentation
Box 595
Virginia Beach, VA 23451
(804) 428-3588

Awareness Center
685 West End Avenue, #17A
New York, NY 10025
Bernard Green, Ph.D.

Center for the Development of
Human Resources
Wainwright House, Milton Point
Rye, NY 10580

Center for Integrative Education
12 Church Street
New Rochelle, NY 10805

Center for the Whole Person
517 South 22nd Street
Philadelphia, PA 19146

Center for the Whole Person
Route 1, Box 84
Mays Landing, NJ 08330

Creativity Laboratories
463 West St.
New York, NY 10014

East West Foundation
359 Boylston Street
Boston, MA 02116

Greenhouse
12 Essex Street
Cambridge, MA 02139

The Hill Center for Psychosynthesis
in Education
Old Walpole Road
Walpole, NH 03608

Hippocrates Health Institute
25 Exeter Street
Boston, MA 02116
(617) 267-9525, 266-1669
Ann Wigmore, Ph.D., Director

Huxley Institute for Bio-Social
Research
56 West 45th Street, Suite 805
New York, NY 10036

Inner Light Consciousness Institute
Box 206
Virginia Beach, VA 23458
(804) 428-4650
The Rev. Paul Solomon, founder

Integral Yoga Institute
500 West End Avenue
New York, NY 10000
(212) 874-7500

Kundalini Research Foundation
10 East 39th Street
New York, NY 10016
(212) 889-3241
Gopi Krishna, founder

Lisle Fellowship
511 Meadow Hall Drive
Rockville, MD 20851
(301) 762-3054

The Mankind Research Foundation
1640 Kalmia NW
Washington, DC 20012
(202) 882-4000

New Haven Center for Human
Relations
400 Prospect Street
New Haven, CT 06511

Quest
4933 Auburn Avenue
Bethesda, MD 20014
(301) 652-0697

Sri Chinmoy Centre, Inc.
Box 32433
Jamaica, NY 11431

Suffolk Growth Center
Box 136
Mount Sinai, NY 11766
(516) 744-4768

Synergos
3920 SW 67 Terrace
Fort Lauderdale, FL 33314

Vedanta Society
34 West 71st Street
New York, NY 10023

Wainwright House
Center for Development of Human
Resources
260 Stuyvesant Avenue
Rye, NY 10580

Yoga Institute of Washington, Inc.
1629 K Street NW, Suite 539A
Washington, DC 20006

Bibliography

THE BIBLIOGRAPHY represents an initial attempt by the editors to select books that appear to be relevant to the burgeoning field of wholistic healing. A bibliography of this type can make no claim to being comprehensive. The primary reason for inclusion of books has been that the editors have found them to be, not only informative, but challenging, stimulating, and thought provoking.

Acupuncture

Austin, Mary. *Acupuncture Therapy*. New York: ASI, 1972.

Houston, F. M. *The Healing Benefits of Acupressure: Acupuncture without Needles*. New Canaan, Conn.: Keats, 1974.

Mann, Felix. *The Ancient Chinese Art of Healing: Acupuncture*. New York: Random House, 1963.

McGarey, William A. *Acupuncture and Body Energies*. Phoenix: Gabriel Press, 1974.

Motoyama, Hiroshi. *Chakra, Nadi of Yoga and Meridians, Points of Acupuncture*. Tokyo: Institute for Religious Psychology, 1972.

Motoyama, Hiroshi. *The Ejection of Energy from the Chakra of Yoga and Meridian Points of Acupuncture*. Tokyo: Institute for Religious Psychology, 1975.

Motoyama, Hiroshi. *How To Measure and Diagnose the Functions of Meridian Points of Acupuncture*. Tokyo: Institute of Religious Psychology, 1975.

Veith, Ilza. "Acupuncture Therapy—Past and Present," *Journal of the American Medical Association*, May 12, 1972.

Anatomy-Pharmacology-Physiology

Anson, Barry J. *Atlas of Human Anatomy*. 5th ed. Philadelphia: W. B. Saunders, 1971.

Conn, Howard F., ed. *Current Therapy 1976*. Philadelphia: W. B. Saunders, 1976.

Davson, Hugh, and Eggleton, Grace, eds. *Starling & Lovatt Evans Principles of Human Physiology*. 14th ed. London: J. & A. Churchill, 1968.

Goodman, Louis S., and Gilman, Alfred, eds. *Pharmacological Basis of Therapeutics*. New York: Macmillan, 1975.

Gray, Henry. *Gray's Anatomy*. 29th American ed. Philadelphia: Lea & Febiger, 1973.

Body Awareness

Alexander, F. Matthias. *The Alexander Technique*. New York: University Press, 1969.

Barlow, Wilfred. *The Alexander Technique*. New York: Knopf, 1973.

Cannon, Walter B. *The Wisdom of the Body*. New York: W. W. Norton, 1963.

Cooper, Kenneth. *Aerobics*. New York: Bantam, 1972.

Downing, George, and Rush, Anne Kent. *The Massage Book*. New York: Random House, 1972.

Feitis, Rosemary. *Ida Rolf Talks About Rolfing and Physical Reality*. New York: Harper and Row, 1978.

Feldenkrais, Moshe. *Awareness through Movement*. New York: Harper and Row, 1972.

Keyes, Ken, Jr. *Loving Your Body*, New York: Frederick Fell, 1974.

Kurtz, Ron, and Prestera, Hector. *The Body Reveals: An Illustrated Guide to the Psychology of the Body*. New York: Harper and Row, 1976.

Lowen, Alexander. *The Betrayal of the Body*. New York: Collier, 1967.

———. *Bioenergetics*. New York: Penguin, 1975.

Rolf, Ida. *Rolfing*. Santa Monica, Calif.: Dennis-Landman, 1977.

Spino, Mike. *Beyond Jogging*. Millbrae, Calif.: Celestial Arts, 1976.

Yoels, Jennifer. *Re-Shape Your Body, Revitalize Your Life*. Englewood Cliffs, N.J.: Prentice-Hall, 1972.

For and about Children

Berends, Polly Berrien. *Whole Child/Whole Parent*. New York: Harper's Magazine Press, 1975.

Briggs, Dorothy Corkille. *Your Child's Self-Esteem*. Garden City, N.Y.: Doubleday, 1975.

Button, Alan D. *The Authentic Child*. New York: Random House, 1969.

Carr, Rachel. *Be a Frog, a Bird or a Tree*. Garden City, N.Y.: Doubleday, 1973.

Freed, Alvyn, *TA for Tots*. Sacramento, Calif.: A. M. Freed, 1973.

Gold, Cybele. *Joyous Childbirth*. Berkeley, Calif.: And-Or Press, 1977.

Hodgson, Joan. *Hullo Sun*. Liss, Hampshire, England: White Eagle Publishing Trust, 1972.

Janov, Arthur. *The Feeling Child*. New York: Simon & Schuster, 1973.

Kent, Howard. *My Fun with Yoga*. London: Hamlyn, 1975.

Khan, Sufi Inayat. *Education from Before Birth to Maturity*. London: Sufi, 1974.

Leboyer, Frederick. *Birth without Violence*. New York: Knopf, 1976.

———. *Loving Hands*. New York: Knopf, 1976.

Lederman, Janet. *Anger and the Rocking Chair*. New York: Viking, 1969.

Milinaire, Caterine. *Birth*. New York: Harmony, 1974.

Montessori, Maria. *The Absorbent Mind*. New York: Dell, 1967.

———. *The Discovery of the Child*. New York: Ballantine, 1974.

Piaget, Jean. *The Early Growth of Logic in the Child*. New York: W. W. Norton, 1969.

Richards, Ruth, and Abrams, Joy. *Let's Do Yoga*. New York: Holt, Rinehart and Winston, 1975.

Rozman, Deborah. *Meditating with Children*. Boulder Creek, Calif.: University of the Trees Press, 1975.

Satchidanda, Sri Swami. *The Mother Is the Baby's First Guru*. Pomfret Center, Conn.: Satchidanda Ashram-Yogaville, 1976.

Urbanowski, Ferris. *Yoga for New Parents*. New York: Balaram, Harper's Magazine Press, 1975.

West, Bill G. *Free to Be Me*. New York: World, 1971.

Consciousness

Carrington, Patricia. *Freedom in Meditation*. Garden City, N.Y.: Doubleday, Anchor, 1977.

Castaneda, Carlos. *A Separate Reality: Further Conversations with Don Juan*. New York: Simon & Schuster, 1971.

———. *Journey to Ixtlan: The Lessons of Don Juan*. New York: Simon & Schuster, 1972.

————. *Tales of Power*. New York: Simon & Schuster, 1974.

Colton, Ann Ree. *Watch Your Dreams*. New York: Arc, 1973.

Faraday, Ann. *The Dream Game*. New York: Harper and Row, 1974.

Ferguson, Marilyn. *The Brain Revolution*. New York: Bantam, 1975.

Franck, Frederick. *The Zen of Seeing: Seeing/Drawing as Meditation*. New York: Vintage, 1973.

Grof, Stanislav. *Realms of the Human Unconscious*. New York: E. P. Dutton, 1976.

Hanson, Virginia. *Approaches to Meditation*. Wheaton, Ill.: Theosophical Publishing House, 1973.

Ichazo, Oscar. *What Is Mind; What Is Reasoning; What Is Consciousness; What Is History, and What Is Arica*. New York: Arica Institute, 1975.

Jacobson, E. *Progressive Relaxation*. Chicago: University of Chicago Press, 1938.

Johnston, William. *Silent Music*. New York: Harper and Row, 1974.

Jung, Carl G. *Memories, Dreams, Reflections*. New York: Vintage, 1963.

————. *Man and His Symbols*. Garden City, N.Y.: Doubleday, 1964.

Krippner, Stanley, and Rubin, Daniel. *The Energies of Consciousness: Explorations in Acupuncture, Auras and Kirlian Photography*. New York: Gordon and Breach Science Publishers, 1975.

Luthe, W., ed. *Autogenic Therapy*. Vol. 1–5. New York: Grune and Stratton, 1969.

————. *Creativity Mobilization Technique*. New York: Grune and Stratton, 1975.

Massy, Robert E. *Hill's Theory of Consciousness*. Boulder Creek, Calif.: University of the Trees Press, 1976.

Metzner, Ralph. *Maps of Consciousness*. London: Collier Macmillan, 1971.

Mishlove, Jeffrey. *The Roots of Consciousness, Psychic Liberation through History, Science and Experience*. New York: Random House, 1975.

Naranjo, Claudio, and Ornstein, Robert E. *On the Psychology of Meditation*. New York: Viking, 1971.

Null, Gary. *Biofeedback, Fasting and Meditation*. New York: Pyramid Communications, 1974.

Ornstein, Robert E. *The Psychology of Consciousness*. San Francisco: W. H. Freeman, 1972.

————, ed. *The Nature of Human Consciousness*. San Francisco: W. H. Freeman, 1973.

Radah, Swami Sivananda. *Divine Light Invocation*. India: Swami Sivananda Radha, 1966.

Reschtschaffen, A.; Kales, A.; Berger, R. J.; Dement, W. C.; Jacobson, A.; Johnson, L. C.; Jouvet, M.; Monroe, L. J.; Oswald, I.; Roffward, H.P.; Roth, B.; and Walter, R. D. *A Manual of Standardized Terminology, Techniques and Scoring System for Sleep Stages of Human Subjects.* Washington, D.C.: U. S. Public Health Service, 1968.

Sayadaw, Mahasi. *Practical Insight Meditation.* San Francisco: Unity Press, 1972.

Schwartz, Gary E., and Shapiro, David. *Consciousness and Self-Regulation.* New York: Plenum, 1976.

Segal, Julius, and Luce, Gay Gaer. *The Third World of the Mind: Sleep.* New York: Coward McCann, 1972.

Shattock, E. H. *An Experiment in Mindfulness.* New York: Samuel Weiser, 1972.

Stone, Justin F. *Meditation for Healing.* Albuquerque, N.M.: Sun Publishing Company, 1977.

Tart, Charles T. *States of Consciousness.* New York: E. P. Dutton, 1975.

———, ed. *Altered States of Consciousness.* Garden City, N.Y.: Doubleday, Anchor, 1969.

Weil, Andrew. *The Natural Mind,* Boston: Houghton Mifflin, 1970.

White, John. *The Highest State of Consciousness.* Garden City, N.Y.: Doubleday, Anchor, 1972.

Zubek, John P., ed. *Sensory Deprivation: Fifteen Years of Research.* New York: Appleton-Century-Crofts, 1969.

On Death and Dying

Becker, E. *The Denial of Death.* New York: Macmillan, 1973.

———. *Escape from Evil.* New York: Macmillan, Free Press, 1975.

Brown, Norman O. *Life against Death.* Middletown, Conn.: Wesleyan University Press, 1959.

Budge, E. A. Wallis. *The Egyptian Book of the Dead.* New York: Dover, 1967.

Choron, J. *Death and Western Thought.* New York: Colliers, 1963.

———. *Death and Modern Man (Modern Man and Mortality).* New York: Collier Macmillan, 1972.

Colton, Ann Ree. *Men in White Apparel.* Glendale, Calif.: Arc, 1961.

Cutler, Donald, et al. *Updating Life and Death.* Boston: Beacon, 1970.

Davitz, L., and Davitz, J. "How Do Nurses Feel When Patients Suffer?" *American Journal of Nursing,* September 1975.

Evans-Wentz, W. Y. *The Tibetan Book of the Dead*. New York: Oxford University Press, 1974.

Garfield, C. "Consciousness Alteration and Fear of Death." *Journal of Trans-Personal Psychology* 7, no. 2 (1975): 147.

Glaser, Barney G., and Strauss, Anselm L. *Awareness of the Dying*. Chicago: Aldine, 1965.

Grollman, Earl A. *Talking about Death*. Boston: Beacon, 1970.

Hutschnecker, Arnold A. *The Will to Live*, New York: Cornerstone Library, 1974.

Jacobson, Nils. *Life without Death*. New York: Delacorte, Dell, 1974.

Jury, Dan. *Gramp*. New York: Grossman, 1975.

Kasten, R. B., and Aisenberg, R. *Psychology of Death*. New York: Springer, 1972.

Kavanaugh, Robert E. *Facing Death*. Baltimore: Benguin, 1974.

Keleman, Stanley. *Living Your Dying*. New York: Random House-Bookworks, 1974.

Kobrzycki, P. "Dying with Dignity at Home." *American Journal of Nursing*, August 1975.

Kubler-Ross, Elizabeth. *On Death and Dying*. New York: Macmillan, 1969.

⸻. *Questions and Answers on Death and Dying*. New York: Macmillan, 1974.

⸻. *Death: The Final Stage of Growth*. Englewood Cliffs, N.J.: Prentice-Hall, 1975.

Mills, Liston A., ed. *Perspectives on Death*. Nashville: Abingdon, 1969.

Noyes, Russel. "The Experience of Dying." *Psychiatry* 35 (May 1972).

Parkes, Colin Murray. *Bereavement*. New York: International University Press, 1972.

Pattison, E. "The Experience of Dying." *The American Journal of Psychotherapy* 21, no. 1 (1967): 32.

Sudnow, David. *Passing On*. Englewood Cliffs, N.J.: Prentice-Hall, 1967.

Switzer, David. *Dynamics of Grief*. Nashville: Abingdon, 1970.

Thielicke, Helmut. *Death and Life*. Philadelphia: Fortress, 1970.

Verwoerdt, Adriaan. *Communication with the Fatally Ill*. Springfield, Ill.: Charles C. Thomas, 1966.

Watson, Lyall. *The Romeo Error: A Matter of Life and Death*. Garden City, N.Y.: Doubleday, 1974.

Weisman, Avery. *On Dying and Denying*. New York: Behavioral Publications, 1970.

Eastern Philosophy and Religion

Baba, Meher. *Beams from Meher Baba on the Spiritual Panorama*. New York: Harper and Row, 1971.

Dass, Ram. *The Only Dance There Is*. Garden City, N.Y.: Doubleday, 1974.

Govinda, Lama Anagarika. *Foundations of Tibetan Mysticism*. New York: Samuel Weiser, 1974.

Kapleau, Philip. *The Three Pillars of Zen*. New York: Harper and Row, 1961.

Organ, T. W. *The Hindu Quest for the Perfection of Man*. Athens, Ohio: Ohio University Press, 1970.

Reifler, Sam. *I Ching: A New Interpretation for Modern Times*. New York: Bantam, 1974.

Sandweiss, Samuel H. *Sai Baba/ The Holy Man and the Psychiatrist*. San Diego: Birth Day, 1975.

Shah, Idries. *The Sufis*. Garden City, N.Y.: Doubleday, 1971.

Singh, Trilochan, et al. *The Sacred Writings of the Sikhs*. New York: Samuel Weiser, 1973.

Siu, R. G. H. *The Portable Dragon: The Western Man's Guide to the I Ching*. Cambridge, Mass.: Massachusetts Institute of Technology Press, 1974.

Suzuki, D. T. *The Field of Zen*. New York: Harper and Row, 1969.

Suzuki, Shunryu. *Zen Mind, Beginner's Mind*. New York: Weatherhill, 1974.

Trungpa, Chogyam. *Cutting through Spiritual Materialism*. Berkeley, Calif.: Shambhala, 1973.

Watts, Alan. *The Spirit of Zen: A Way of Life, Work, and Art in the Far East*. New York: Grove, 1958.

Wilhelm, R. *The I Ching*. Bollingen Series 19. Princeton, N.J.: Princeton University Press, 1967.

Yogananda, Paramahansa. *Autobiography of a Yogi*. Los Angeles: Self-Realization Fellowship, 1969.

Ethnic Healing Systems

Boyd, Doug. *Rolling Thunder*. New York: Random House, 1974.

Chow, Effie Poy Yew. *Acupuncture: Its History and Its Educational Significance to Western Health Practices in the USA*. Santa Barbara, Calif.: The Fielding Institute, 1975.

Dash, Vd. Bhagwan. *Ayurvedic Treatment for Common Diseases*. New Delhi: Delhi Diary Publishers, 1974.

Dimond, E. Grey. More Than Herbs and Acupuncture. New York: W. W. Norton, 1975.

Djukanovic, V., and Mach, E. P. *Alternative Approaches to Meeting Basic Health Needs in Developing Countries.* Geneva, Switzerland: World Health Organization, 1975.

Erdoes, Richard, and Lame Deer, John (Fire). *Lame Deer: Seeker of Visions.* New York: Simon & Schuster, 1972.

Huang Ti Nei Ching Su Wen. *The Yellow Emperor's Classic of Internal Medicine,* translated by Ilza Veith. Berkeley and Los Angeles: University of California Press, 1966.

Huard, Pierre, and Wong, Ming. *Chinese Medicine.* New York: McGraw-Hill, 1968.

Lewis, J. H. *The Biology of the Negro.* Chicago: University of Chicago Press, 1942.

Namikoshi, Tokujiro. *Shiatsu: Japanese Finger Pressure Therapy.* San Francisco: Japan Publications, 1974.

Palos, Stephan. *The Chinese Art of Healing.* New York: Herder & Herder, 1963.

Reitzes, D. C. *Negroes and Medicine.* Cambridge, Mass.: Harvard University Press, 1958.

Rinpoche, Rechung. *Tibetan Medicine.* Berkeley and Los Angeles: University of California Press, 1973.

Steiger, Brad. *Medicine Power.* Garden City, N.Y.: Doubleday, 1974.

Storm, Hyemeyohsts. *Seven Arrows.* New York: Ballantine, 1972.

Thakkur, Chandrasekhar G. *Introduction to Ayurveda: The Science of Life.* New York: ASI, 1974.

Vogel, Virgil J. *American Indian Medicine.* New York: Ballantine, 1970.

Wallnoffer, Henrich, and von Rottauscher, Ann. *Chinese Folk Medicine.* New York: Crown, 1971.

Walters, Frank. *Book of the Hopi.* New York: Ballantine, 1963.

Weslager, C. A. *Magic Medicines of the Indians.* Wallingford, Pa.: The Middle Atlantic Press, 1973.

Williams, Richard A. *Textbook of Black-Related Diseases.* New York: McGraw-Hill, 1975.

Medicine-Surgery

Ackerman, Lauren V. *Surgical Pathology.* 3d ed. St. Louis: C. V. Mosby, 1964.

Artz, Curtis P., and Hardy, James D. *Complications in Surgery and Their Management,* Philadelphia: W. B. Saunders, 1961.

Cooper, Philip. *The Craft of Surgery*. 3 vols. 2d ed. Boston: Little, Brown, 1971.

Gell, P. G. H., Coombs, R. R. A., and Lachmann, P. J. *Clinical Aspects of Immunology*. 3d ed. Oxford: Blackwell Scientific, 1975.

Gross, Robert E. *Surgery of Infancy and Childhood*. Philadelphia: W. B. Saunders, 1953.

Moore, Francis D. *Metabolic Care of the Surgical Patient*. Philadelphia: W. B. Saunders, 1959.

Nelson, Waldo E. *Textbook of Pediatrics*. 10th ed. Philadelphia: W. B. Saunders, 1975.

Natural Remedies

Airola, Paavo. *How to Get Well*, Phoenix: Health Plus, 1974.

————. *Health Secrets from Europe*. New York: Arco, 1975.

Bates, W. H. *Better Eyesight without Glasses*. New York: Henry Holt, 1940/1943.

Blackie, Dr. Margery G. *The Patient, Not the Cure*. Great Britain: MacDonald and Co., Ltd., 1976.

Blattacharyya, A. K. *Septenate Mixtures in Homeopathy*. Calcutta: Firma K. L. Mukhopadhyay, 1972.

Bolton, Brett. *Edgar Cayce Speaks of Food, Beverages and Physical Health*. New York: Avon, 1969.

Carey, George W. *The Biochemic System of Medicine*. Calcutta: Haren & Brother, 1971.

Clark, Linda. *Help Yourself to Health*, New York: Pyramid, 1972.

————. *The Best of Linda Clark*. New Canaan, Conn.: Keats, 1976.

Garten, M. O. *The Health Secrets of a Naturopathic Doctor*. West Nyack, N.Y.: Parker, 1967.

Jarvis, D. C. *Folk Medicine*. New York: Holt, Rinehart & Winston, 1958.

Kloss, Jethro. *Back to Eden*. Riverside, Calif.: Lifeline, 1973.

Meyers, Clarence. *American Folk Medicine*. New York: Crowell, 1973.

Taylor, Renee. *Hunza Health Secrets*. New York: Award, 1964.

Wilkens, Emily. *Secrets from the Super Spas*. New York: Grosset & Dunlap, 1976.

Wolf, Adolf H. *Good Medicine: Life in Harmony with Nature*. B. C.: Good Medicine, 1970.

Yaller, Robert, and Yaller, Raye. *The Health Spas*. Santa Barbara, Calif.: Woodbridge, 1974.

Nutrition

Abrahamson, E. M., and Pezet, E. W. *Body, Mind and Sugar*. New York: Henry Holt, 1951.

Ballentine, Rudolph. *Diet and Nutrition: A Holistic Approach*. Honesdale, PA: Himalayan International Institute, 1978.

Bieler, Henry G. *Food Is Your Best Medicine*. New York: Vintage, 1965.

Davis, Adelle. *Let's Eat Right to Keep Fit*. New York: Harcourt, Brace, Jovanovich, 1954.

Dovring, Folke. "Soybeans." *Scientific American* 230 (1974): 14–22.

Hawkins, David, and Pauling, Linus. *Orthomolecular Psychiatry*. San Francisco: W. W. Freeman,

Kelsay, J. L. "A Compendium of Nutritional Status Studies and Dietary Evaluation Studies Conducted in the United States, 1957–1967," *Journal of Nutrition* 99, supplement 1, part 2: 123–66.

Lappe, Frances M. *Diet for a Small Planet*. New York: Friends of the Earth/ Ballantine, 1971.

Norman, Philip. "Fundamentals of Nutrition for Physicians and Dentists." *Oral Surgery* 33: 780–85.

Pauling, Linus. *Vitamin C and the Common Cold*. San Francisco: W. W. Freeman, 1970.

Pfeiffer, Carl C. *Mental and Elemental Nutrients*. New Canaan, Conn.: Keats, 1975.

Taylor, Renee. *Hunza Health Secrets for Long Life and Happiness*. Englewood Cliffs, N.J.: Prentice-Hall, 1966.

Watson, George. *Nutrition and Your Mind*. New York: Harper and Row, 1972.

Watt, B., and Merrill, A. *Composition of Foods*. Washington, D.C.: U.S. Government Printing Office, 1963.

Parapsychology

Bolton, Brett. *Edgar Cayce Speaks*. New York: Avon, 1969.

Cerminara, G. *Many Mansions*. New York: New American Library, 1972.

Colton, Ann Ree. *Ethical ESP*. Glendale, Calif.: ARC, 1971.

Hardy, Alister, et al. *The Challenge of Chance*. New York: Random House, 1973.

Krippner, S. *Galaxies of Life*. New York: Interface, 1973.

Mitchell, Edgar D. *Psychic Exploration*. New York: Putnam, 1974.

Moss, Thelma. *The Probability of the Impossible*. New York: New American Library, 1974.

Motoyama, Hiroshi. *The Present Situation of Parapsychology in the World*. Tokyo: The Institute of Religious Psychology, 1969.

————, ed. *Research for Religion and Parapsychology*. Tokyo: International Association for Religion and Parapsychology, 1976.

Ostrander, S., and Schroeder, L. *Psychic Discoveries behind the Iron Curtain*. New York: Prentice Hall, 1971.

————. *Handbook of PSI Discoveries*. New York: Berkeley, 1974.

Regush, June, and Regush, Nicholas. *PSI: The Other World Catalogue*. Toronto: Longman Canada, 1974.

Rhine, J. B. *Extrasensory Perception*, Boston: Branden Press, 1973.

Rhine, J. B., and Associates. *Parapsychology: From Duke to FRNM*. Durham, N.C.: Parapsychology Press, 1965.

Rhine, J. B. *Progress in Parapsychology*. Durham, Parapsychology Staff, 1973.

Rhine, Louisa E. *ESP in Life and Lab: Tracing Hidden Channels*. New York: Macmillan, 1973.

Roberts, Jane. *How to Develop Your ESP Power*. New York: Frederick Fell, 1974.

Ryzl, Milan. *Parapsychology: A Scientific Approach*. New York: Hawthorn, 1970.

Sherman, Harold. *How to Make ESP Work for You*. New York: Fawcett Crest, 1964.

Wilson, Colin. *The Occult*. New York: Random House, 1973.

Perception and Visualization

Arnheim, Rudolf. *Visual Thinking*. Berkeley and Los Angeles: University of California Press, 1969.

Babbitt, Edwin S. *The Principles of Light and Color: The Healing Power of Color*. New Hyde Park, N.Y.: University Books, 1967.

Birren, Faber. *Color in Your World*, London: Collier Macmillan, 1974.

————. *Color Psychology and Color Therapy*. New Hyde Park, N.Y.: University Books, 1974.

Clark, Linda. *The Ancient Art of Color Therapy*. Old Greenwich, Conn.: Devin-Adair, 1975.

Graham, F. Lanier. *The Rainbow Book*. Berkeley, Calif.: Shambhala, 1975.

Heline, Corinne. *Color and Music in the New Age*, La Canada, Calif.: New Age Press, 1974.

————. *Healing and Regeneration through Color*. La Canada, Calif.: New Age Press, 1975.

Huxley, Aldous. *The Art of Seeing*. Seattle: Montana Books, 1942.

Kelley, Charles R. *New Techniques of Vision Improvement, Energy and Character*, Santa Monica, Calif.: Interscience Research Institute, 1971.

Keyes, Laurel E. *Toning: The Creative Power of the Voice*. Santa Monica, Calif.: DeVorss, 1973.

Mayer, Gladys. *Color and Healing*. Sussex: New Knowledge, 1974.

Ott, John N. *Health and Light*. Old Greenwich, Conn.: Devin-Adair, 1974.

Samuels, Nancy, and Samuels, Mike. *Seeing with the Mind's Eye*. New York: Random House Bookworks, 1975.

Personal Growth and Lifestyle

Adler, Nathan. *New Life Styles and the Antinomian Personality: The Underground Stream*. New York: Harper and Row, 1972.

Alder, Vera S. *The Fifth Dimension: The Future of Mankind*. New York: Samuel Weiser, 1970.

Carnegie, Dale. *How to Win Friends and Influence People*. New York: Pocket Books, 1936.

Dubois, Renee. *Man Adapting*. New Haven, Conn.: Yale University Press, 1965.

Henderson, C. William. *Awakening: Ways to Psycho-Spiritual Growth*. Englewood Cliffs, N.J.: Prentice-Hall, 1975.

Keyes, Ken, Jr. *Handbook to Higher Consciousness*. Berkeley, Calif.: Living Love Center, 1974.

Krishnamurti, J. *Think of These Things*. New York: Harper and Row, 1970.

Lande, Nathaniel. *Mindstyles/Lifestyles*. Los Angeles: Price/Stern/Sloan, 1976.

Maltz, Maxwell. *Psycho-Cybernetics*. New York: Essandess Special Edition, 1967.

McCamy, John C., and Presley, James. *Human Life Styling*. New York: Harper and Row, 1972.

Otto, Herbert A., and Mann, John. *Ways of Growth*. New York: Ballantine, 1971.

Peale, Norman Vincent. *The Power of Positive Thinking*. New York: Fawcett, 1974.

Peterson, Severin. *A Catalog of the Ways People Grow*. New York: Ballantine, 1971.

Peterson, Severin, and Pines, Maya. *Health and Disease*. New York: Time/Life Science Library, 1965.

Rahe, R. H. "Subjects' Recent Life Changes and Their Near-Future Illness Reports." *Annals of Clinical Research* 4 (1972): 250–65.

Roberts, Oral. *Better Health and Miracle Living*. Tulsa, Okla.: Oral Roberts Evangelistic Assn., 1976.

Rose, Anthony L., and Auw, Andre. *Growing Up Human*. New York: Harper and Row, 1974.

Tournier, Paul. *The Meaning of Persons*. New York: Harper and Row, 1957.

———. *The Whole Person in a Broken World*. New York: Harper and Row, 1965.

Willing, C. A. *The Impersonal Life*. Albuquerque, N.M.: Sun, 1975.

Philosophy

Campbell, Joseph. *The Masks of God: Creative Mythology*. New York: Viking, 1970.

Frankl, Viktor E. *Man's Search for Meaning*. New York: Washington Square Press, 1959.

Lilly, John C. *The Center of the Cyclone*. New York: Bantam, 1973.

———. *The Human Biocomputer*. New York: Bantam, 1974.

Ouspensky, P. D. *The Fourth Way*. New York: Random House, 1971.

Teilhard de Chardin, Pierre. *The Phenomenon of Man*. New York: Harper and Row, 1965.

———. *The Future of Man*. New York: Harper and Row, 1969.

Walker, Kenneth. *A Study of Gurdjieff's Teaching*. London: Jonathan Cape, 1957.

Physiology

Barber, Theodore, et al., eds. *Biofeedback and Self-Control*. Chicago: Aldine-Atherton, 1970.

Benson, Herbert. *The Relaxation Response*. New York: Morrow, 1975.

"Biofeedback in Action." *Medical World News* 14 (March 9, 1973): 47.

Birk, Lee. *Biofeedback: Behavior Medicine*. New York: Grune & Stratton, 1973.

Brown, Barbara B. *Stress and the Art of Biofeedback*. New York: Harper and Row, 1977.

Burr, Harold S. *The Fields of Life: Our Links with the Universe*. New York: Ballantine, 1973.

Cain, Michael Peter. *TM: Discovering Inner Energy and Overcoming Stress*. New York: Delacorte, 1975.

Funderburk, James. *Science Studies Yoga*. Chicago: Himalayan International Institute, 1977.

Geba, Bruno H. *Breathe Away Your Tension*. Berkeley, Calif.: Bookworks, 1973.

Gentry, W. Doyle; Shows, W. Derek; and Thomas, Michael. "Chronic Low Back Pain: A Psychological Profile." *Psychosomatic Medicine* 15 (1974): 174.

Hymes, Alan C.; Raab, D. E.; Yonehira, E. G.; Nelson, G. D.; and Printy, A. L. "Acute Pain Control by Electrostimulation: A Preliminary Report." *Advances in Neurological Sciences* (1974): 761.

Jonas, Gerald. *Visceral Learning: Toward a Science of Self-Control*. New York: Viking, 1974.

Luce, Gay Gaer. *Body Time*. New York: Pantheon, 1971.

McCrady, Richard E., and McCrady, Jean B. *Biofeedback: An Annotated Bibliography of Published Research with Human Subjects Since 1960*. Pomona, Calif.: Behavioral Instrument Company, 1975.

Melzack, R., and Wall, P. D. "Pain Mechanisms: A New Theory." *Science* 150 (1965): 971.

Miller, Neal E., et al. *Biofeedback and Self-Control 1973*. Chicago: Aldine, 1974.

Ostfeld, A. M., and Shekelle, R. B. "Psychological Variables and Blood Pressure." In *The Epidemiology of Hypertension*, edited by J. Stamler, R. Stamler, and T. N. Pullman, pp. 321-31. New York: Grune and Stratton, 1967.

Patel, C. H. "Yoga and Biofeedback in the Management of Hypertension." *Lancet* 2 (1973): 1053-55.

Ramacharaka, Yogi. *Science of Breath*. Fort: D. B. Taraporevala, 1960.

Robbins, P. R. "Personality and Psychosomatic Illness; A Selective Review of Research." *Genetic Psychology Monographs* 80 (1969): 51-90.

Sargent, Joseph D., Green, Elmer E., and Walters, Dale E. "The Use of Autogenic Feedback Training in a Pilot Study of Migraine and Tension Headaches." *Headache* 12 (1972): 120.

Selye, Hans. *Stress without Distress*. Philadelphia: Lippincott, 1974.

Shapiro, David; Tursky, Bernard; Gershon, Elliot; and Stern, Melvin. "Effects of Feedback and Reinforcement on the Control of Human Systolic Blood Pressure." *Science* 163 (1969): 588.

Sokolow, M.; Klais, B. L.; Harris, R. E.; and Bennett, L. F. "Personality and Predisposition to Essential Hypertension." In *The Pathogenesis of Essential Hypertension*, Proceedings of the Prague Symposium, edited by J. H. Cort, pp. 143-53. Prague: State Medical Publishing House, 1961.

Stoyva, Johann, ed. *Biofeedback and Self-Regulation*. New York: Plenum, 1976.

Sugi, Y., and Akutsu, K. "Studies on Respiration and Energy-Metabolism During Sitting in Zazen." *Research Journal of Physical Education* 12 (1968): 190–206.

Tart, C. T. "Patterns of Basal Skin Resistance During Sleep." *Psychophysiology* 4 (1967): 35–39.

Thomas, C. B. "The Psychological Dimensions of Hypertension." In *The Epidemiology of Hypertension*, edited by J. Stamler, R. Stamler, and T. N. Pullman, pp. 332–39. New York: Grune and Stratton, 1967.

Thommen, George. *Is This Your Day? (Biorhythm)*. New York: Award, 1964.

Timmons, B., and Kamiya, J. "The Psychology and Physiology of Meditation and Related Phenomena: A Bibliography." *Journal of Transpersonal Psychology* 1 (1970).

Tinbergen, N. "Ethnology and Stress Diseases." *Science* 185 (1974): 20–27.

Wallace, R. K. "Physiological Effects of Transcendental Meditation." *Science* 167 (1970): 1751–54.

Wallace, R. K., and Benson, H. "The Physiology of Meditation." *Scientific American* 226 (1972): 84–90.

Wickramasekera, Ian. *Biofeedback, Behavior Therapy and Hypnosis*. Chicago: Nelson-Hall, 1976.

Psychology, Counseling and Psychotherapy

Assagioli, Roberto. *Psychosynthesis*. New York: Viking, 1965.

———. *The Act of Will*. Baltimore: Penguin, 1974.

Bateson, Gregory. *Steps to an Ecology of Mind*. New York: Ballantine, 1972.

Berne, Eric. *A Layman's Guide to Psychiatry and Psychoanalysis*. New York: Simon & Schuster, 1968.

Frankl, Viktor E. *Psychotherapy and Existentialism*. New York: Simon & Schuster, 1967.

Jung, Carl. *Memories, Dreams and Reflections*. New York: Random House, 1963.

Maltz, Maxwell. *Psycho-Cybernetics*. Englewood Cliffs, N.J.: Prentice-Hall, 1960.

Schultz, William C. *Elements of Encounter: A Bodymind Approach*. Big Sur, Calif.: Joy Press, 1973.

Shapiro, Evelyn, ed. *PsychoSources: A Psychology Resource Catalog*. New York: Communications Research Machines, 1973.

Tart, Charles T., ed. *Transpersonal Psychologies*. New York: Harper and Row, 1975.

Watts, Alan W. *Psychotherapy East and West*. New York: Ballantine, 1974.

Religious and Theological

Addington, Jack Ensign. *The Time for Miracles Is Now*. New York: Dodd, Mead, 1973.

Frankl, Viktor E. *The Unconscious God*. New York: Simon & Schuster, 1975.

Johnston, W. *Christian Zen*. New York: Harper and Row, 1971.

Needleman, J. *The New Religions*. Garden City, N.Y.: Doubleday, 1970.

Perlman, Eric, ed. *Spiritual Community Guide for North America*. San Rafael, Calif.: Spiritual Community Publications, 1974.

Simons, William, ed. *A Pilgrim's Guide to Planet Earth*. San Rafael, Calif.: Spiritual Community Publications, 1974.

Steiner, Rudolf. *Theosophy: An Introduction*. New York: Anthroposophic, 1971.

————. *Occult Science: An Outline*. New York: Anthroposophic, 1972.

Stewart, Leland P., ed. *International Cooperation Council Directory, 1977*. Beverly Hills, Calif.: International Cooperation Council, 1977.

Spiritual and Psychic Healing

Bailes, Frederick. *Hidden Power for Human Problems*. Englewood Cliffs, N.J.: Prentice-Hall, 1957.

Edwards, Harry. *The Evidence for Spirit Healing*. London: Spiritualist Press, 1953.

Fuller, John G. *Arigo: Surgeon of the Rusty Knife*. New York: Simon & Schuster, 1975.

Goldsmith, Joel S. *The Art of Spiritual Healing*. New York: Harper and Row, 1959.

Grad, Bernard, et al. "The Influence of an Unorthodox Method of Treatment on Wound Healing in Mice." *International Journal of Parapsychology* 3 (Spring 1961): 5–24.

Hammond, Sally. *We Are All Healers*. New York: Harper and Row, 1973.

Krieger, Dolores. "The Response of In-Vivo Human Hemoglobin to an Active Healing Therapy by Direct Laying-On of Hands." *Human Dimensions* 1 (Autumn 1972): 12–15.

Krippner, Stanley, and Villoldo, Alberto. *The Realms of Healing*. Millbrae, Calif.: Celestial Arts, 1976.

Leadbeater, C. W. *Invisible Helpers*. Madras: The Theosophical Publishing House, 1973.

Ponder, Catherine. *The Healing Secret of the Ages*. West Nyack, N.Y.: Parker, 1964.

Rorvik, D. M. "The Healing Hand of Mr. E." *Esquire* 81 (February 1974): 70, 154, 156, 159–160.

Sanford, Agnes. *The Healing Power of the Bible*. Philadelphia: Lippincott, 1969.

Sherman, Harold. *Your Power to Heal*. New York: Harper and Row, 1972.

Stelter, Alfred. *PSI–Healing*. New York: Bantam, 1976.

Sugrue, Thomas. *There Is a River: The Story of Edgar Cayce*. New York: Dell, 1970.

Turner, Gordon. *Outline of Spiritual Healing*. New York: Warner, 1972.

Valentine, Tom. *Psychic Surgery*. New York: Pocket Books, 1975.

Worrall, Ambrose, and Worrall, Olga. *The Gift of Healing*. New York: Harper and Row, 1976.

Wholistic Healing

Bennett, Hal Z., and Samuels, Mike. *Be Well*. New York: Random House, 1974.

———. *The Well Body Book*. New York: Random House, 1974.

Daemion, Jonathan. *Path-ways to Wholeness: A Healing Guide*. Berkeley, Calif.: Clear Life Publications, 1975.

Inglis, Brian. *Fringe Medicine*. New York: Putnam, 1969.

Kritzer, J. Haskel. *Text-Book of Iridiagnosis*. Chicago: Press of John F. Higgins, 1921.

Loomis, Evarts G., and Paulson, J. Sig. *Healing for Everyone: Medicine of the Whole Person*. New York: Hawthorn, 1975.

Majno, Guido. *The Healing Hand: Man and Wound in the Ancient World*. Cambridge, Mass.: Harvard University Press, 1975.

Miller, Don E. *BodyMind: The Whole Person Health Book*. London: Prentice-Hall International, 1974.

Miller, Stuart, et al. *Dimensions of Humanistic Medicine*. San Francisco: The Institute for the Study of Humanistic Medicine, 1975.

Muramoto, Naboru. *Healing Ourselves*. New York: Avon, 1973.

Pelletier, Kenneth R. *Mind as Healer, Mind as Slayer*. New York: Dell, 1977.

Shealy, C. Norman. *90 Days to Self-Health*. New York: Dial, 1977.

Thiel, Peter Johannes. *The Diagnosis of Disease by Observation of the Eye.*
    Part 2, vol. 1. 1918. Reprint. Mokelumne Hill, Calif.: Health Research,
    1974.

Yoga

Acharya, Pundit. *Breath, Sleep, the Heart, and Life.* Lower Lake, Calif.: Dawn
    Horse, 1975.
Chaudhuri, Haridas. *Integral Yoga–The Concept of Harmonious and Creative
    Living.* Wheaton, Ill.: Theosophical Publishing House, 1974.
Devi, Indra. *Yoga for Americans.* Englewood Cliffs, N.J.: Prentice-Hall, 1959.
Haich, Elisabeth, and Yesudian, Selvarajan. *Yoga and Health.* New York:
    Harper, 1953.
Hittleman, Richard. *Introduction to Yoga.* New York: Bantam, 1969.
Iyengar, B. K. S. *Light on Yoga.* New York: Shocken, 1974.
Mishra, Rammurti S. *Fundamentals of Yoga.* Garden City, N. Y.: Doubleday,
    Anchor, 1974.
"Neurophysiology." *Journal of the Indian Medical Association.* 48 (1967):
    167–70.
Rama, Swami, et al. *Yoga and Psychotherapy: The Evolution of Consciousness.*
    Glenview, Ill.: Himalayan Institute, 1976.
Saraswati, Swami Shivananda. *Yogic Therapy.* Calcutta: Brahmachari Yoges-
    war Umachal Yogashram, 1969.
Satchidananda. *Integral Yoga Hatha.* New York: Holt Paperback, 1970.
Satprem. *Sri Aurobindo, or the Adventure of Consciousness.* New York: Harper
    and Row, 1968.
Wood, Ernest. *Yoga.* Baltimore: Penguin, 1968.

Index